Neural Stem Cells: Therapies

Neural Stem Cells: Therapies

Edited by **Jose Clark**

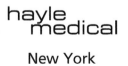

hayle
medical

New York

Published by Hayle Medical,
30 West, 37th Street, Suite 612,
New York, NY 10018, USA
www.haylemedical.com

Neural Stem Cells: Therapies
Edited by Jose Clark

International Standard Book Number: 978-1-63241-285-0 (Hardback)

The publisher's policy is to use permanent paper from mills that operate a sustainable forestry policy. Furthermore, the publisher ensures that the text paper and cover boards used have met acceptable environmental accreditation standards.

Trademark Notice: Registered trademark of products or corporate names are used only for explanation and identification without intent to infringe.

Printed in the United States of America.

Contents

Preface VII

Neural Stem Cells and Therapy 1

Chapter 1 Noncoding RNAs in Neural Stem Cell Development 3
Shan Bian and Tao Sun

Chapter 2 Neural Stem/Progenitor Cell Clones as Models for
Neural Development and Transplantation 21
Hedong Li, He Zhao, Xiaoqiong Shu and Mei Jiang

Chapter 3 Neural Stem Cells: Exogenous
and Endogenous Promising Therapies for Stroke 47
M. Guerra-Crespo, A.K. De la Herrán-Arita,
A. Boronat-García, G. Maya-Espinosa, J.R. García-Montes,
J.H. Fallon and R. Drucker-Colín

Chapter 4 Endogenous Neural Stem/Progenitor Cells and
Regenerative Responses to Brain Injury 93
Maria Dizon

Chapter 5 Ischemia-Induced Neural Stem/Progenitor Cells
Within the Post-Stroke Cortex in Adult Brains 105
Takayuki Nakagomi and Tomohiro Matsuyama

Chapter 6 Assessing the Influence of Neuroinflammation on
Neurogenesis: *In Vitro* Models Using Neural Stem Cells and
Microglia as Valuable Research Tools 121
Bruno P. Carreira, Maria Inês Morte,
Caetana M. Carvalho and Inês M. Araújo

Chapter 7 Immune System Modulation of Germinal and
Parenchymal Neural Progenitor Cells in
Physiological and Pathological Conditions 151
Chiara Rolando, Enrica Boda and Annalisa Buffo

Chapter 8   **Mesenchymal Stromal Cells and Neural Stem Cells
Potential for Neural Repair in Spinal Cord Injury and
Human Neurodegenerative Disorders**   179
Dasa Cizkova, Norbert Zilka, Zuzana Kazmerova,
Lucia Slovinska, Ivo Vanicky, Ivana Novotna-Grulova,
Viera Cigankova, Milan Cizek and Michal Novak

Permissions

List of Contributors

Preface

This book is a collection of research work by international veterans in the neural stem cell field and includes the characterization of adult and embryonic neural stem cells in both vertebrates as well as invertebrates. Specifically, this book provides techniques and also describes the challenges of employing neural stem cells for therapy of neurological disorders and spinal cord as well as brain injuries. It is intended for basic readers, doctors, students and researchers who are interested in comprehending the principles and novel discoveries in neural stem cells and therapy.

Significant researches are present in this book. Intensive efforts have been employed by authors to make this book an outstanding discourse. This book contains the enlightening chapters which have been written on the basis of significant researches done by the experts.

Finally, I would also like to thank all the members involved in this book for being a team and meeting all the deadlines for the submission of their respective works. I would also like to thank my friends and family for being supportive in my efforts.

Editor

Neural Stem Cells and Therapy

Noncoding RNAs in
Neural Stem Cell Development

Shan Bian and Tao Sun
Department of Cell and Developmental Biology
Cornell University Weill Medical College
USA

1. Introduction

Neural stem cells and neural progenitors/precursors (NSCs/NPs) are identified in both embryonic and adult central nervous system (CNS). NSCs can self-renew and give rise to neurons and glia. The development of NSCs is controlled by precisely orchestrated gene expression regulation. Recently, emerging evidence has shown the importance of noncoding RNA regulation in NSC self-renewal, proliferation, survival and differentiation. In this chapter, we will present new research of noncoding RNA functions in NSC development. We will highlight the future directions of applying noncoding RNAs in stem cell-based therapy for neurological diseases.

2. Noncoding RNAs

Noncoding RNAs (ncRNAs) are functional RNA molecules that do not show protein translation capability. ncRNAs consist of ribosomal RNAs (rRNAs), transfer RNAs (tRNAs), piwi-interacting RNAs (piRNAs), microRNAs (miRNAs), and long noncoding RNAs (lncRNAs) and so on. ncRNAs have shown to play distinct but also conserved roles in normal development in invertebrates and vertebrates.

2.1 piRNAs

piRNAs are a group of small RNAs with size between 26-31 nucleotides (nt), which are only found in male and female germlines of invertebrates and within testes in mammalians (Houwing et al., 2007; 2009; Lander et al., 2001; Lau et al., 2006; Seto et al., 2007). piRNAs interact with piwi proteins to form RNA-protein complexes (Das et al., 2008; Houwing et al., 2007). The piRNA-protein complexes have been shown to silence transcription, specifically transposons (Brennecke et al., 2008; Das et al., 2008). Since piRNAs are mainly expressed during the germline stem cell development, they will not be discussed further in this chapter.

2.2 miRNAs

miRNAs are ~22 nt highly conserved small noncoding RNAs found in almost all eukaryotic cells (Khraiwesh et al., 2010) (Fig. 1). Like coding genes, miRNAs are mainly transcribed by the

RNA Polymerase II (Pol II) into long primary miRNA transcripts (pri-miRNAs). Pri-miRNAs are next cleaved by Drosha, a class 2 RNase III enzyme, to produce short hairpin stem-loop structures, known as precursor miRNAs (pre-miRNAs) (Ambros, 2008; Gregory et al., 2006). Pre-miRNAs are then processed into about 20-25 nt double-stranded mature miRNAs by RNase III enzyme Dicer (Lund and Dahlberg, 2006). The duplex undergoes unwinding and the strand with the weakest base pairing at its 5′ terminus, together with Dicer and many associated proteins including Argonaute proteins, form an active RNA-induced silencing complex (RISC) (Neilson and Sharp, 2008; Rana, 2007). A miRNA recognizes and binds to the 3′ untranslated region (3′ UTR) of target messenger RNAs (mRNAs) by imperfect complementary sequence recognition (Neilson and Sharp, 2008; Wang et al., 2004). Once bound, the RISC can negatively regulate miRNA targets by degrading the mRNA or repressing its translation (Khraiwesh et al., 2010; Pratt and MacRae, 2009) (Fig. 1).

miRNAs are classified into intergenic and intragenic miRNAs, depending on their genomic location (Lagos-Quintana et al., 2001; Lau et al., 2001; Lee and Ambros, 2001). Intergenic miRNAs are located at intergenic regions (between genes) in the genome. These miRNAs are usually transcribed using their own promoters. Intragenic miRNAs normally lie in intronic regions of coding genes with the same orientation. They are often transcribed together with the host genes.

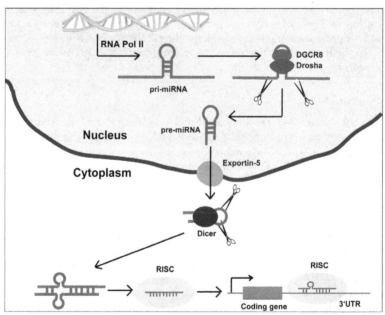

Fig. 1. A scheme of microRNA biogenesis. microRNAs silence target coding genes by binding to the 3′ untranslated region (3′ UTR).

2.3 lncRNAs

The majority of the human genome has previously been considered as "junk" DNA, since only about 1.5% of the human genome, which occupies over 3 billion DNA base pairs, consists of protein-coding genes (Lander et al., 2001). A recent study of a large-scale complementary DNA (cDNA) sequencing project has shown that four fifths of transcripts of the human genome are RNA transcripts that don't encode proteins (Kapranov et al., 2007). These RNA transcripts are normally longer than 200 nt, thus they are called long noncoding RNAs. Except no open reading frame (ORF) found within lncRNAs, they share many features with coding mRNAs such as 5' capping. lncRNAs usually contain exons and introns (Carninci et al., 2005).

lncRNAs display different features of genomic location and orientation in the genome. Emerging evidence has demonstrated potential functions of lncRNAs in many biological events. lncRNAs have been shown to modulate gene transcription via different mechanisms. For example, some *cis*-antisense lncRNAs complementary to protein-coding transcripts regulate expression of the coding genes (Feng et al., 2006; Kotake et al., 2010; Pasmant et al., 2007; Tochitani and Hayashizaki, 2008; Yu et al., 2008); some lncRNAs modulate transcription factors by acting as co-regulators (Feng et al., 2006; Nguyen et al., 2001; Shamovsky et al., 2006; Wang et al., 2008; Willingham et al., 2005; Yang et al., 2001). Moreover, some studies have shown that lncRNAs are involved in epigenetic regulations such as chromatin and histone modification, and X-chromosome inactivation (Denisenko et al., 1998; Mancini-Dinardo et al., 2006; Mazo et al., 2007; Rinn et al., 2007; Sanchez-Elsner et al., 2006; Tsai et al., 2010; Wutz et al., 2002).

3. Noncoding RNAs and neural stem cell development

Noncoding RNAs such as miRNAs and lncRNAs participate gene expression regulation in many ways. The underlying mechanisms of noncoding RNA functions in normal development are beginning to be uncovered. In this book chapter, we will focus on reviewing functions of miRNAs and lncRNAs in neural stem cell development, such as NSC self-renewal, cell fate determination and survival.

3.1 miRNAs and self-renewal and proliferation of NSCs

The ability of self-renewal is essential for NSCs/NPs to perpetuate themselves to maintain an undifferentiated status during the embryonic stage and even in the adulthood (Gage, 2000; Shi et al., 2008; Temple, 2001). NSC proliferation and self-renewal are modulated by a complicated regulation network that consists of growth factors, epigenetic regulators, transcription factors and extrinsic signaling molecules from the NSC niche. Recent discovers have indicated that ncRNAs also play important roles in NSC self-renewal through a post-transcriptional regulation mechanism (Doe, 2008; Shi et al., 2008).

miRNAs have been shown to play essential roles in regulating NSC proliferation. Since Dicer is the key enzyme in miRNA processing, several studies have reported the global effects of miRNAs in NSC development by ablating *Dicer* and in turn blocking biogenesis of all miRNAs in the CNS using tissue specific Cre lines. Conditional deletion of *Dicer* from the mouse cerebral cortex using the *Emx1-Cre* line results in a significant reduction in cortical size and the cortical NP pool (De Pietri Tonelli et al., 2008; Kawase-Koga et al., 2010; Kawase-Koga et al., 2009). *Dicer* ablation from the mouse CNS using the *Emx1-Cre* and *Nestin-Cre* line causes a reduction of NSC numbers and abnormal differentiation (Andersson et al., 2010; Kawase-Koga et al., 2009) (Fig. 2A). *Dicer*-deficient NSCs display apoptosis when mitogens are withdrawn from the culture medium (Fig. 2A). Because Dicer is also involved in maintaining the heterochromatin assembly, the defects of NSCs in *Dicer* knockout mice need to be carefully interpreted (Fukagawa et al., 2004; Kanellopoulou et al., 2005). Examining functions of individual miRNAs will help reveal precise roles of miRNAs in the NSC self-renewal and proliferation (Fig. 3).

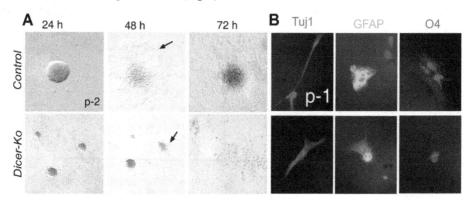

Fig. 2. A. *Dicer*-deficient (*Dicer-Ko*) neural stem cells (NSCs) did not survive well in a differentiation culture medium without mitogens. Most *Dicer-Ko* neurospheres died after 48 hours in culture. Many differentiated cells (arrows) migrated away from the control neurosphere but not from the *Dicer-Ko* neurospheres. B. Under the differentiation condition without mitogens, passaged (p-1) *Dicer-Ko* NSCs gave rise to cells expressing neuronal (Tuj1+) and glial (GFAP+ and O4+) markers. However, their morphology was abnormal, as shown with shorter neurites and processes than controls (Kawase-Koga et al., 2010).

let-7, the first identified miRNA (Reinhart et al., 2000), has been shown to regulate NSC proliferation and differentiation by targeting the nuclear receptor TLX and the cell cycle regulator cyclin D1 (Zhao et al., 2010a) (Fig. 3). Overexpression of *let-7b* inhibits NSC proliferation and enhances differentiation, while knockdown of *let-7b* promotes NSC proliferation (Zhao et al., 2010a). It appears that the expression levels of let-7 in NSCs are controlled by a feedback regulation of Lin-28, a pluripotency factor that controls miRNA processing in NSCs (Rybak et al., 2008). Lin-28 binds to the *let-7* precursor and inhibits its processing by Dicer. On the other hand, the expression of Lin-28 is repressed by let-7 and miR-125, allowing the maturation of let-7 (Fig. 4A). This feedback loop reveals an autoregulation between miRNA let-7 and miR-125, and transcription factor Lin-28 during NSC development (Rybak et al., 2008).

miR-124 is identified as a CNS-enriched miRNA and its expression is upregulated during neuronal differentiation (Lagos-Quintana et al., 2002) (Fig. 3). In the adult brain, NSCs are identified in the subventricular zone (SVZ). In cultured adult NSCs derived from the SVZ and in the SVZ *in vivo*, knocking down *miR-124* results in an increase of NSC proliferation and a decrease of differentiation, while overexpressing *miR-124* reduces the number of dividing precursors and enhances neuronal differentiation (Cheng et al., 2009). Moreover, miR-124 modulates NSC proliferation and differentiation by suppressing Sox9 expression in adult NSCs (Cheng et al., 2009). A recent study has shown that miR-124 regulates neuronal differentiation through a mutual inhibition mechanism of Ephrin-B1 (Arvanitis et al., 2010). In addition, miR-124 promotes differentiation of NPs by modulating a network of nervous system-specific alternative splicing through suppressing expression of PTBP1, which encodes a global repressor of alternative pre-mRNA splicing (Makeyev et al., 2007). Together, miR-124 plays a general role in promoting differentiation of embryonic and adult NSCs and NPs. It appears that miR-124 executes its function through repressing various targets.

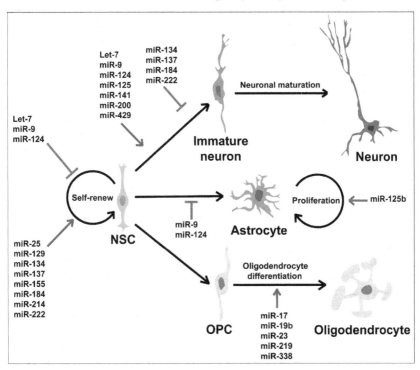

Fig. 3. Many miRNAs are involved in neural stem cell (NSC) self-renewal and differentiation into neurons, astrocytes and oligodendrocyte precursor cells (OPCs) and oligodendrocytes.

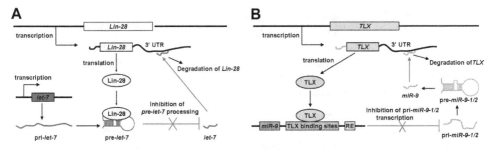

Fig. 4. Feedback loop regulation of miRNAs and their target genes. A. Let-7 processing is inhibited by Lin-28, and the 3' untranslated region (3' UTR) of Lin-28 has binding sites for Let-7. B. TLX inhibits miR-9 expression, while miR-9 displays silencing effects on TLX.

miR-9 is another CNS-enriched miRNA. miR-9 is shown to inhibit NSC proliferation but promote differentiation through a feedback regulation of a nuclear receptor TLX (Zhao et al., 2009) (Fig. 4B). In human embryonic stem cell (ESC) derived NPs, miR-9 is shown to have a positive effect on proliferation but a negative effect on migration by directly targeting Stmn1, which increases microtubule instability (Delaloy et al., 2010). The opposite effect of miR-9 on proliferation is perhaps caused by differential physical contacts of miR-9 with target genes and the different culture systems.

In the CNS of *Xenopus*, miR-9 knockdown promotes the proliferation of NPs in the hindbrain, leads to an increased expression of *cyclin D1* and a downregulation of *p27Xic1* (Bonev et al., 2011). miR-9 targets *Hairy1* and regulates proliferation of NPs (Bonev et al., 2011). In zebrafish, miR-9 promotes differentiation of NPs that give rise to neurons at the midbrain-hindbrain domain and controls the organization of the midbrain-hindbrain boundary by targeting several genes in the Fibroblast growth factor (Fgf) signaling, such as *fgf8-1* and *fgfr1* (Leucht et al., 2008). In the chick spinal cord, miR-9 specifies a subtype of motor neurons that project axons to the axial muscles from motor neuron progenitors by specifically targeting transcription factor FoxP1 (Otaegi et al., 2011).

In the mouse brain, miR-9 function is demonstrated by the generation of *miR-9-2* and *miR-9-3* double knockout mice. *miR-9* double mutants show reduced cortical layers, disordered migration of interneurons, and misrouted thalamocortical axons and cortical axon projections, suggesting an important role of miR-9 in NP proliferation, differentiation and migration during brain development (Shibata et al., 2011). Moreover, it appears that miR-9 regulates multiple target genes, including Foxg1, Pax6 and Gsh2, which have shown to be essential in cortical development (Shibata et al., 2011). Therefore, miR-9 plays an important role in controlling differentiation of NSCs/NPs in different regions in the CNS (Fig. 3).

The major role of let-7, miR-124 and miR-9 is to inhibit NSC/NP proliferation and to induce their differentiation into specific cell types. miRNAs that promote proliferation of NSCs and NPs have also been identified (Fig. 3). miR-134 plays a role in enhancing proliferation of cortical NPs by targeting doublecortin (Dcx) and/or Chordin-like 1 (Chrdl-1) (Gaughwin et al., 2011). miR-25 is shown to be a major player in the miR-106-25 cluster in neural development. Overexpression of *miR-25* but not *miR-106b* and *miR-93* promotes adult NP proliferation (Brett et al., 2011). Interestingly, the expression of the miR-106-25 cluster is regulated by FoxO3, a transcription factor maintaining the NSC population (Renault et al., 2009).

During the retina development, *otx2* and *vsx1* genes are shown to control the division of retinal precursors and differentiation into bipolar retina neurons. In early retinal precursors, the expression of *otx2* and *vsx1* is inhibited, accompanied with a rapid precursor division. miR-129, miR-155, miR-214, and miR-222, which are highly expressed in the embryonic retina, have been identified to target and repress translation of *otx2* and *vsx1*, by which they promote proliferation of retinal precursors (Decembrini et al., 2009).

miRNA expression is also controlled by epigenetic regulators in the NSC development. The expression of miR-137 is regulated by DNA methyl-CpG-binding protein (MeCP2) and transcription factor Sox2. miR-137 modulates adult NSC proliferation and cell fate determination by targeting Ezh2, a histone methyltransferase and polycomb group protein (Szulwach et al., 2010). Ectopic expression of *miR-137* in adult NSCs enhances proliferation, while knockdown of *miR-137* promotes differentiation of adult NSCs (Szulwach et al., 2010).

In addition, miR-184 expression is suppressed by methyl-CpG binding protein 1 (MBD1) and miR-184 promotes adult NSC proliferation by repressing the expression of Numb-like (Numbl) (Liu et al., 2010).

3.2 lncRNAs and proliferation of NSCs

The lncRNAs may also play a role in controlling NSC proliferation, even though studies of lncRNAs in NSC development are still sparse. Sox2 is a transcription factor and plays a key role in the maintenance of the undifferentiating state of embryonic and adult NSCs (Pevny and Placzek, 2005). *Sox2 overlapping transcript* (*Sox2OT*) is a lncRNA containing *Sox2* gene and shares the same transcriptional orientation with *Sox2* (Fig. 5A). Similar to *Sox2*, *Sox2OT* is stably expressed in mouse embryonic stem cells and down-regulated during differentiation. *Sox2OT* is expressed in the neurogenic regions of the adult mouse brain including olfactory bulb (OB), rostral migratory stream (RMS) and SVZ, and is dynamically regulated during vertebrate CNS development, implying its role in regulating NSC self-renewal and neurogenesis (Amaral et al., 2009; Mercer et al., 2008).

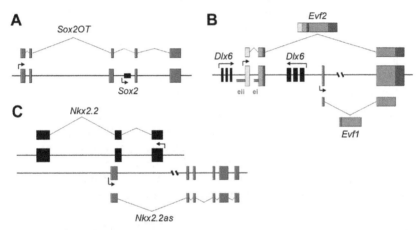

Fig. 5. Genomic location and potential functions of long noncoding RNAs (lncRNAs) (Bian and Sun, 2011). A. *Sox2 overlapping transcript Sox2OT* is a lncRNA containing *Sox2* gene and shares the same transcriptional orientation with *Sox2*. B. *Evf2* is transcribed from the intergenic region between the *Dlx-5* and *Dlx-6* loci, and is overlapped with *Dlx-5/6* enhancer i (ei) and enhancer ii (eii) sequences. *Evf2* acts as a transcriptional co-activator of Dlx-2 and activates the *Dlx5/6* enhancer. C. *Nkx2.2 antisense* (*Nkx2.2as*) is an antisense lncRNA to *Nkx2.2* gene and promotes *Nkx2-2* expression.

3.3 Summary

Taken together, self-renewal and differentiation of NSCs and NPs are controlled by complex gene regulation networks that consist of both protein coding genes and noncoding miRNAs. During proliferation and differentiation of NSCs and NPs, one miRNA can have multiple target genes and features a feedback regulation with their targets (Figs. 3 and 4). The availability of physical contacts and the binding affinity of a miRNA and its targets perhaps determine interactions of the miRNA with the specific targets. The interactions of miRNAs and their target genes eventually produce proper protein output of key factors that directly control self-renewal, proliferation and differentiation of NSCs/NPs.

3.4 NSC survival controlled by noncoding RNAs

Several reports have shown that miRNAs play a general role in controlling cell survival. Conditional deletion of *Dicer* from neural crest cells using *Wnt1-Cre* mouse line results in an increased apoptosis of neural crest-derived cells (Zehir et al., 2010). Ablation of *Dicer* from postmitotic neurons in the cortex and the hippocampus using *calmoduln kinase II* (*CaMKII*) promoter-driven *Cre* transgenic mice results in smaller cortex, enhanced cortical cell death (Davis et al., 2008). *Emx1-Cre Dicer* conditional knockout mice have shown an increased apoptosis, especially in the ventricular zone (VZ) and SVZ (De Pietri Tonelli et al., 2008). Our own work of cortical NSCs of *Emx1-Cre Dicer* conditional knockout mice using proteomic analysis by mass spectrometry and bioinformatic assays has indicated that *Dicer* deletion results in an increase of pro-cell-death and a decrease of pro-survival proteins in *Dicer*-deficient NSCs (Kawase-Koga et al., 2010) (Fig. 2A). Interestingly, an upregulation of fragile X mental retardation protein (FMRP), a proven target for miR-124, and Caspase3, a key cell apoptosis molecule, are observed in *Dicer*-deficient NSCs. On the other hand, proteins such as transforming growth factor-beta receptor type II (TGFβR2) and SOD1 are downregulated in *Dicer*-deficient NSCs (Kawase-Koga et al., 2010). These observations suggest that miRNAs perhaps control survival of NSCs by modulating the balance of protein output of genes regulating apoptosis and survival.

Neurotrophins and their receptors play important roles in the NSC proliferation, survival and differentiation. miR-128 is shown to target the truncated non-catalytic form of the human neurotrophin-3 receptor (NTRK3), which affects membrane remodeling and cytoskeletal reorganization. Overexpression of *miR-128* in neuroblastoma cells leads to round cell body and shorter neurites, which is similar to knockdown of truncated NTRK3. miR-128 overexpression causes altered expression of genes involved in cell proliferation and apoptosis such as antiapoptotic factor Bcl-2, suggesting an important role of miR-128 on cell survival (Guidi et al., 2010). Moreover, miR-134 is shown to be required for inhibiting apoptosis initiated by Chrdl-1 in cortical progenitors (Gaughwin et al., 2011). Studies on an ethanol teratogenic culture model by exposing embryonic cortex-derived NPs in ethanol have revealed different roles of miRNAs during this pathological process (Sathyan et al., 2007). In NP cultures, miR-21 is suppressed by the ethanol exposure and the reduction of miR-21 causes cell apoptosis, suggesting an anti-apoptotic effect of miR-21 (Sathyan et al., 2007).

The BH3-only family is a group of pro-apoptotic regulators, including Bim, Hrk, Bmf, Puma and N-Bak, which induce cytochrome c release from mitochondria (Giam et al., 2008). Overexpression of miR-29b in neurons inhibits endogenous BH3-only proteins Bim, Puma and Bmf, and promotes neuronal survival (Giam et al., 2008; Kole et al., 2011). In the brain of the calorie-restricted mice, expression of three miRNAs, miR-181a-1*, miR-30e and miR-34a, is significantly downregulated with a corresponding upregulation of their target gene Bcl-2, a decrease of pro-apoptotic factor Bax and cleavage of Caspases (Khanna et al., 2011). Overexpressing these three genes results in an increased cell apoptosis, accompanied with a decrease in Bcl-2 expression (Khanna et al., 2011).

miRNAs also play an important role in neural tissue growth and organ development by regulating cell survival. In *Drosophila*, the Hippo pathway together with Yorkie transcriptional activator contribute to the regulation of tissue growth by stimulating cell proliferation and inhibiting apoptosis (Saucedo and Edgar, 2007). Recent studies have shown that Yorkie not only activates cyclin E and apoptosis inhibitor DIAP1, but also triggers the expression of *bantam* miRNA to promote proliferation and cell survival (Huang et al., 2005; Thompson and Cohen, 2006). A downregulation of *bantam* miRNA is found in dying Rim cells at the eye margin, and restoration of *bantam* miRNA to higher levels prevents apoptosis of these cells, suggesting a role of *bantam* miRNA in enhancing cell survival in eye development (Thompson and Cohen, 2006). In addition, as the largest miRNA family in *Drosophila*, miR-2/6/11/13/308 are required for inhibiting embryonic apoptosis by suppressing pro-apoptotic factors hid, grim, reaper and sickle (Leaman et al., 2005).

In the forebrain of *Xenopus*, miR-9 deletion results in apoptosis of NPs due to increased expression of p53 (Bonev et al., 2011). In addition, miR-24a is expressed in the retina of *Xenopus* (Walker and Harland, 2009). Overexpression of *miR-24a* in retinal cells prevents cells from death, while knockdown of *miR-24a* causes a reduction in eye size due to an increased apoptosis (Walker and Harland, 2009). miR-24a controls cell survival by a negative regulation of pro-apoptotic factors caspase9 and apaf1.

In summary, miRNAs play critical roles in regulating survival of both NSCs/NPs and postmitotic neurons. miRNAs either promote cell survival or lead to apoptosis, depending on functions of their target genes.

3.5 NSC differentiation and cell fate determination mediated by noncoding RNAs

In the mammalian CNS, different neural cell types arise and migrate in a precise temporospatial manner. In the developing mouse brain, neurons arise first by embryonic day 12 (E12), neurogenesis peaks at E14 and ceases by E18. Astrocytes appear around E18, with their numbers peaking in the postnatal period. Oligodendrocytes are generated after birth when the neurogenesis is almost complete. Studies have shown that ncRNAs play an important role in regulating both neurogenesis and gliogenesis.

3.5.1 Cell fate determination controlled by miRNAs

miRNAs play essential roles in NSC differentiation and the cell fate switch between neurons and glia (Cuellar et al., 2008; Hebert et al., 2010; Zheng et al., 2010). We have found that *Dicer*-deficient NSCs display abnormal differentiation, with shorter neurites in neurons and fewer processes in glial cells (Kawase-Koga et al., 2010) (Fig. 2B). Conditional deletion of *Dicer* from the mouse forebrain neurons using *CamKII-Cre* line results in neuronal degeneration and an increase in glial fibrillary acidic protein (GFAP)-positive astrocytes (Hebert et al., 2010). *Dicer* ablation in the dopaminoceptive neurons in the basal ganglia using a *dopamine receptor-1 (DR-1)-Cre* line leads to astrogliogenesis, but not neurodegeneration (Cuellar et al., 2008). Interestingly, in the mouse spinal cord, conditional deletion of *Dicer* using *Olig1-Cre* line disrupts production of both oligodendrocytes and astrocytes (Zheng et al., 2010). These observations suggest that global loss of miRNAs in specific precursor cells affects production of distinct cell types.

miRNA expression profiling studies have shown that some miRNAs are preferentially expressed in neurons or glia. For example, miR-124 and miR-128 are highly expressed in neurons, while miR-23 is restrictively expressed in astrocytes. miR-26 and miR-29 display higher expression in astrocytes than in neurons; and miR-9 and miR-125 are evenly expressed in neurons and astrocytes (Smirnova et al., 2005). Overexpressing *miR-124* in cultured NSCs and in embryonic cortical NPs using lenti-virus and *in utero* electroporation, respectively, promotes neurogenesis and stimulates cortical progenitor migration (Maiorano and Mallamaci, 2009). In cultured adult NSCs, overexpressing *miR-124* enhances neuronal differentiation (Cheng et al., 2009). Ectopic expression of miR-124a and miR-9 in the embryonic stem cell-derived NPs results in a great reduction of GFAP-positive astrocytes compared to the control groups, while knockdown of miR-9, but not miR-124a, switches differentiation of NPs from neurogenesis to astrogliogenesis (Krichevsky et al., 2006). miR-124 and miR-9 promotes neurogenesis by targeting phospholated signal transducer and activator of transcription 3 (STAT3), a transcription factor normally initiating astrogliogenesis (Bonni et al., 1997; Krichevsky et al., 2006).

miR-200 family members, including miR-200a, miR-200b, miR-200c, miR-141 and miR-429, are highly expressed in the developing olfactory bulb. Loss of function of the *miR-200* family prevents normal differentiation of olfactory precursors into mature neurons (Choi et al., 2008). Foxg1, Zfhx1 and Lfng have been identified as the targets of the miR-200 family that affect neurogenesis of the olfactory bulb.

Specific miRNAs that promote gliogenesis have also been identified. Brain-enriched miR-125b is up-regulated in cultured interleulin-6 (IL-6)-induced human astrocytes. Loss of function of *miR-125b* causes an impaired proliferation of astrocytes, accompanied by an upregulation of a miR-125b target cyclin-dependent kinase inhibitor 2A (CDKN2A), which is a negative modulator for cell proliferation (Pogue et al., 2010). The *miR-17-92* cluster displays enriched expression in cultured oligodendrocytes. Specific deletion of the *miR-17-92* cluster from oligodendrocyte precursor cells (OPCs) results in a decreased number of Olig2-positive oligodendrocytes in the mouse brain (Budde et al., 2010). Overexpression of *miR-17* and *miR-19b* in cultures increases the number of oligodendrocytes. The *miR-17-92* cluster regulates oligodendrocyte development by targeting tumor suppressor *Pten* and activating its downstream Akt signaling pathway.

Moreover, *miR-219* and *miR-338* are identified in the oligodendrocyte lineage in the mouse spinal cord and brain. Overexpression of *miR-219* and *miR-338* in cultured OPCs and in the embryonic chick neural tube promotes differentiation of oligodendrocytes, while knockdown of these two miRNAs in OPC cultures and knockdown of *miR-219* in zebrafish abolish oligodendrocyte maturation (Zhao et al., 2010b). Oligodendrocyte differentiation inhibitors Sox6 and Hes5 are identified as targets of miR-219 and miR-338 during oligodendrocyte development (Zhao et al., 2010b).

Lamin B1 (LMNB1) is reported to be associated with autosomal domination leukodystrophy disease (ADLD), a CNS demyelination disorder (Padiath et al., 2006). Overexpression of Lamin B1 represses expression of oligodendrocyte-specific genes such as myelin basic protein (MBP) and myelin oligodendrocyte glycoprotein (MOG), and leads to impaired oligodendrocyte maturation. A recent study has shown that Lamin B1 is post-transcriptionally regulated by miR-23, a glia-specific miRNA. Overexpression of *miR-23* results in significantly increased number of oligodendrocytes and rescues the defects of oligodendrocyte differentiation caused by Lamin B1 (Lin and Fu, 2009).

3.5.2 Cell fate determination regulated by lncRNAs

Studies of lncRNA functions on NSC differentiation are emerging. Dlx-6 is a homeobox containing transcription factor and plays an important role in forebrain neurogenesis (Wang et al., 2010). *Embryonic ventral forebrain-1 (Evf1)* is a 2.7 kb lncRNA transcribed upstream of the mouse *Dlx-6* gene (Kohtz and Fishell, 2004). As an alternatively spliced form of *Evf1*, *Evf2* is transcribed from the intergenic region between the *Dlx-5* and *Dlx-6* loci, and is overlapped with the conserved *Dlx-5/6* intergenic enhancer (Feng et al., 2006; Zerucha et al., 2000) (Fig. 5B). Induced by the Sonic hedgehog (Shh) signaling pathway, *Evf2* has been proven to function as a transcriptional co-activator of Dlx-2 and activates the *Dlx5/6* enhancer during forebrain development (Feng et al., 2006). Deletion of *Evf2* results in a reduction of GABAergic interneurons and impaired synaptic inhibition in the developing hippocampus (Bond et al., 2009).

Nkx2.2 antisense (Nkx2.2as) is an antisense lncRNA to *Nkx2.2* gene, which is expressed in the developing mammalian forebrain and is required for oligodendrocyte development (Price et al., 1992) (Fig. 5C). Ectopic expression of *Nkx2.2as* in cultured NSCs induces oligodendrocyte differentiation through an upregulation of the *Nkx2.2* mRNA level, suggesting that *Nkx2.2as* regulates NSC differentiation and promotes gliogenesis by modulating protein coding gene *Nkx2.2* expression (Tochitani and Hayashizaki, 2008).

Retinal noncoding RNA 2 (RNCR2), an intergenic lncRNA also known as *Gomafu* and *Miat*, is an abundant polyadenylated RNA in the developing retina (Blackshaw et al., 2004). *RNCR2* is highly expressed in both mitotic and postmitotic retinal progenitors. Knockdown of *RNCR2* leads to an increase of amacrine cells and Müller glial cells in postnatal retina. Mislocalization of *RNCR2* from nuclear to cytoplasm photocopies the effects caused by *RNCR2* knockdown, suggesting that *RNCR2* is required for retinal precursor cell specification (Rapicavoli et al., 2010).

4. Noncoding RNAs as a tool for stem cell-based therapy

Because of the features of self-renewal and the ability to differentiate into many cell types in the CNS, applying NSCs for the treatment of neurological disorders, especially neurodegeneration diseases and injuries in the CNS, has become promising. Directing NSCs into specific cell types and transplanting these cells to replace damaged cells in the CNS have been proven to be successful in some mouse models (Kim and de Vellis, 2009).

Transplantation of NSCs into aged triple transgenic Alzheimer's disease mouse model (3×Tg-AD) rescues the spatial learning and memory defects in these mice (Blurton-Jones et al., 2009). Parkinson's disease (PD) results from a loss of dopaminergic neurons in the substantia nigra. It involves abnormalities in movement variably accompanied by sensory, mood and cognitive changes. Transplantation of undifferentiated human NSCs into PD primate models causes a significant behavioral improvement (Redmond et al., 2007). Directed differentiation of mouse ventral midbrain NSCs in the presence of Shh, FGF8 and Wnt5a produce 10-fold more dopaminergic neurons *in vitro* (Parish et al., 2008).

Transplantation of these pre-differentiated dopaminergic neurons into the brain of PD mouse models results in functional recovery (Parish et al., 2008). Implantation of human NSCs in the rat model of Huntington's disease (HD) is shown improved motor function (McBride et al., 2004). Furthermore, delayed transplantation of adult mouse NSCs surrounding the lesion site of the spinal cord promotes remyelination and functional recovery after spinal cord injuries in rats (Karimi-Abdolrezaee et al., 2006).

Stem cell-based therapeutic applications for neurological disorders also face problems. First, the molecular mechanisms that control NSC proliferation and differentiation into distinct cell types are still unclear. Second, to succeed in clinical applications, transplanting sufficient numbers of NSCs and specific neuronal cell types is critical. Third, to achieve functional recovery from neurological disorders, transplanted cells need to acquire connections with neighbor neurons and restore neural circuitry. Although little studies of using ncRNAs for therapeutic treatment have been done, the emerging reports of ncRNA functions in NSC proliferation and cell fate determination have shown promising future directions. Moreover, due to the technical advances in ncRNA *in vitro* synthesis and delivery, particularly miRNAs, manipulating ncRNA expressions in NSCs will provide a new means for stem cell based therapies for neurological diseases.

5. Acknowledgment

We thank members of the Sun lab for providing thoughtful comments. Owing to space limitations, we apologize for being unable to cite many excellent papers in this field. This work was supported by the Ellison Medical Foundation (T. S.), an award from the Hirschl/Weill-Caulier Trust (T. S.) and an R01-MH083680 grant from the NIH/NIMH (T. S.).

6. References

Amaral PP, Neyt C, Wilkins SJ, Askarian-Amiri ME, Sunkin SM, Perkins AC, et al. Complex architecture and regulated expression of the Sox2ot locus during vertebrate development. *RNA* 2009; 15: 2013-27.

Ambros V. The evolution of our thinking about microRNAs. *Nat Med* 2008; 14: 1036-40.

Andersson T, Rahman S, Sansom SN, Alsio JM, Kaneda M, Smith J, et al. Reversible block of mouse neural stem cell differentiation in the absence of dicer and microRNAs. *PLoS One* 2010; 5: e13453.

Arvanitis DN, Jungas T, Behar A, Davy A. Ephrin-B1 reverse signaling controls a posttranscriptional feedback mechanism via miR-124. Mol Cell Biol 2010; 30: 2508-17.

Bian S, Sun T. Functions of Noncoding RNAs in Neural Development and Neurological Diseases. *Mol Neurobiol* 2011; 44: 359-73.

Blackshaw S, Harpavat S, Trimarchi J, Cai L, Huang H, Kuo WP, et al. Genomic analysis of mouse retinal development. *PLoS Biol* 2004; 2: E247.

Blurton-Jones M, Kitazawa M, Martinez-Coria H, Castello NA, Muller FJ, Loring JF, et al. Neural stem cells improve cognition via BDNF in a transgenic model of Alzheimer disease. *Proc Natl Acad Sci U S A* 2009; 106: 13594-9.

Bond AM, Vangompel MJ, Sametsky EA, Clark MF, Savage JC, Disterhoft JF, et al. Balanced gene regulation by an embryonic brain ncRNA is critical for adult hippocampal GABA circuitry. *Nat Neurosci* 2009; 12: 1020-7.

Bonev B, Pisco A, Papalopulu N. MicroRNA-9 reveals regional diversity of neural progenitors along the anterior-posterior axis. *Dev Cell* 2011; 20: 19-32.

Bonni A, Sun Y, Nadal-Vicens M, Bhatt A, Frank DA, Rozovsky I, et al. Regulation of gliogenesis in the central nervous system by the JAK-STAT signaling pathway. *Science* 1997; 278: 477-83.

Brennecke J, Malone CD, Aravin AA, Sachidanandam R, Stark A, Hannon GJ. An epigenetic role for maternally inherited piRNAs in transposon silencing. *Science* 2008; 322: 1387-92.

Brett JO, Renault VM, Rafalski VA, Webb AE, Brunet A. The microRNA cluster miR-106b~25 regulates adult neural stem/progenitor cell proliferation and neuronal differentiation. *Aging (Albany NY)* 2011; 3: 108-24.

Budde H, Schmitt S, Fitzner D, Opitz L, Salinas-Riester G, Simons M. Control of oligodendroglial cell number by the miR-17-92 cluster. *Development* 2010; 137: 2127-32.

Carninci P, Kasukawa T, Katayama S, Gough J, Frith MC, Maeda N, et al. The transcriptional landscape of the mammalian genome. *Science* 2005; 309: 1559-63.

Cheng LC, Pastrana E, Tavazoie M, Doetsch F. miR-124 regulates adult neurogenesis in the subventricular zone stem cell niche. *Nat Neurosci* 2009; 12: 399-408.

Choi PS, Zakhary L, Choi WY, Caron S, Alvarez-Saavedra E, Miska EA, et al. Members of the miRNA-200 family regulate olfactory neurogenesis. *Neuron* 2008; 57: 41-55.

Cuellar TL, Davis TH, Nelson PT, Loeb GB, Harfe BD, Ullian E, et al. Dicer loss in striatal neurons produces behavioral and neuroanatomical phenotypes in the absence of neurodegeneration. *Proc Natl Acad Sci U S A* 2008; 105: 5614-9.

Das PP, Bagijn MP, Goldstein LD, Woolford JR, Lehrbach NJ, Sapetschnig A, et al. Piwi and piRNAs act upstream of an endogenous siRNA pathway to suppress Tc3 transposon mobility in the Caenorhabditis elegans germline. *Mol Cell* 2008; 31: 79-90.

Davis TH, Cuellar TL, Koch SM, Barker AJ, Harfe BD, McManus MT, et al. Conditional loss of Dicer disrupts cellular and tissue morphogenesis in the cortex and hippocampus. *J Neurosci* 2008; 28: 4322-30.

De Pietri Tonelli D, Pulvers JN, Haffner C, Murchison EP, Hannon GJ, Huttner WB. miRNAs are essential for survival and differentiation of newborn neurons but not for expansion of neural progenitors during early neurogenesis in the mouse embryonic neocortex. *Development* 2008; 135: 3911-21.

Decembrini S, Bressan D, Vignali R, Pitto L, Mariotti S, Rainaldi G, et al. MicroRNAs couple cell fate and developmental timing in retina. *Proc Natl Acad Sci U S A* 2009; 106: 21179-84.

Delaloy C, Liu L, Lee JA, Su H, Shen F, Yang GY, et al. MicroRNA-9 coordinates proliferation and migration of human embryonic stem cell-derived neural progenitors. *Cell Stem Cell* 2010; 6: 323-35.

Denisenko O, Shnyreva M, Suzuki H, Bomsztyk K. Point mutations in the WD40 domain of Eed block its interaction with Ezh2. *Mol Cell Biol* 1998; 18: 5634-42.

Doe CQ. Neural stem cells: balancing self-renewal with differentiation. *Development* 2008; 135: 1575-87.

Feng J, Bi C, Clark BS, Mady R, Shah P, Kohtz JD. The Evf-2 noncoding RNA is transcribed from the Dlx-5/6 ultraconserved region and functions as a Dlx-2 transcriptional coactivator. *Genes Dev* 2006; 20: 1470-84.

Fukagawa T, Nogami M, Yoshikawa M, Ikeno M, Okazaki T, Takami Y, et al. Dicer is essential for formation of the heterochromatin structure in vertebrate cells. *Nat Cell Biol* 2004; 6: 784-91.

Gage FH. Mammalian neural stem cells. *Science* 2000; 287: 1433-8.

Gaughwin P, Ciesla M, Yang H, Lim B, Brundin P. Stage-Specific Modulation of Cortical Neuronal Development by Mmu-miR-134. *Cereb Cortex* 2011.

Giam M, Huang DC, Bouillet P. BH3-only proteins and their roles in programmed cell death. *Oncogene* 2008; 27 Suppl 1: S128-36.

Gregory RI, Chendrimada TP, Shiekhattar R. MicroRNA biogenesis: isolation and characterization of the microprocessor complex. *Methods Mol Biol* 2006; 342: 33-47.

Guidi M, Muinos-Gimeno M, Kagerbauer B, Marti E, Estivill X, Espinosa-Parrilla Y. Overexpression of miR-128 specifically inhibits the truncated isoform of NTRK3 and upregulates BCL2 in SH-SY5Y neuroblastoma cells. *BMC Mol Biol* 2010; 11: 95.

Hebert SS, Papadopoulou AS, Smith P, Galas MC, Planel E, Silahtaroglu AN, et al. Genetic ablation of Dicer in adult forebrain neurons results in abnormal tau hyperphosphorylation and neurodegeneration. *Hum Mol Genet* 2010; 19: 3959-69.

Houwing S, Kamminga LM, Berezikov E, Cronembold D, Girard A, van den Elst H, et al. A role for Piwi and piRNAs in germ cell maintenance and transposon silencing in Zebrafish. *Cell* 2007; 129: 69-82.

Huang J, Wu S, Barrera J, Matthews K, Pan D. The Hippo signaling pathway coordinately regulates cell proliferation and apoptosis by inactivating Yorkie, the Drosophila Homolog of YAP. *Cell* 2005; 122: 421-34.

Kanellopoulou C, Muljo SA, Kung AL, Ganesan S, Drapkin R, Jenuwein T, et al. Dicer-deficient mouse embryonic stem cells are defective in differentiation and centromeric silencing. *Genes Dev* 2005; 19: 489-501.

Kapranov P, Cheng J, Dike S, Nix DA, Duttagupta R, Willingham AT, et al. RNA maps reveal new RNA classes and a possible function for pervasive transcription. *Science* 2007; 316: 1484-8.

Karimi-Abdolrezaee S, Eftekharpour E, Wang J, Morshead CM, Fehlings MG. Delayed transplantation of adult neural precursor cells promotes remyelination and functional neurological recovery after spinal cord injury. *J Neurosci* 2006; 26: 3377-89.

Kawase-Koga Y, Low R, Otaegi G, Pollock A, Deng H, Eisenhaber F, et al. RNAase-III enzyme Dicer maintains signaling pathways for differentiation and survival in mouse cortical neural stem cells. *J Cell Sci* 2010; 123: 586-94.

Kawase-Koga Y, Otaegi G, Sun T. Different timings of Dicer deletion affect neurogenesis and gliogenesis in the developing mouse central nervous system. *Dev Dyn* 2009; 238: 2800-12.

Khanna A, Muthusamy S, Liang R, Sarojini H, Wang E. Gain of survival signaling by down-regulation of three key miRNAs in brain of calorie-restricted mice. *Aging (Albany NY)* 2011; 3: 223-36.

Khraiwesh B, Arif MA, Seumel GI, Ossowski S, Weigel D, Reski R, et al. Transcriptional control of gene expression by microRNAs. *Cell* 2010; 140: 111-22.

Kim SU, de Vellis J. Stem cell-based cell therapy in neurological diseases: a review. *J Neurosci Res* 2009; 87: 2183-200.

Kohtz JD, Fishell G. Developmental regulation of EVF-1, a novel non-coding RNA transcribed upstream of the mouse Dlx6 gene. *Gene Expr Patterns* 2004; 4: 407-12.

Kole AJ, Swahari V, Hammond SM, Deshmukh M. miR-29b is activated during neuronal maturation and targets BH3-only genes to restrict apoptosis. *Genes Dev* 2011; 25: 125-30.

Kotake Y, Nakagawa T, Kitagawa K, Suzuki S, Liu N, Kitagawa M, et al. Long non-coding RNA ANRIL is required for the PRC2 recruitment to and silencing of p15(INK4B) tumor suppressor gene. *Oncogene* 2010; 30: 1956-62.

Krichevsky AM, Sonntag KC, Isacson O, Kosik KS. Specific microRNAs modulate embryonic stem cell-derived neurogenesis. *Stem Cells* 2006; 24: 857-64.

Lagos-Quintana M, Rauhut R, Lendeckel W, Tuschl T. Identification of novel genes coding for small expressed RNAs. *Science* 2001; 294: 853-8.

Lagos-Quintana M, Rauhut R, Yalcin A, Meyer J, Lendeckel W, Tuschl T. Identification of tissue-specific microRNAs from mouse. *Curr Biol* 2002; 12: 735-9.

Lander ES, Linton LM, Birren B, Nusbaum C, Zody MC, Baldwin J, et al. Initial sequencing and analysis of the human genome. *Nature* 2001; 409: 860-921.

Lau NC, Lim LP, Weinstein EG, Bartel DP. An abundant class of tiny RNAs with probable regulatory roles in Caenorhabditis elegans. *Science* 2001; 294: 858-62.

Lau NC, Seto AG, Kim J, Kuramochi-Miyagawa S, Nakano T, Bartel DP, et al. Characterization of the piRNA complex from rat testes. *Science* 2006; 313: 363-7.

Leaman D, Chen PY, Fak J, Yalcin A, Pearce M, Unnerstall U, et al. Antisense-mediated depletion reveals essential and specific functions of microRNAs in Drosophila development. *Cell* 2005; 121: 1097-108.

Lee RC, Ambros V. An extensive class of small RNAs in Caenorhabditis elegans. *Science* 2001; 294: 862-4.

Leucht C, Stigloher C, Wizenmann A, Klafke R, Folchert A, Bally-Cuif L. MicroRNA-9 directs late organizer activity of the midbrain-hindbrain boundary. *Nat Neurosci* 2008; 11: 641-8.

Lin ST, Fu YH. miR-23 regulation of lamin B1 is crucial for oligodendrocyte development and myelination. *Dis Model Mech* 2009; 2: 178-88.

Liu C, Teng ZQ, Santistevan NJ, Szulwach KE, Guo W, Jin P, et al. Epigenetic regulation of miR-184 by MBD1 governs neural stem cell proliferation and differentiation. *Cell Stem Cell* 2010; 6: 433-44.

Lund E, Dahlberg JE. Substrate selectivity of exportin 5 and Dicer in the biogenesis of microRNAs. *Cold Spring Harb Symp Quant Biol* 2006; 71: 59-66.

Maiorano NA, Mallamaci A. Promotion of embryonic cortico-cerebral neuronogenesis by miR-124. *Neural Dev* 2009; 4: 40.

Makeyev EV, Zhang J, Carrasco MA, Maniatis T. The MicroRNA miR-124 promotes neuronal differentiation by triggering brain-specific alternative pre-mRNA splicing. *Mol Cell* 2007; 27: 435-48.

Mancini-Dinardo D, Steele SJ, Levorse JM, Ingram RS, Tilghman SM. Elongation of the Kcnq1ot1 transcript is required for genomic imprinting of neighboring genes. *Genes Dev* 2006; 20: 1268-82.

Mazo A, Hodgson JW, Petruk S, Sedkov Y, Brock HW. Transcriptional interference: an unexpected layer of complexity in gene regulation. *J Cell Sci* 2007; 120: 2755-61.

McBride JL, Behrstock SP, Chen EY, Jakel RJ, Siegel I, Svendsen CN, et al. Human neural stem cell transplants improve motor function in a rat model of Huntington's disease. *J Comp Neurol* 2004; 475: 211-9.

Mercer TR, Dinger ME, Sunkin SM, Mehler MF, Mattick JS. Specific expression of long noncoding RNAs in the mouse brain. *Proc Natl Acad Sci U S A* 2008; 105: 716-21.

Neilson JR, Sharp PA. Small RNA regulators of gene expression. *Cell* 2008; 134: 899-902.

Nguyen VT, Kiss T, Michels AA, Bensaude O. 7SK small nuclear RNA binds to and inhibits the activity of CDK9/cyclin T complexes. *Nature* 2001; 414: 322-5.

Otaegi G, Pollock A, Hong J, Sun T. MicroRNA miR-9 modifies motor neuron columns by a tuning regulation of FoxP1 levels in developing spinal cords. *J Neurosci* 2011; 31: 809-18.

Padiath QS, Saigoh K, Schiffmann R, Asahara H, Yamada T, Koeppen A, et al. Lamin B1 duplications cause autosomal dominant leukodystrophy. *Nat Genet* 2006; 38: 1114-23.

Parish CL, Castelo-Branco G, Rawal N, Tonnesen J, Sorensen AT, Salto C, et al. Wnt5a-treated midbrain neural stem cells improve dopamine cell replacement therapy in parkinsonian mice. *J Clin Invest* 2008; 118: 149-60.

Pasmant E, Laurendeau I, Heron D, Vidaud M, Vidaud D, Bieche I. Characterization of a germ-line deletion, including the entire INK4/ARF locus, in a melanoma-neural system tumor family: identification of ANRIL, an antisense noncoding RNA whose expression coclusters with ARF. *Cancer Res* 2007; 67: 3963-9.

Pevny L, Placzek M. SOX genes and neural progenitor identity. *Curr Opin Neurobiol* 2005; 15: 7-13.

Pogue AI, Cui JG, Li YY, Zhao Y, Culicchia F, Lukiw WJ. Micro RNA-125b (miRNA-125b) function in astrogliosis and glial cell proliferation. *Neurosci Lett* 2010; 476: 18-22.

Pratt AJ, MacRae IJ. The RNA-induced silencing complex: a versatile gene-silencing machine. *J Biol Chem* 2009; 284: 17897-901.

Price M, Lazzaro D, Pohl T, Mattei MG, Ruther U, Olivo JC, et al. Regional expression of the homeobox gene Nkx-2.2 in the developing mammalian forebrain. *Neuron* 1992; 8: 241-55.

Rana TM. Illuminating the silence: understanding the structure and function of small RNAs. *Nat Rev Mol Cell Biol* 2007; 8: 23-36.

Rapicavoli NA, Poth EM, Blackshaw S. The long noncoding RNA RNCR2 directs mouse retinal cell specification. *BMC Dev Biol* 2010; 10: 49.

Redmond DE, Jr., Bjugstad KB, Teng YD, Ourednik V, Ourednik J, Wakeman DR, et al. Behavioral improvement in a primate Parkinson's model is associated with multiple homeostatic effects of human neural stem cells. *Proc Natl Acad Sci U S A* 2007; 104: 12175-80.

Reinhart BJ, Slack FJ, Basson M, Pasquinelli AE, Bettinger JC, Rougvie AE, et al. The 21-nucleotide let-7 RNA regulates developmental timing in Caenorhabditis elegans. *Nature* 2000; 403: 901-6.

Renault VM, Rafalski VA, Morgan AA, Salih DA, Brett JO, Webb AE, et al. FoxO3 regulates neural stem cell homeostasis. *Cell Stem Cell* 2009; 5: 527-39.

Rinn JL, Kertesz M, Wang JK, Squazzo SL, Xu X, Brugmann SA, et al. Functional demarcation of active and silent chromatin domains in human HOX loci by noncoding RNAs. *Cell* 2007; 129: 1311-23.

Rybak A, Fuchs H, Smirnova L, Brandt C, Pohl EE, Nitsch R, et al. A feedback loop comprising lin-28 and let-7 controls pre-let-7 maturation during neural stem-cell commitment. *Nat Cell Biol* 2008; 10: 987-93.

Sanchez-Elsner T, Gou D, Kremmer E, Sauer F. Noncoding RNAs of trithorax response elements recruit Drosophila Ash1 to Ultrabithorax. *Science* 2006; 311: 1118-23.

Sathyan P, Golden HB, Miranda RC. Competing interactions between micro-RNAs determine neural progenitor survival and proliferation after ethanol exposure: evidence from an ex vivo model of the fetal cerebral cortical neuroepithelium. *J Neurosci* 2007; 27: 8546-57.

Saucedo LJ, Edgar BA. Filling out the Hippo pathway. *Nat Rev Mol Cell Biol* 2007; 8: 613-21.

Seto AG, Kingston RE, Lau NC. The coming of age for Piwi proteins. *Mol Cell* 2007; 26: 603-9.

Shamovsky I, Ivannikov M, Kandel ES, Gershon D, Nudler E. RNA-mediated response to heat shock in mammalian cells. *Nature* 2006; 440: 556-60.

Shi Y, Sun G, Zhao C, Stewart R. Neural stem cell self-renewal. *Crit Rev Oncol Hematol* 2008; 65: 43-53.

Shibata M, Nakao H, Kiyonari H, Abe T, Aizawa S. MicroRNA-9 regulates neurogenesis in mouse telencephalon by targeting multiple transcription factors. *J Neurosci* 2011; 31: 3407-22.

Smirnova L, Grafe A, Seiler A, Schumacher S, Nitsch R, Wulczyn FG. Regulation of miRNA expression during neural cell specification. *Eur J Neurosci* 2005; 21: 1469-77.

Szulwach KE, Li X, Smrt RD, Li Y, Luo Y, Lin L, et al. Cross talk between microRNA and epigenetic regulation in adult neurogenesis. *J Cell Biol* 2010; 189: 127-41.

Temple S. The development of neural stem cells. *Nature* 2001; 414: 112-7.

Thompson BJ, Cohen SM. The Hippo pathway regulates the bantam microRNA to control cell proliferation and apoptosis in Drosophila. *Cell* 2006; 126: 767-74.

Tochitani S, Hayashizaki Y. Nkx2.2 antisense RNA overexpression enhanced oligodendrocytic differentiation. *Biochem Biophys Res Commun* 2008; 372: 691-6.

Tsai MC, Manor O, Wan Y, Mosammaparast N, Wang JK, Lan F, et al. Long noncoding RNA as modular scaffold of histone modification complexes. *Science* 2010; 329: 689-93.

Walker JC, Harland RM. microRNA-24a is required to repress apoptosis in the developing neural retina. *Genes Dev* 2009; 23: 1046-51.

Wang X, Arai S, Song X, Reichart D, Du K, Pascual G, et al. Induced ncRNAs allosterically modify RNA-binding proteins in cis to inhibit transcription. *Nature* 2008; 454: 126-30.

Wang XJ, Reyes JL, Chua NH, Gaasterland T. Prediction and identification of Arabidopsis thaliana microRNAs and their mRNA targets. *Genome Biol* 2004; 5: R65.

Wang Y, Dye CA, Sohal V, Long JE, Estrada RC, Roztocil T, et al. Dlx5 and Dlx6 regulate the development of parvalbumin-expressing cortical interneurons. *J Neurosci* 2010; 30: 5334-45.

Willingham AT, Orth AP, Batalov S, Peters EC, Wen BG, Aza-Blanc P, et al. A strategy for probing the function of noncoding RNAs finds a repressor of NFAT. *Science* 2005; 309: 1570-3.

Wutz A, Rasmussen TP, Jaenisch R. Chromosomal silencing and localization are mediated by different domains of Xist RNA. *Nat Genet* 2002; 30: 167-74.

Yang Z, Zhu Q, Luo K, Zhou Q. The 7SK small nuclear RNA inhibits the CDK9/cyclin T1 kinase to control transcription. *Nature* 2001; 414: 317-22.

Yu W, Gius D, Onyango P, Muldoon-Jacobs K, Karp J, Feinberg AP, et al. Epigenetic silencing of tumour suppressor gene p15 by its antisense RNA. *Nature* 2008; 451: 202-6.

Zehir A, Hua LL, Maska EL, Morikawa Y, Cserjesi P. Dicer is required for survival of differentiating neural crest cells. *Dev Biol* 2010; 340: 459-67.

Zerucha T, Stuhmer T, Hatch G, Park BK, Long Q, Yu G, et al. A highly conserved enhancer in the Dlx5/Dlx6 intergenic region is the site of cross-regulatory interactions between Dlx genes in the embryonic forebrain. *J Neurosci* 2000; 20: 709-21.

Zhao C, Sun G, Li S, Lang MF, Yang S, Li W, et al. MicroRNA let-7b regulates neural stem cell proliferation and differentiation by targeting nuclear receptor TLX signaling. *Proc Natl Acad Sci U S A* 2010a; 107: 1876-81.

Zhao C, Sun G, Li S, Shi Y. A feedback regulatory loop involving microRNA-9 and nuclear receptor TLX in neural stem cell fate determination. *Nat Struct Mol Biol* 2009; 16: 365-71.

Zhao X, He X, Han X, Yu Y, Ye F, Chen Y, et al. MicroRNA-mediated control of oligodendrocyte differentiation. *Neuron* 2010b; 65: 612-26.

Zheng K, Li H, Zhu Y, Zhu Q, Qiu M. MicroRNAs are essential for the developmental switch from neurogenesis to gliogenesis in the developing spinal cord. *J Neurosci* 2010; 30: 8245-50.

2

Neural Stem/Progenitor Cell Clones as Models for Neural Development and Transplantation

Hedong Li, He Zhao, Xiaoqiong Shu and Mei Jiang
West China Developmental & Stem Cell Institute,
Department of Obstetric & Gynecologic/Pediatric,
Key Laboratory of Obstetric & Gynecologic,
Pediatric Diseases and Birth Defects of Ministry of Education,
West China Second University Hospital,
Sichuan University, Chengdu, Sichuan Province,
P.R. China

1. Introduction

Neural stem cells (NSCs) are somatic stem cells, capable of giving rise to all the mature cell types of the adult nervous system. NSCs are generally "simple" in their cell shape, and acquire much more complex morphology as they differentiate into mature cell types. Morphological changes are not the only phenomena, both genetic and epigenetic alterations also mark the NSC differentiation, allowing development of series of genetic and immunological markers to identify and isolate certain cell types from developing neural tissue. During early phase of the development of central nervous system (CNS), NSCs occupy the newly formed neural tube as a thin layer of cells (called neuroepithelium), which later become thicker and more complex in cellular architecture by the process of cell proliferation, differentiation, migration and maturation in a precisely organized fashion. The underlying mechanisms of these processes are always the attraction to neurobiologists.

NSC differentiation does not occur overnight; rather, it occurs in a progressive manner hypothesized by the lineage-restriction theory. As development proceeds, NSCs acquire additional features (demonstrated by markers) and become regionally diversified under the influence of gradients of growth factors and cytokines. These cells still proliferate, but their differentiation potential may be limited capable of giving rise to fewer cell types as they divide. This group of dividing cells at any CNS developmental stages is often referred as "neural progenitor pool" (Fig. 1). Lineage restriction hypothesis indicates that NSCs undergo progressive loss of differentiation potential (i.e. the number of cell types that they can give rise to) as neural development proceeds. In support of this notion, certain cell surface markers (e.g. A2B5 and 5A5) have been found to label and fractionate lineage-restricted progenitors of the developing spinal cord in a non-overlapping manner (Mayer-Proschel et al., 1997). However, lineage restriction is not the only mechanism of NSC development. For example, Noble examined the expression patterns of A2B5 and 5A5 in the developing forebrain and identified a population of neural progenitors expressing both markers suggesting that NSC differentiation is a much more complicated process in the brain than in the spinal cord (Noble et al., 2003). Therefore, the original lineage-restriction theory based on the expression of A2B5 and 5A5 may be an oversimplified one and can not be generalized to explain NSC differentiation in the entire developing CNS. Nevertheless, it initiated a logical prediction, which will be modified or corrected by more upcoming results from different area of the developing CNS.

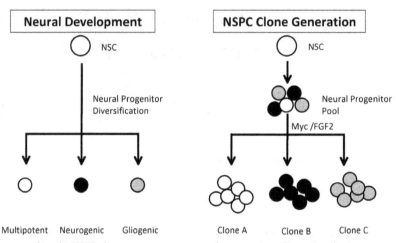

Fig. 1. Immortalized NSPC clones represent neural progenitor diversity during development.

NSCs differentiate at different rate and direction, which creates a diversity of neural progenitors at any given period of CNS development. One way to reveal neural progenitor diversity is to generate neural progenitor clones (Fig. 1). Over the past decades, numerous NSC and neural progenitor clones have been generated, and they have proven to be great models in delineating mechanisms of NSC differentiation. Many of these clones have also been transplanted into animal models of various neurological diseases and trauma, and demonstrated their great usefulness for obtaining mechanistic insights on how exogenous NSCs interact with host tissues and promising effects in animal's behavioural recovery. In our laboratory, we also took this approach and generated various neural stem/progenitor cell (NSPC) clones from rat embryonic forebrains. In this book chapter, we will review more recent discoveries with these "old" and more recently generated neural progenitor clones as in vitro models to unravel NSC differentiation mechanisms as well as cellular tools for testing their therapeutic potentials in paradigms of transplantation. In the era of translational research, we would like to stress on the need for neurobiologists to take on the mission seriously and format our thinking to materialize the transition from bench to bedside.

2. Generation of neural stem/progenitor cell clones

Neural cell lines have been generated by numerous approaches including isolation from spontaneous or induced neural tumors and somatic cell fusion with immortal cells. These cell lines have been widely used as in vitro models, some of which we are still experimenting on today such as Neuro-2a, PC12 cells. More recently, with the advance of our understanding on genetic networks controlling cell proliferation, the "purpose-driven" generation of NSPC clones has been systematically performed. Both growth factor stimulation (epigenetic) and viral introduction of immortalizing genes such as oncogenes (genetic) have proven to be efficient in generating NSPC clones. In this section, we will summarize genetic functions of commonly used immortalizing genes (Myc, neu, large T-antigen, adenoviral E1A, Tert and p53) in promoting cell proliferation and growth factor dependency of the resulting NSPC clones including human NSPC clones (summarized in Table 1 below).

2.1 Immortalizing genes

Myc has been most extensively studied in cancer research since its deregulation relates many different types of tumors (Grandori et al., 2000). Myc also plays a critical role in stem cell biology and development where its expression is tightly controlled (Laurenti et al., 2009). As such, many cancers have been suggested to derive from stem cells during development where Myc expression persists or is deregulated into the adulthood. Myc has various cellular functions ranging from proliferation, cell growth and differentiation to apoptosis. Thirty years after its discovery, the exact molecular mechanisms of Myc mediating these functions still remain elusive. As an immortalizing tool, however, Myc has been widely used to generate cell lines from different lineages, especially neural cell lines, some of which are still widely applied in neuroscience research.

Myc encodes a transcription factor that binds to E-box sequence CACGTG on genomic DNA. Myc protein dimerizes with another bHLH transcription factor Max through its bHLH/LZ domain, and its transregulatory domain can interact with numerous co-factors to execute its transcriptional activity on target genes including the transcription activator E2F-1 (Fig. 2). The critical function domains of Myc proteins have been mapped to their N- and C-terminus, which contain the transregulatory domain and the basic-helix-loop-helix-leucine zipper (bHLH/LZ) domain, respectively (Farina et al., 1992; Min et al., 1993; Min and Taparowsky, 1992).

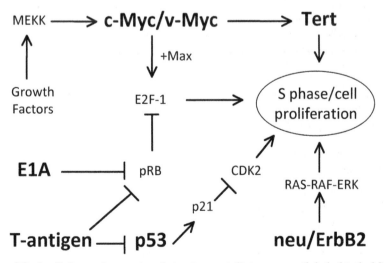

Fig. 2. Simplified cellular pathways involving immortalizing genes (labeled in bold).

V-Myc, the viral homologue of cellular Myc (c-Myc), was first discovered from a transforming retrovirus MC29 from chicken with spontaneous myelocytomatosis and subsequently cloned and sequenced (Alitalo et al., 1983; Reddy et al., 1983; Watson et al., 1983). V-Myc is expressed as a fusion protein Gag-Myc in MC29 and other related retroviruses. Although the Gag portion of the fusion protein seems to be dispensable in its transforming activity (Shaw et al., 1985), the first generation of v-Myc containing retrovirus for immortalization was created as fusion of v-Myc with part of Gag protein (Villa et al., 2000). Myc genes carry mutations, some of which potentiate their transforming activity. A frequently detected mutation Thr58 on c-Myc, which is equivalent to Thr61 on v-Myc, is often found in Burkitt's lymphomas where c-Myc was first discovered (Albert et al., 1994). A Thr58 to Ala substitution (T58A) in c-Myc has been found to promote its proliferative effect in NSCs, and a resulting NSC line immortalized by this mutant c-Myc exhibited enhanced cell proliferation compared with NSC line generated by the wild type gene (De Filippis et al., 2008).

Large T antigen is another popular immortalizing gene used to generate NSC lines. Numerous NSC lines have been derived by utilizing different forms of large T antigen (e.g. temperature-sensitive and N-terminally truncated mutants) from different regions of the developing CNS (Whittemore and Snyder, 1996). SV40 large T antigen is one of the early gene products during viral infection by polyomavirus SV40. SV40 is a double-stranded DNA virus first identified in 1960 and is responsible for formation of solid tumors upon infection. Large T antigen is involved in viral genome replication after infection and regulation of host cell cycle mainly through its perturbation of tumor suppressor protein p53 and the retinoblastoma protein (pRB) (Fig. 2), although several other cellular factors, including the transcriptional co-activators p300 and CBP, may also contribute to its transformation function (Ahuja et al., 2005).

p53 is a tumor suppressor protein and its function is involved in preventing cancer formation. P53 plays many cellular roles in its anti-cancer function, which include cell cycle regulation, apoptosis and genome stability. Upon activation, p53 can initiate a cell cycle arrest to allow DNA repair to take place, or signal cells to go on apoptosis if the DNA damage is unfixable. One mechanism of such function of p53 protein is that, upon activation, it can turn on the expression of p21, which forms complex with cyclin-dependent kinase 2 (CDK2) and inhibits its promoting activity in G1/S transition in the cell cycle (Wierod et al., 2008) (Fig. 2). Gene knockout of p53 or mutations that affect p53 binding to DNA results in unavailability of p21 to act as a stop signal in cell cycle. As such, cell will continue to divide and in some cases will form tumors. The inactivation of p53 can transform cells, and this also provides a way to immortalize cells. Indeed, NSPC clones have been reported to derive from p53 knockout mice (Tominaga et al., 2005; Yamada et al., 1999), but cautions have to be practiced in using these cells in transplantation since they are supposed to be sensitive to DNA mutations and therefore more likely to develop tumors in vivo.

E1A is one of the early gene products of adenoviruses and has also been reported to immortalize neural progenitor cells. The primary cellular target of E1A is pRB (Nevins, 1992). The tumor suppressor protein pRB prevents cell proliferation by inhibiting cell cycle progression. Dysfunction of pRB is often detected in many types of cancer. pRB is a member of pocket protein family and can bind and inhibit E2F-1 transcription activator, thereby preventing cell cycle from entering S phase. Upon adenoviral infection, E1A binds tumor suppressor protein pRB (Fig. 2) and transforms cells with the help of another early gene product E1B, which binds p53.

The oncogene neu was first discovered in a neural tumor, and later was found to share the same sequence with human epidermal growth factor receptor 2 (HER2) and avian erythroblastosis oncogene B2 (ErbB2). HER2/neu is an oncogene that is involved in many types of cancer (Dougall et al., 1994). HER2/neu is a transmembrane receptor tyrosine kinase, and it clusters with other members of the EGFR family and initiates signal transduction pathways that lead to cell proliferation and differentiation. The downstream signaling pathways include the RAS-RAF-MAP kinase, the phosphatidyl inositol 3-kinase (PI3K), and the Akt pathways, where RAS-RAF-MAP kinase pathway plays a more important role to cell cycle progression, thus neural progenitor immortalization when HER2/neu is overexpressed (Fig. 2). Immortalization with neu has been reported (Frederiksen et al., 1988; Sherman et al., 1999), but rare.

Telomerase (Tert) is a reverse transcriptase that adds DNA sequence repeats ("TTAGGG" in all vertebrates) to the 3'-end of DNA strands in the telomere regions of chromosome. In nearly all dividing mammalian cells, telomere shortening is prevented by the activity of Tert, which ensures the sufficient DNA replication during cell division. The decreased expression level of Tert accompanied by telomere shortening of chromosome is often observed in cells that lose the capacity of cell division and become senescence. Overexpression of Tert often leads to cancer formation and also provides a tool for immortalization of neural progenitors (Bai et al., 2004; Roy et al., 2004; Schwob et al., 2008) (Table 1).

hNSPC clone	Tissue origin	Immortalizing gene	Reference
B4, C2, C10 and others	13 wks, brain	Tet-off v-Myc	(Sah et al., 1997)
HNSC.100	10-10.5 wks, diencephalic and telencephalic regions	v-Myc	(Villa et al., 2000)
hSC11V-TERT	9-13 wks, spinal cord	hTERT	(Roy et al., 2004)
hNS2	10 wks, forebrain	v-Myc	(Villa et al., 2004)
hNPC-TERT	fetal SVZ (age?)	hTERT	(Bai et al., 2004)
CTX0E03	first trimester, brain	c-MycER, conditional	(Pollock et al., 2006)
hc-NSC-F7b and others	8-9 wks, cortex	v-Myc	(Cacci et al., 2007)
ReNcell VM	10 wks, midbrain	v-Myc	(Donato et al., 2007)
ReNcell CX	14 wks, cortex	c-Myc	(Donato et al., 2007)
T-IhNSC	10.5 wks, diencephalic and telencephalic tissue	c-Myc (T58A) mutant	(De Filippis et al., 2008)
hVM1	10 wks, ventral mesencephalon	v-Myc	(Villa et al., 2009)
HB2.G2	11–14 wks, telencephalic tissue	Tet-on v-Myc	(Kim et al., 2011)

Table 1. Summary of immortalized human NSPC clones.

2.2 Growth factor dependency

Genetic modification such as overexpressing an oncogene in a cell is expected to bypass growth factor stimulation and thus make possible the cell cycle progression. In reality, however, many neural progenitor cell lines generated by oncogenes mentioned above are heavily dependent on growth factors for their in vitro proliferation. Upon removal of these growth factors, progenitor cells cease proliferation and go on with differentiation towards mature cell types in correlation with the drastic down-regulation of the oncogene expression (such as in the case of v-Myc). Although the mechanism of this phenomenon (oncogene down-regulation upon growth factor withdrawal) is still unclear (perhaps some type of feedback loop system is controlling the exogenous oncogene expression), it provides an extremely important safety prerequisite in using these immortalized cells especially in a transplantation scenario, since the primary phenotypes of a tumorigenetic cell are growth factor independency and loss of contact-inhibition.

Although some of the early generated neural progenitor lines were propagated in mediums containing fetal calf serum (FCS) and sometimes in combination with growth factors, more defined serum-free medium has been widely applied in culturing these cells and FCS has been used as inducing reagent for differentiation into certain neural cell types such as astroglia. Growth factors such as fibroblast growth factor 2 (FGF2) and epidermal growth factor (EGF) have been shown to promote proliferation of immortalized neural progenitors (Kitchens et al., 1994) and are commonly used in serum-free medium as mitogens to promote neural progenitor cell division. In combination of growth factor stimulation and immortalizing genes, NSCs can be expanded in large quantity without obvious phenotypic abnormalities. Then, upon growth factor withdrawal, NSCs simultaneously differentiate along distinct cell lineages. Differentiation inducing factors such as cytokines and neurotrophic factors can be applied to facilitate differentiation and survival of certain cell types. For example, neurotrophin 3 (NT3) and brain-derived neurotrophic factor (BDNF) induce neuronal differentiation and promote neurite outgrowth, while bone morphogenic proteins (BMPs) and leukymia inhibitory factor (LIF) induce astroglial differentiation by upregulating expression of astrocytic marker, glial fibrillary acidic protein (GFAP). Sonic hedgehog homolog (SHH) and platelet-derived growth factor (PDGF) are mitogens to subpopulations of neural progenitors and favor differentiation towards oligodendrocyte lineage.

3. Neural stem/progenitor cell clones as in vitro models

As in vitro models, immortalized neural progenitor clones possess advantages over primary cells isolated from tissue. Firstly, one can produce large quantity of immortalized cells because of the activity of exogenously introduced oncogenes that keep cell proliferation almost infinitely in the presence of appropriate growth factors. Secondly, in vitro expanded immortalized progenitors have cellular homogeneity of higher degree than primary cells since most of these progenitor clones reported are clonal. Lastly, probably because of their promoted cell cycle properties, immortalized progenitor clones are more assessable to genetic modification and more likely to maintain gene expression over passages. There are excellent reviews in the past categorizing most of these clones and describing scientific insights resulted from them (Martinez-Serrano and Bjorklund, 1997; Vescovi and Snyder, 1999; Whittemore and Snyder, 1996). In this section, we will review more recent works on these clones and new clones generated from our lab and others, and focus on their value as in vitro models.

3.1 Models of neural progenitor development

Neural progenitors exhibit spatiotemporal diversity during CNS development (Li and Shi, 2010). To model neural progenitor development, immortalized clones have been isolated from different regions of the CNS at different developmental stages (Whittemore and Snyder, 1996).

Hippocampus plays pivotal roles in learning and memory, and is one of the few sites in adult CNS that retain the capacity of neurogenesis. Therefore, the proliferation and differentiation of hippocampal neural progenitor are of great interests to neurobiologists. HiB5 was isolated as a hippocampal neuronal progenitor from E16 rat (Renfranz et al., 1991), and has been used to model hippocampal neurogenesis. It was found that activation of RARgamma promotes proliferation of HiB5 cells in vitro (Chung et al., 2000). When HiB5 cells were treated with all-trans- or 9-cis-retinoic acid (RA), a significantly increased proportion of these cells were found in S-phase. This was accompanied by increased level of bcl-2 mRNA, while the level of bax mRNA was not affected, which suggests that retinoid treatment increases viable cells by enhancing proliferation rather than suppressing cell death. Furthermore, the proliferation promoting effect of retinoid on HiB5 cells can be mimicked by RARgamma-selective agonist and blocked by its antagonist (Chung et al., 2000). HiB5 cells can model differentiation of hippocampal neurons as well. To give an example, PKA signalling pathway was examined for its role in hippocampal neuronal differentiation process. Kim G et al. demonstrated that treatment of HiB5 cells by cyclic AMP (cAMP) in a serum-free medium containing N2 supplement induced drastic neurite outgrowth of these cells and inhibition of their proliferation (Kim et al., 2002). Phosphorylation of cAMP responsive element binding protein (CREB) was observed accompanied by increased expression of neuronal markers including neurofilaments and decreased expression of glial markers such as nestin and GFAP. Furthermore, overexpression of a GFP-fused protein kinase A (PKA) catalytic subunit alpha protein induced neurite outgrowth in HiB5 cells. Altogether, the authors demonstrated the critical involvement of PKA pathway in hippocampal neuronal differentiation using HiB5 clone as an in vitro model. More recently, another Korean group applied a traditional Korean medicine, Scutellaria baicalensis extract, in the culture of HiB5 cells and showed that it enhanced cell survival of HiB5 and increased their differentiation into choline acetyltransferase (ChAT) positive cholinergic neurons. Along with in vivo data, the authors suggested that Scutellaria baicalensis extract might be used as a neuroprotective medicine in cerebral ischemia (Heo et al., 2009).

Hippocampus maintains on-going neurogenesis in the adult CNS, and yet many of the newborn hippocampal neurons die shortly after birth especially when brain insults occur. Using HiB5 as a model cell, Cacci E et al. were able to show that increased cytokine release by activated microglia may contribute to the death of hippocampal neurons (Cacci et al., 2005). When TNFalpha, as well as conditioned medium from activated microglia, was added to the culture medium, HiB5 cells quickly ceased proliferation and underwent significant cell death. Both HiB5 and microglia express TNF receptors, TNF-R1 and TNF-R2, which may mediate this effect. Hippocampus is vulnerable to different types of insults that lead to neuronal cell death in this brain region. Glucocorticoid (GC), a steroid hormone, participates in normal glucose metabolism. However, when high hippocampal GC level is prolonged, for example in prolonged stressed condition, hippocampal neurons undergo apoptosis. Heat shock protein Hsp27 has been shown to antagonize GC-evoked apoptosis in HiB5 cells (Son et al., 2005). When HiB5 cells were treated with dexamethasone (DEX), a synthetic GC, apoptosis occurred. Interestingly, expression of Hsp27 was also induced upon this treatment. To evaluate possible function of Hsp27 in this process, Son GH et al. overexpressed several constructs in HiB5 cells before DEX treatment and demonstrated that Hsp27 protects hippocampal neurons from GC-induced apoptosis (Son et al., 2005). The same research group also demonstrated that another heat shock protein Hsp25 is involved in neuroprotective effect in hippocampal neurons as well. Furthermore, phosphorylation of Hsp25 mediated by MAPK and ERK signalling is important for its translocation from cytoplasma to nucleus, where it protects nuclear structure, thereby preventing neuronal cell death (Geum et al., 2002). P62, a ubiquitously expressed phosphoprotein, is implied to play a role in protecting hippocampal neuronal survival. When overexpressed in HiB5 cells, p62 not only reduces cell death, but also promotes neuronal differentiation of the cells (Joung et al., 2005). In addition, pre-treatment by vitamin D3 substantially reduced the degree of DEX-induced apoptosis in HiB5 and primary hippocampal neurons suggesting a cross-talk between vitamin D3 and GC pathways (Obradovic et al., 2006).

Isolated from rat E14 striatum, neural progenitor clone ST14A has been used as a model for striatum-derived neurons (Cattaneo and Conti, 1998). The availability of large number of cells made it possible and convenient to examine signalling pathways in these cells. Wnt signalling has been shown to involve in NSC differentiation by expressing necessary Wnt receptors (Lange et al., 2006). ST14A cells express JAK/STAT signalling components and are susceptible to cytokine stimulation leading to cell proliferation (Cattaneo et al., 1996). Ventrally born neurons such as cortical interneurons reach neocortex by tangential migration. The migratory property of ST14A has been realized and used as a model of neuronal migration in vitro. Hepatocyte growth factor /scatter factor (HGF/SF) has been involved in migration and proliferation in many types of epithelial cells. HGF/SF and its receptor Met are also present in the developing CNS as well as ST14A cells. When ST14A cells were exposed to HGF/SF in culture, the cells quickly changed morphology and increased cell motility, a process that involves PI3-K pathway as revealed by pharmacological blocking analysis (Cacci et al., 2003). The cytoskeletal rearrangement including actin network and dissociation of beta-catenin from N-cadherin were also observed in ST14A cells upon treatment of HGF/SF, but not nerve growth factor (NGF), BDNF, NT3 and ciliary neurotrophic factor (CNTF) (Soldati et al., 2008). ErbB family proteins play important function in neuronal migration. Gambarotta et al. demonstrated that ErbB4, but not ErbB1-3, is a crucial receptor of neuregulin1 (Nrg1) in activating migration of ST14A cells (Gambarotta et al., 2004). By gene expression profiling analysis, the same group subsequently identified the epidermal growth factor receptor pathway substrate 8 (Eps8), a multimodular regulator of actin dynamics, as a key mediator of Nrg1/ErbB4 induced neuronal migration (Fregnan et al., 2011).

Radial glia (RG) is a transient cell type during CNS development. It is known by their unique bipolar radial morphology, which is important for its function of supporting neuronal migration. Later, RG has been shown to give rise to neurons and probably the major neuronal precursors throughout the developing CNS (Noctor et al., 2002). We generated first RG clones by v-myc immortalization and demonstrated their properties in vitro including expression of RG specific markers and ability to support neuronal migration. Because of their transient nature, isolation and propagation of RG in vitro have been unsuccessful. The v-myc immortalized RG clones (RG3.6 and L2.3) showed high proliferation rate in the presence of FGF2 and maintained RG markers over many passages, which provides an in vitro model system to allow examination and manipulation on this cell type (Hasegawa et al., 2005; Li et al., 2004). We did observe a gradual change in expression of certain markers in cultured RG clones during passage. For example, brain lipid binding protein (BLBP), a specific RG marker, decreases while a marker for GRPs, A2B5, increases. This initial observation eventually led us to discover a transition from RG to restricted precursors during embryonic forebrain development (Li et al., 2004; Li and Grumet, 2007). To further stablize RG in culture, we introduced actived form of Notch1 into clone L2.3 by retroviral infection. We found that active Notch1 signalling inhibited GRP marker expression and enhanced RG morphology and gene expression (Li et al., 2008a).

Among series of neural progenitor clones generated in our lab, clone L2.2 showed neuronal restricted differentiation in vitro. Moreover, L2.2 gives rise to exclusively GABAergic neuronal subtype upon FGF2 withdrawal as evaluated by their expression of TuJ1, GADs, Dlxs and calretinin (Li et al., 2008b). Neurons derived from L2.2 fire action potential in culture, and this functional differentiation is accelerated when cocultured with RG clone RG3.6 probably through a cell-cell contact mechanism, because the conditioned medium from RG3.6 was not able to exert the same effect. The neuronal progeny of RG clone identified by TuJ1 positivity exhibits projection neuron phenotypes, e.g., bipolar simple morphology, and the majority ($87.4 \pm 1.5\%$) of which are glutamate immunoreactive. Based on our gene expression analysis, L2.3 differentiated culture also expressed T-brain-1 (Tbr-1) transcription factor, which, along with Pax-6 and Tbr-2, is an essential marker for projection neuron differentiation in vivo (Hevner, 2006). During cortical neurogenesis, most, if not all, of glutamatergic projection neurons come from RG, which later differentiate into glial cells. Therefore, clone L2.2 and L2.3 (or RG3.6) generate interneurons and projection neurons, respectively in culture, and they may serve as in vitro models to study interaction between these different neuronal subtypes during cortical development.

3.2 Gene profiling and high-throughput analysis

The availability of large quantity of cells by in vitro expansion of immortalized neural progenitors made large-scale analysis possible. For example, gene expression profiling experiment using ST14A cells overexpressing GDNF has revealed upregulated genes that are involved in neural differentiation and migration (Pahnke et al., 2004). ST14A cells overexpressing CNTF demonstrated increased proliferation, metabolic activity and resistance to stress during early differentiation (Weinelt et al., 2003). Similarly, gene expression profiling analysis confirmed this observation by showing upregulated genes that are involved in stress response pathway of this CNTF-ST14A cells (Bottcher et al., 2003). By overexpressing activated Notch1 gene in RG clone L2.3, we generated a new clone NL2.3 that exhibits enhanced RG marker expression and exaggerated RG morphology (Li et al., 2008a). To explore genes that are responsible for RG phenotype, we conducted gene expression comparison between NL2.3 and its parental clone L2.3. As expected, RG related genes such as BLBP, nestin, tenasin and vimentin were upregulated in NL2.3, and surprisingly we also found that cell adhesion molecules, especially nidogen1 (showing 50 fold increase comparing to L2.3), were upregulated, which may explain the better attachment of NL2.3 cells on laminin-coated substrate. We further confirmed the functional role of nidogen1 in mediating cell adhesion by antibody blocking experiments, and revealed a previously unrecognized link between Notch1 signalling and cell adhesion. In addition, we showed that primary RG cells also express nidogen1 in a secreted fashion demonstrating the physiological significance of this result (Li et al., 2008a).

Proteomics in NSCs is still in its early stage. Nevertheless, large quantity of cells from immortalized progenitors is well suited for this type of analysis. Clone ST14A and an immortalized human NSC clone ReNcell VM have been applied in 2-DE proteomic profiling leading to meaningful discoveries (Beyer et al., 2007; Hoffrogge et al., 2007). Another significant application of expandable neural progenitor cells is high throughput (HTP) screening. Beside drug screening in neural progenitors in pharmaceutical industry, there is also an increasing demand for HTP protocol for genetic analysis on a genome scale. Park JY et al. developed two HTP-optimized expression vector systems that allow generation of red fluorescent protein (RFP)-tagged target proteins (Park et al., 2007). Using these systems, the authors screened sixty representative human C2 domains for their neuronal promoting effect, and identified two C2 domains for their further study. This is another good example for taking advantages of large quantity of cells from immortalized NSC clones.

3.3 Models for neurological diseases

NSC clones are capable not only to facilitate research on NSC differentiation, but also provide model systems for neurological diseases. Here, we give an example on clone ST14A. Derived from embryonic striatum, ST14A cells have been used as in vitro model for Huntingtin's disease (HD). In fact, it has been shown that under serum-free condition, ST14A cells were able to differentiate into DARPP-32-positive medium spiny neurons spontaneously and displayed electrophysiological properties similar to those of medium spiny neurons (Ehrlich et al., 2001). Protein aggregation is the hallmark of neurodegenerative diseases including HD. Ossato G et al. developed a so-called number and brightness method to monitor aggregation of Huntingtin exon 1 protein directly in live ST14A cells and found that the mutant protein underwent a two-step aggregation process, an initial phase of monomer accumulation and oligomer formation followed by protein inclusion depleting monomers in the cytoplasma (Ossato et al., 2010). The pathology of HD has been well documented, and yet its underlying molecular mechanisms still remain elusive. Using the same clone, Sadri-Vakili G et al. demonstrated that epigenetic regulation plays a role in HD progression (Sadri-Vakili et al., 2007). It was found that despite no change in overall acetylated histone levels, histone H3 was hypo-acetylated at the promoter regions of certain down-regulated genes in ST14A cells as well as in R6/2 mice, an animal model for HD. Furthermore, histone deacetylase (HDAC) inhibitor treatment increased level of acetylated histones and seemed to correct expression of misregulated genes, suggesting a potential therapeutic application of HDAC inhibitors for HD (Sadri-Vakili et al., 2007). Altered cholesterol biosynthetic pathway has been reported to involve in HD. The expression level of several key genes in the cholesterol pathway is severely disrupted in brain tissues of HD mice and human patients (Valenza et al., 2005). Mutant Huntingtin was introduced into ST14A cells and it significantly reduced total cellular cholesterol mass. By adding cholesterol back to the cells, the authors were able to prevent cell death of mutant ST14A in a dose-dependent manner. This report uncovered the cholesterol pathway as a novel player in HD, which could be used as a potential target for HD treatments. Phosphorylation of Huntingtin protein appears to be protective in HD, which is mediated by phosphatase calcineurin and phosphokinase Akt. Regulator of calcineurin (RCAN1-1L) is suppressed in HD patient samples, and overexpression of RCAN1-1L in ST14A cells that contain mutant Huntingtin gene increases phophorylation of Huntingtin and reduces ST14A cell death (Ermak et al., 2009). Therefore, the authors claim that RCAN1-1L might be a mediator for HD progression and offer an alternative avenue for drug treatments.

3.4 Testing biomaterials

Biomaterial science has been a fast-growing field providing promising materials for tissue engineering. Biocompatibility of these materials is a big issue since they will be in contact with human cells and tissue. Large quantity of cells, especially cells derived from immortalized neural progenitors are well suited to test toxicity of biomaterials to cells in culture, because in many cases, transplantation of neural progenitor cells is accompanied by biomaterials in the hope that the latter can potentiate stem cell differentiation and migration. The biocompatibility of a variety of biomaterials including polymers and nanofibers were tested using immortalized progenitor cells as first step towards biological applications. Poly(lactic-co-glycolic acid) (PLGA) was compared with other types of polymers in culturing with clone HiB5, where it performed the best in terms of supporting cell viability and neurite outgrowth. This result provided evidence that PLGA could be used as a scaffold for NSC transplantation for nerve regeneration (Bhang et al., 2007). Polymers can also be created to have different patterns and dimensions by various means. Electrospun poly(l-lactide) (PLLA) fibers with different parameters were tested in culture with NSPC clone C17.2. The cells displayed significantly different growth and differentiation depending on fiber pattern and dimension they adhered (He et al., 2010). PLLA can also be modified by tethering laminin-deirved peptides through a cross-linking reagent, and the modified PLLA showed significant improvement in supporting cell survival and neurite outgrowth of C17.2 cells (He et al., 2009). A UV pre-irradiation followed by UV grafting technique can create gradients of carboxyl group on poly(acrylic acid) (PAA) substrates. It was shown that C17.2 cells adhered to these substrates and appeared to respond the carboxyl gradient by directionally sending out neurites (Li et al., 2005). Polymers modified to be electronic affected seeding density of C17.2 cells and may have effects on stem cell differentiation as well (Salto et al., 2008). This report provided an alternative electronic control over NSC differentiation.

Nanotechnology has revolutionized the biomaterial field. Polymers and scaffolds produced at nano-scale have proven to be superior than other material in biological applications. Biomaterials made by nanopolymers possess high surface-to-volume ratio and offer a variety of topographic features that may promote cellular behavior. Nanofibrous scaffolds fabricated with different ratios of poly(epsilon-caprolactone) (PCL) and gelatin were tested in their ability to promote neuronal differentiation of C17.2 cells, and the PCL/gelatin 70:30 ratio generated the best biomaterial suited for nerve regeneration (Ghasemi-Mobarakeh et al., 2008). Similar cell culture tests were also performed on electroconductive polymeric nanowire templates showing that polypyrrole coating improved their effects on cell adhesion and proliferation (Bechara et al., 2011).

4. Neural stem/progenitor cell clones for transplantation

The promise for stem cells including NSCs is someday they may be used as therapeutic cures for diseases. In animal models, there are numerous reports that support this promise and demonstrate great potential of these cells in tissue protection, replacing lost cells and restoring behavioural function when transplanted in a variety of diseases and trauma. Immortalized NSCs provide unlimited cell number and maintain stem cell characteristics such as differentiation potentials to certain cell lineages, and therefore are outstanding candidates for this purpose. Attempts have been made for NSCs to go into human patients hoping they behave similarly to transplanted cells in animals. However, the major concern is the safety of these cells. NSCs derived from either primary tissue or immortalized counterparts have tendency to form tumors upon transplantation since their cell cycle dynamics have been altered by stimulation of growth factors and/or exogenous oncogenes in the case of immortalized NSCs. Although researchers have claimed that some of the oncogenes are non-transforming (e.g. Myc) and their expression is drastically reduced after NSC differentiation and transplantation in vivo, precautionary measures have to be taken into practice to ensure the safety of these cells in clinical settings. In this section, we will review up-to-date reports from others' work on transplantation using immortalized neural progenitor clones in normal and diseased CNS. We will also describe our work using neural progenitor clones to treat spinal cord injury in rat. Finally, we will touch on tumor inhibition, an unexpected property of NSCs revealed by studies using immortalized NSPC clones.

4.1 Transplantation into normal CNS

In order for NSCs to fulfil neural reparative goal, a key property is to be able to differentiate into mature cell types in regions of transplantation. Neurogenesis and neuronal differentiation are already completed in most regions of the adult brain. Therefore, it is a bit of challenge for transplanted cells to differentiate under this "mature" environment. Surprisingly, however, permissive cues must be still present in neonatal and adult CNS allowing neuronal differentiation to occur. Immortalized NSCs have been transplanted first into normal animals and tested in their survival, migration and differentiation potentials under in vivo environments. For example, RN33B, a conditionally immortalized neural progenitor clone derived from E13 rat medullary raphe nucleus (Whittemore and White, 1993), was transplanted into various regions of neonatal and adult brains. In cerebral cortex and hippocampus formation, RN33B cells survived up to 24 weeks and differentiate with morphologies similar to pyramidal neurons, granule neurons and polymorphic neurons in a region-specific manner (Shihabuddin et al., 1995). Electron microscopy and immunohistochemistry demonstrated that differentiated RN33B cells received synapses from host neurons. In striatum, transplanted RN33B cells survived, integrated and differentiated into neurons and glia, some of which displayed morphological and phenotypic properties of medium-sized spiny neurons. These neurons were also found to form connections with primary striatal target, the globus pallidus, by retrograde tracing analysis (Lundberg et al., 1996). Furthermore, GFP-labelled RN33B cells transplanted into hippocampus exhibited remarkable neuronal morphology and were capable of firing action potentials and receiving synaptic inputs of both excitatory and inhibitory nature (Englund et al., 2002). In contrast to neuronal differentiation mentioned above, RN33B cells transplanted in the mesencephalon predominantly differentiated into astroglia (Lundberg et al., 2002). These observations suggest that regional cues are still present in the adult brain that can direct differentiation of transplanted neural progenitors into certain cell types, which can integrate into local tissue structures, although it has been shown that neonatal brains have greater capacity to encourage differentiation, especially neuronal differentiation, of transplanted cells than adult brains suggesting a decline of permissive cues during CNS development (Shihabuddin et al., 1995).

On the other hand, immortalized progenitors derived from one region of the brain can differentiate into cell types specific to the other indicating plasticity of these cells that may broaden their reparative application in different areas of the CNS. Indeed, when RN33B, along with another NSPC clone C17.2 derived from postnatal cerebellum, was transplanted into adult retina, they survived up to 4 weeks and differentiate into both neurons and glia in all major retinal cell layers including retinal pigment epithelium (Warfvinge et al., 2001). Intrinsic molecular natures of individual progenitor clones have to be considered when applying them into transplantation therapies. They all may be multipotent in culture, but have limited potentials to differentiate in vivo. For example, two weeks after transplantation into adult striatum, unlike RN33B cells to become both neurons and glia, clones HiB5 and ST14A differentiate mostly into glial cells (Lundberg et al., 1996), indicating their distinct intrinsic properties including possible distinct responsiveness to the local host environment. Worthy of noting is that these NSC-derived astroglia functionally integrated into host by showing reactive phenotype in response to brain damage (Lundberg and Bjorklund, 1996). By using immortalized NSC clones, the above mentioned results demonstrated the plasticity of NSCs to differentiate into distinct cell types by responding to local cues, and the fact that adult brains still retain, to a certain degree, the ability to direct differentiation of exogenous neural progenitor cells. C17.2 cells were also transplanted into lumbar region of normal spinal cord where they differentiated into nonmyelinating ensheathing cells. In addition, they appeared to induce host axons to form de novo tracts aiming at graft site probably through the action of their secreted neurotrophic factors, suggesting NSCs may also trigger regenerative potentials of host tissue needing for repair (Yan et al., 2004).

4.2 Neurodegenerative diseases

Neurodegenerative diseases are caused by region-specific, progressive cell death and include Parkinson's disease (PD), HD, Alzheimer's disease (AD) and amyotrophic lateral sclerosis (ALS). This is an area where cell replacement therapies are on high demand. We will take PD as an example to highlight the value of immortalized progenitors in testing effects of NSCs in PD animal models in terms of neuroprotection and differentiation into desired neuronal cell type. The common pathology of PD patients is the progressive loss of dopaminergic neurons in the substantial nigra that normally project axons onto striatum. As a result, dopamine level in the striatum greatly reduced, which is believed to induce PD symptoms such as dystonic cramps and dementia (Weidong et al., 2009). Attempts have been made to restore dopamine level by various means, which seem to alleviate symptoms to a certain degree, but they can not prevent PD progression and replenish the lost neurons.

Clone C17.2 has been transplanted into normal and lesioned striatum of the adult rat brain in testing their behaviour in local environment where dopaminergic neurons reside. Consistent with the notion mentioned above, these cells were able to turn on neuronal markers and tyrosine hydroxylase (TH), an enzyme critical to dopamine systhesis, suggesting that local cues are still present and powerful enough to direct multipotent immortalized NSCs to differentiate into local neuronal subtypes (Yang et al., 2002). Efforts have also been made to reinforce dopaminergic differentiation of transplanted progenitors to maximize their effects in PD animal models. For example, C17.2 cells have been genetically modified to overexpress enzymes (e.g. TH and GTP cyclohydrolase 1) (Ryu et al., 2005), Nuclear receptor related 1 protein (NURR1) (Li et al., 2007) and secreted factors (e.g. neurturin) (Liu et al., 2007) towards the goal of getting more dopaminergic neurons. Both TH and GTP cyclohydrolase 1 are required for efficient L-DOPA synthesis, since HPLC assays demonstrated that L-DOPA released from C17.2 cells that are transduced with both genes (C17.2-THGC) is 760-fold higher than that from C17.2 cells transduced with TH gene alone (C17.2-TH). Following transplantation into striatum of PD rats, C17.2-THGC was able to promote animals' behavioural improvement when compared with transplants with parental C17.2 cells (Ryu et al., 2005). NURR1 has been shown to induce downstream target genes such as TH and facilitate dopaminergic differentiation. When overexpressed in C17.2 cells, NURR1 enhanced cell differentiation into dopaminergic neurons and even promoted behavioural recovery to a certain extent (Li et al., 2007). Unlike in normal CNS, transplanted neural progenitors have to overcome unfavourable environment in diseased tissue to survive and differentiate. Therefore, manipulations that mitigate local environment may prove to facilitate beneficial outcomes. Neurturin is a secreted factor that belongs to glial cell-derived neurotrophic factor (GDNF) family. Like GDNF, neurturin exerted neuroprotective effects on host dopaminergic neurons after transplantation into lesioned striatum. In addition, neurturin also promoted dopaminergic differentiation of C17.2 cells when overexpressed, and animal behaviour as well (Liu et al., 2007). Similarly, interleukin-10 overexpression in C17.2 lowered immune response of host tissue to create a beneficial microenvironment for cell survival and differentiation (Wang et al., 2007). In addition, treatment of melatonin in combination with C17.2 showed neuroprotection in PD models (Sharma et al., 2007).

4.3 Brain and spinal cord injury

Traumatic brain injury (TBI), also called acquired brain injury or simply head injury, occurs when a sudden trauma causes damage to the brain. TBI can result when the head suddenly and violently hits an object, or when an object pierces the skull and enters brain tissue. Symptoms of a TBI can be mild, moderate, or severe, depending on the extent of the damage to the brain. Besides direct damage of brain tissue by trauma, secondary damage in TBI results from toxic effects of a variety of modulators that magnify the initial traumatic damage. Among these modulators are the excitatory transmitter glutamate, the intracellular messenger calcium, and the intercellular messenger nitric oxide. Glutamate-induced toxicity, also called excitotoxicity, occurs from excess glutamate release following trauma. Because of the very limited capacity of the brain for self-repair, cellular transplantation has been explored to improve repair. The goal of many studies has been to replace the lost neurons (Bjorklund, 2000; Gage, 2000; Lie et al., 2004; McKay, 1997). Although instructive cues for neuronal differentiation in normal adult brains seem still exist (albeit declining comparing to neonatal brains), the local environment around the injured brain region could be very different. Transplanted cells have to overcome extra hurdles such as glutamte excitotoxicity and high concentration of released cytokines to survive and differentiate. Nevertheless, studies in the past have shown that immortalized progenitors can survive and differentiate upon transplantation in TBI. C17.2 cells were injected into adult mouse brains at 3 days after lateral controlled cortical impact injury (Riess et al., 2002). The study demonstrated cell survival of C17.2 as long as 13 weeks post-transplantation and significant improvement in motor behavior of C17.2 transpalnted animals as compared with those received human embryonic kidney cells. It was also found in this study that C17.2 cells implanted contralateral to the impact side differentiated into mostly neurons, while the cells implanted ipsilateral to the impact side differentiated into astroglial cells as well as neurons consistent with the notion that injured environment favors glial differentiation of transplanted NSCs (Riess et al., 2002). In order to improve the efficacy of NSC mediated beneficial effects in TBI treatemnt, immortalized progenitors engineered to express neurotrophic factors have been utilized. As expected, these genetically modified cells showed neuroprotective effects and improved functional recovery of the animals. For example, C17.2 overexpressing GDNF (GDNF-C17.2) improved survival of transplanted cells, enhanced neuronal differentiation of these cells and promoted learning behavior of the TBI rats at 6 weeks after transplantation comparing to parental C17.2 cells (Bakshi et al., 2006). Similarly, HiB5 progenitor clone engineered to secrete NGF (NGF-HiB5), when transplanted peripheral to the TBI site, decreased apoptosis of the host hippocampal neurons and improved motor and cognitive function comparing to controls (Philips et al., 2001).

Spinal cord injury (SCI) is a severe CNS injury often resulting in long-term disability. Immediately after contusion there is limited histological evidence of damage followed by neuronal death (hours), and that is followed by macrophage infiltration, Wallerian degeneration and astrogliosis (days-weeks). Similarly to TBI, physical disruption of spinal cord causes membrane depolarization and results in massive glutamate release, which is not only excitotoxic to injured cells themselves but surrounding cells. Several weeks after contusion injury in humans as well as in rats (but not in mice), cystic cavities develop surrounded by gliotic scars associated with extracellular matrix including chondroitin sulfate proteoglycans (CSPG), which is not hospitable to axonal regeneration (Busch and Silver, 2007).

Advances in cell characterization and isolation are opening new opportunities for cell transplantation to repair tissue damage by replacing cells that restore lost function (Gage, 2000). Numerous immortalized NSCs have been implanted into SCI to test their differentiation potentials and efficacy on functional recovery. Embryonic raphe nucleus-derived progenitor clone RN33B morphologically differentiated into multipolar neurons resembling nearby endogenous ones when transplanted into gray matter of normal spinal cord. However, only relatively undifferentiated RN33B cells with bipolar morphology could be found at 2 weeks after transplantation into rat spinal cords with various types of injuries with depletion of endogenous neurons due to the lesions. The authors suggested that cell-cell contact mechanisms contribute to instructive local cues for permissive neuronal differentiation of transplanted progenitors, and that molecules released from the injury site may also have prevented these cells from becoming neurons (Onifer et al., 1997; Whittemore, 1999). On the other hand, implanted neural progenitors secrete neurotrophic factors themselves, which may alter the microenvironment they encounter inside the CNS tissue. Clone C17.2 cells have been shown to naturally express and secrete several trophic factors including NGF, BDNF and GDNF both in vitro and in vivo after transplantation (Lu et al., 2003). When implanted into adult rat spinal cords with cystic dorsal column lesion, C17.2 cells promoted extensive growth of endogenous axons. Elevated expression of one factor NT3 by genetic modification in C17.2 expanded this promoting effect (Lu et al., 2003), and improved C17.2 cell survival near the lesion site and functional recovery analyzed by Basso-Beattie-Bresnahan (BBB) scoring (Zhang et al., 2007). We reported that an immortalized neural progenitor clone sharing properties with NSPC and radial glia (RG3.6) migrated extensively in the injured rat spinal cord and improved open field walking when transplanted acutely following contusive SCI (Hasegawa et al., 2005). The transplanted RG3.6 cells partially protected the rat spinal cord against several aspects of secondary injury including loss of axons and myelin as well as accumulation of CSPG and macrophages (Hasegawa et al., 2005).

Patients with SCI not only lose motor function below the injury site, but often develop debilitating neuropathic pain (allodynia) over time (Siddall et al., 1999), which diminishes the quality of their lives. The mechanisms underlying allodynia may be very complex and many possible factors contribute to these symptoms (Hulsebosch, 2005). One direct factor is the loss or reduction of inhibitory tone in the spinal cord sensory processing due to injury. Therapeutic strategies that prevent induction of allodynia, such as cell transplants that release anti-nociceptive substances, can be used to enhance the endogenous descending inhibitory neurotransmitter systems, such as GABA and serotonin (5HT). Immortalized progenitor RN33B cells were therefore used as a vehicle to deliver GABA in SCI. RN33B cells overexpressing GAD67, an enzyme critical for GABA synthesis, were transplanted into lumbar subarachnoid space of the rat spinal cord with chronic constraint injury (CCI) (Eaton et al., 1999b). Seven weeks after transplantation, RN33B cells were found on the pial surface of the spinal cord, and the animals that received these cells showed significantly reduction of both tactile and temperature allodynia comparing to those that received control cells. In the same CCI injury model, RN33B cells overexpressing BDNF or galanin have also been shown to have beneficial effects in reducing allodynia (Cejas et al., 2000; Eaton et al., 1999a). When C17.2 NSCs were transplanted into injured spinal cord, they primarily differentiated into astrocytes, which may result in sprouting of dorsal horn nociceptive neurons and in turn allodynia of the animals. GDNF, when overexpressed in transplanted C17.2 cells, reduced nociceptive fiber sprouting and allodynia to a certain extent suggesting a protective or analgesic effect of GDNF on injury-induced neuropathic pain (Macias et al., 2006). We have isolated cortical GABAergic interneuron progenitor clones from rat embryonic forebrains and demonstrated their restricted interneuronal differentiation in culture. We are further testing these intrinsic GABAergic progenitor clones in vitro and after transplanation in SCI, hoping that the cells can differentiate into neurons with GABAergic phenotype in SCI, not only to release GABA to reduce allodynia, but also to integrate into local neuronal circuitry and permanently eliminate the pain-like syndrome. Towards that goal, we have demonstrated that one such clone exhibited spontaneous synaptic activity when cocultured with E17 hippocampal neurons (Li et al., 2011).

4.4 Tumor inhibition

One surprising and yet interesting feature of NSCs when implanted in vivo is their ability to target tumorous tissues and inhibit their growth. For example, immortalized neural progenitor clones isolated from different regions of the embryonic brain, HiB5 (hippocampus) and ST14A (striatum primordium), were transplanted into nucleus Caudatus of Fisher rats along with N29 glioma cells. Both progenitors exhibited anti-tumor activity and prolonged animal's survival. Clone HiB5 was also shown to inhibit an additional tumor type and even be effective when transplanted 1 week after tumor cells inoculation (Staflin et al., 2004). Clone C17.2 was also tested in their tumor-tropic capacities in a similar paradigm, and the results showed that these cells were able to inhibit tumors of both neural and nonneural origin (Brown et al., 2003). Furthermore, C17.2 cells were able to migrate into the tumor mass even when injected via peripheral vasculatures showing great homing capacity of these cells that can be used to deliver therapeutic agents. The mechanism of the NSC homing phenomena towards tumor is not very clear. C17.2 chemotactic migration was tested in vitro by conditioned medium prepared from glioma culture as well as 13 different tumor-associated growth factors (Heese et al., 2005). The results showed that scatter factor/hepatocyte growth factor (SF/HGF) was the most potent one in attracting C17.2 cells in culture. In addition, antibody against SF/HGF was able to block the migratory behaviour of these cells stimulated by glioma-conditioned medium. Furthermore, Allport JR et al. showed tumor-targeting acivity of C17.2 in vivo and identified two other factors that are involved in this NSC homing event (Allport et al., 2004). This study showed that C17.2 cells that were transduced to express luciferase (C17.2-luc) accumulated onto tumors in mice carrying Lewis lung carcinomas. In vitro analysis showed that accumulation of C17.2-luc cells on tumor-derived endothelium (TEC) can be inhibited by functional blocking antibodies against SDF-1alpha and CD49d suggesting the involvement of SDF-1alpha/CXCR4 receptor and alpha4-integrin in the recruitment of C17.2-luc cells (Allport et al., 2004).

Unlike C17.2, HiB5 cells have not been able to show homing capacity towards tumors, even though HiB5 cells exhibited growth-inhibitory effect when they were cotransplanted with tumor cells into animals. Honeth et al. introduced the chemokine receptor CXCR3 to HiB5 cells and demonstrated its functionality by responding to ligand stimulation and activating downstream signaling pathways such as ERK and SAPK/JNK (Honeth et al., 2006). Upon transplantation, these modified cells showed enhanced migration towards glioma that expressed CXCR3 ligands, IP-10 and I-TAC, in comparison with parental HiB5 cells. This study provided proof-of-concepts that immortalized progenitors can be genetically modified and acquire homing capacity towards tumor to either inhibit tumor growth on its own or deliver therapeutic agents for local treatments. Among good examples of this notion is the study that was carried out by Barresi V and colleagues, where they genetically engineered neural progenitor clone ST14A to express cytosine deaminase (CD), by which 5-fluorocytosine (5-FC) can be converted into 5-fluorouracil (5-FU) to suppress tumor growth. DiI prelabeled CD-expressing ST14A cells were cotransplanted into rat brains with C6 glioma. The data showed that ST14A cells survived inside C6 tumor mass for at least 10 days and significantly reduced the size of tumor comparing to controls presumably through the action of 5-FU (Barresi et al., 2003).

5. Conclusions and perspectives

NSCs hold enormous promises for treating neurological diseases. However, at the present time, we are still facing many hurdles, one of which is how to direct these multipotent cells to become the desired cell types for a certain disease. NSPC clones proliferate rapidly in culture and maintain certain important characteristic properties after passages, therefore provide invaluable models for in vitro studies and transplantable tools for testing hypothesis in treating neurological disorders. Immortalized neural progenitor clones are potentially tumorigenic since they are engineered to express oncogenes such as Myc. Even though many reports have demonstrated that Myc expression is growth factor-dependent and can be down-regulated to an undetectable level after FGF2 withdrawal both in vitro and after transplantation, cautions have been taken to ensure the shutdown of oncogene expression upon cell differentiation. For example, modified immortalizing oncogenes such as the temperature-sensitive mutant of large T antigen, tsA58, have been used to generate a series of neural progenitor clones from the developing CNS. The tsA58 gene product is stable at permissive temperature (33°C), but rapidly degraded when temperature goes higher such as body temperature in culture as well as after transplantation into animals. Generation of neural progenitor clones using controllable-Myc expression may provide another solution to the same problem. Human NSPC clones (summarized in Table 1) have been generated by tetracycline-controllable v-Myc (Kim et al., 2011; Sah et al., 1997) and c-MycER[TAM] transgene (Pollock et al., 2006). On the other hand, functions of promoting proliferation and tumorigenesis can be uncoupled in an experimental setting (Johnson et al., 2008). Therefore, dissecting out functional domains of oncogenes that enable sufficient expansion of neural stem cells and limit (or eliminate) their tumorigenic activity will be advantageous to generate newer version of immortalizing reagents (Harvey et al., 2007; Truckenmiller et al., 2002). A recent report on induced pluripotent stem cells (iPSCs) indicated that L-Myc, a Myc gene isoform, promoted iPSC generation with little transformation activity (Nakagawa et al., 2010). These safety-oriented designs in generation of immortalized progenitors will prove to be crucial in minimizing tumorigenc potential of exogenous oncogenes, and more research should be performed to optimize NSC immortalizing techniques especially in regard to safety for future clinical applications.

Oncogenes that are frequently used for NSC "immortalizations" such as Myc, carry mutations and are prone to spontaneous mutation as well. Some of these mutations potentiate their ability of transformation and tumorigenesis. Therefore, the culturing conditions for in vitro expansion of immortalized NSC clones need to be optimized and controlled in the goal of less stress so that spontaneous mutations can be minimized. The low oxygen culture condition, which many researchers have applied in their human stem cell culture, would fit in this type of precaution in addition to the fact that NSCs grow and differentiate better under this condition. Furthermore, a "quality check" protocol needs to be developed to screen out and eliminate cells with such mutations and tumor-like growth patterns in the case where mutations do occur. Stem cell replacement therapy is at its "transforming" stage. We are very hopeful for its future, but a lot more work needs to be done before it can go on to clinic, especially in regard to safety. Nevertheless, immortalized NSPC clones will for certain be the milestones in the road towards the ultimate goal of stem cell replacement therapy and, in some instances, may very well become therapeutics themselves (Thomas et al., 2009).

6. Acknowledgments

This work was supported by grants from West China Second University Hospital Research Fund, National Natural Science Foundation of China (30971633) , Program for Changjiang Scholars and Innovative Research Team in University (PCSIRT) (IRT0935) and New Jersey Commission on Spinal Cord Research.

7. References

Ahuja, D., Saenz-Robles, M. T. and Pipas, J. M. (2005). SV40 large T antigen targets multiple cellular pathways to elicit cellular transformation. *Oncogene* 24, 7729-45.

Albert, T., Urlbauer, B., Kohlhuber, F., Hammersen, B. and Eick, D. (1994). Ongoing mutations in the N-terminal domain of c-Myc affect transactivation in Burkitt's lymphoma cell lines. *Oncogene* 9, 759-63.

Alitalo, K., Bishop, J. M., Smith, D. H., Chen, E. Y., Colby, W. W. and Levinson, A. D. (1983). Nucleotide sequence to the v-myc oncogene of avian retrovirus MC29. *Proc Natl Acad Sci U S A* 80, 100-4.

Allport, J. R., Shinde Patil, V. R. and Weissleder, R. (2004). Murine neuronal progenitor cells are preferentially recruited to tumor vasculature via alpha4-integrin and SDF-1alpha-dependent mechanisms. *Cancer Biol Ther* 3, 838-44.

Bai, Y., Hu, Q., Li, X., Wang, Y., Lin, C., Shen, L. and Li, L. (2004). Telomerase immortalization of human neural progenitor cells. *Neuroreport* 15, 245-9.

Bakshi, A., Shimizu, S., Keck, C. A., Cho, S., LeBold, D. G., Morales, D., Arenas, E., Snyder, E. Y., Watson, D. J. and McIntosh, T. K. (2006). Neural progenitor cells engineered to secrete GDNF show enhanced survival, neuronal differentiation and improve cognitive function following traumatic brain injury. *Eur J Neurosci* 23, 2119-34.

Barresi, V., Belluardo, N., Sipione, S., Mudo, G., Cattaneo, E. and Condorelli, D. F. (2003). Transplantation of prodrug-converting neural progenitor cells for brain tumor therapy. *Cancer Gene Ther* 10, 396-402.

Bechara, S., Wadman, L. and Popat, K. C. (2011). Electroconductive polymeric nanowire templates facilitates in vitro C17.2 neural stem cell line adhesion, proliferation and differentiation. *Acta Biomater* 7, 2892-901.

Beyer, S., Mix, E., Hoffrogge, R., Lunser, K., Volker, U. and Rolfs, A. (2007). Neuroproteomics in stem cell differentiation. *Proteomics Clin Appl* 1, 1513-23.

Bhang, S. H., Lim, J. S., Choi, C. Y., Kwon, Y. K. and Kim, B. S. (2007). The behavior of neural stem cells on biodegradable synthetic polymers. *J Biomater Sci Polym Ed* 18, 223-39.

Bjorklund, A. (2000). Cell replacement strategies for neurodegenerative disorders. *Novartis Found Symp* 231, 7-15.

Bottcher, T., Mix, E., Koczan, D., Bauer, P., Pahnke, J., Peters, S., Weinelt, S., Knoblich, R., Strauss, U., Cattaneo, E. et al. (2003). Gene expression profiling of ciliary neurotrophic factor-overexpressing rat striatal progenitor cells (ST14A) indicates improved stress response during the early stage of differentiation. *J Neurosci Res* 73, 42-53.

Brown, A. B., Yang, W., Schmidt, N. O., Carroll, R., Leishear, K. K., Rainov, N. G., Black, P. M., Breakefield, X. O. and Aboody, K. S. (2003). Intravascular delivery of neural stem cell lines to target intracranial and extracranial tumors of neural and non-neural origin. *Hum Gene Ther* 14, 1777-85.

Busch, S. A. and Silver, J. (2007). The role of extracellular matrix in CNS regeneration. *Curr Opin Neurobiol* 17, 120-7.

Cacci, E., Claasen, J. H. and Kokaia, Z. (2005). Microglia-derived tumor necrosis factor-alpha exaggerates death of newborn hippocampal progenitor cells in vitro. *J Neurosci Res* 80, 789-97.

Cacci, E., Salani, M., Anastasi, S., Perroteau, I., Poiana, G., Biagioni, S. and Augusti-Tocco, G. (2003). Hepatocyte growth factor stimulates cell motility in cultures of the striatal progenitor cells ST14A. *J Neurosci Res* 74, 760-8.

Cacci, E., Villa, A., Parmar, M., Cavallaro, M., Mandahl, N., Lindvall, O., Martinez-Serrano, A. and Kokaia, Z. (2007). Generation of human cortical neurons from a new immortal fetal neural stem cell line. *Exp Cell Res* 313, 588-601.

Cattaneo, E. and Conti, L. (1998). Generation and characterization of embryonic striatal conditionally immortalized ST14A cells. *J Neurosci Res* 53, 223-34.

Cattaneo, E., De Fraja, C., Conti, L., Reinach, B., Bolis, L., Govoni, S. and Liboi, E. (1996). Activation of the JAK/STAT pathway leads to proliferation of ST14A central nervous system progenitor cells. *J Biol Chem* 271, 23374-9.

Cejas, P. J., Martinez, M., Karmally, S., McKillop, M., McKillop, J., Plunkett, J. A., Oudega, M. and Eaton, M. J. (2000). Lumbar transplant of neurons genetically modified to secrete brain-derived neurotrophic factor attenuates allodynia and hyperalgesia after sciatic nerve constriction. *Pain* 86, 195-210.

Chung, J. J., Cho, S., Kwon, Y. K., Kim, D. H. and Kim, K. (2000). Activation of retinoic acid receptor gamma induces proliferation of immortalized hippocampal progenitor cells. *Brain Res Mol Brain Res* 83, 52-62.

De Filippis, L., Ferrari, D., Rota Nodari, L., Amati, B., Snyder, E. and Vescovi, A. L. (2008). Immortalization of human neural stem cells with the c-myc mutant T58A. *PLoS One* 3, e3310.

Donato, R., Miljan, E. A., Hines, S. J., Aouabdi, S., Pollock, K., Patel, S., Edwards, F. A. and Sinden, J. D. (2007). Differential development of neuronal physiological responsiveness in two human neural stem cell lines. *BMC Neurosci* 8, 36.

Dougall, W. C., Qian, X., Peterson, N. C., Miller, M. J., Samanta, A. and Greene, M. I. (1994). The neu-oncogene: signal transduction pathways, transformation mechanisms and evolving therapies. *Oncogene* 9, 2109-23.

Eaton, M. J., Karmally, S., Martinez, M. A., Plunkett, J. A., Lopez, T. and Cejas, P. J. (1999a). Lumbar transplant of neurons genetically modified to secrete galanin reverse pain-like behaviors after partial sciatic nerve injury. *J Peripher Nerv Syst* 4, 245-57.

Eaton, M. J., Plunkett, J. A., Martinez, M. A., Lopez, T., Karmally, S., Cejas, P. and Whittemore, S. R. (1999b). Transplants of neuronal cells bioengineered to synthesize GABA alleviate chronic neuropathic pain. *Cell Transplant* 8, 87-101.

Ehrlich, M. E., Conti, L., Toselli, M., Taglietti, L., Fiorillo, E., Taglietti, V., Ivkovic, S., Guinea, B., Tranberg, A., Sipione, S. et al. (2001). ST14A cells have properties of a medium-size spiny neuron. *Exp Neurol* 167, 215-26.

Englund, U., Bjorklund, A., Wictorin, K., Lindvall, O. and Kokaia, M. (2002). Grafted neural stem cells develop into functional pyramidal neurons and integrate into host cortical circuitry. *Proc Natl Acad Sci U S A* 99, 17089-94.

Ermak, G., Hench, K. J., Chang, K. T., Sachdev, S. and Davies, K. J. (2009). Regulator of calcineurin (RCAN1-1L) is deficient in Huntington disease and protective against mutant huntingtin toxicity in vitro. *J Biol Chem* 284, 11845-53.

Farina, S. F., Huff, J. L. and Parsons, J. T. (1992). Mutations within the 5' half of the avian retrovirus MC29 v-myc gene alter or abolish transformation of chicken embryo fibroblasts and macrophages. *J Virol* 66, 2698-708.

Frederiksen, K., Jat, P. S., Valtz, N., Levy, D. and McKay, R. (1988). Immortalization of precursor cells from the mammalian CNS. *Neuron* 1, 439-48.

Fregnan, F., Petrov, V., Garzotto, D., De Marchis, S., Offenhauser, N., Grosso, E., Chiorino, G., Perroteau, I. and Gambarotta, G. (2011). Eps8 involvement in neuregulin1-ErbB4 mediated migration in the neuronal progenitor cell line ST14A. *Exp Cell Res* 317, 757-69.

Gage, F. H. (2000). Mammalian neural stem cells. *Science* 287, 1433-8.

Gambarotta, G., Garzotto, D., Destro, E., Mautino, B., Giampietro, C., Cutrupi, S., Dati, C., Cattaneo, E., Fasolo, A. and Perroteau, I. (2004). ErbB4 expression in neural progenitor cells (ST14A) is necessary to mediate neuregulin-1beta1-induced migration. *J Biol Chem* 279, 48808-16.

Geum, D., Son, G. H. and Kim, K. (2002). Phosphorylation-dependent cellular localization and thermoprotective role of heat shock protein 25 in hippocampal progenitor cells. *J Biol Chem* 277, 19913-21.

Ghasemi-Mobarakeh, L., Prabhakaran, M. P., Morshed, M., Nasr-Esfahani, M. H. and Ramakrishna, S. (2008). Electrospun poly(epsilon-caprolactone)/gelatin nanofibrous scaffolds for nerve tissue engineering. *Biomaterials* 29, 4532-9.

Grandori, C., Cowley, S. M., James, L. P. and Eisenman, R. N. (2000). The Myc/Max/Mad network and the transcriptional control of cell behavior. *Annu Rev Cell Dev Biol* 16, 653-99.

Harvey, B. K., Chen, G. J., Schoen, C. J., Lee, C. T., Howard, D. B., Dillon-Carter, O., Coggiano, M., Freed, W. J., Wang, Y., Hoffer, B. J. et al. (2007). An immortalized rat ventral mesencephalic cell line, RTC4, is protective in a rodent model of stroke. *Cell Transplant* 16, 483-91.

Hasegawa, K., Chang, Y. W., Li, H., Berlin, Y., Ikeda, O., Kane-Goldsmith, N. and Grumet, M. (2005). Embryonic radial glia bridge spinal cord lesions and promote functional recovery following spinal cord injury. *Exp Neurol* 193, 394-410.

He, L., Liao, S., Quan, D., Ma, K., Chan, C., Ramakrishna, S. and Lu, J. (2010). Synergistic effects of electrospun PLLA fiber dimension and pattern on neonatal mouse cerebellum C17.2 stem cells. *Acta Biomater* 6, 2960-9.

He, L., Liao, S., Quan, D., Ngiam, M., Chan, C. K., Ramakrishna, S. and Lu, J. (2009). The influence of laminin-derived peptides conjugated to Lys-capped PLLA on neonatal mouse cerebellum C17.2 stem cells. *Biomaterials* 30, 1578-86.

Heese, O., Disko, A., Zirkel, D., Westphal, M. and Lamszus, K. (2005). Neural stem cell migration toward gliomas in vitro. *Neuro Oncol* 7, 476-84.

Heo, H., Shin, Y., Cho, W., Choi, Y., Kim, H. and Kwon, Y. K. (2009). Memory improvement in ibotenic acid induced model rats by extracts of Scutellaria baicalensis. *J Ethnopharmacol* 122, 20-7.

Hevner, R. F. (2006). From radial glia to pyramidal-projection neuron: transcription factor cascades in cerebral cortex development. *Mol Neurobiol* 33, 33-50.

Hoffrogge, R., Beyer, S., Hubner, R., Mikkat, S., Mix, E., Scharf, C., Schmitz, U., Pauleweit, S., Berth, M., Zubrzycki, I. Z. et al. (2007). 2-DE profiling of GDNF overexpression-related proteome changes in differentiating ST14A rat progenitor cells. *Proteomics 7*, 33-46.

Honeth, G., Staflin, K., Kalliomaki, S., Lindvall, M. and Kjellman, C. (2006). Chemokine-directed migration of tumor-inhibitory neural progenitor cells towards an intracranially growing glioma. *Exp Cell Res 312*, 1265-76.

Hulsebosch, C. E. (2005). From discovery to clinical trials: treatment strategies for central neuropathic pain after spinal cord injury. *Curr Pharm Des 11*, 1411-20.

Johnson, S. A., Dubeau, L. and Johnson, D. L. (2008). Enhanced RNA polymerase III-dependent transcription is required for oncogenic transformation. *J Biol Chem 283*, 19184-91.

Joung, I., Kim, H. J. and Kwon, Y. K. (2005). p62 modulates Akt activity via association with PKCzeta in neuronal survival and differentiation. *Biochem Biophys Res Commun 334*, 654-60.

Kim, G., Choe, Y., Park, J., Cho, S. and Kim, K. (2002). Activation of protein kinase A induces neuronal differentiation of HiB5 hippocampal progenitor cells. *Brain Res Mol Brain Res 109*, 134-45.

Kim, K. S., Lee, H. J., Jeong, H. S., Li, J., Teng, Y. D., Sidman, R. L., Snyder, E. Y. and Kim, S. U. (2011). Self-renewal induced efficiently, safely, and effective therapeutically with one regulatable gene in a human somatic progenitor cell. *Proc Natl Acad Sci U S A 108*, 4876-81.

Kitchens, D. L., Snyder, E. Y. and Gottlieb, D. I. (1994). FGF and EGF are mitogens for immortalized neural progenitors. *J Neurobiol 25*, 797-807.

Lange, C., Mix, E., Rateitschak, K. and Rolfs, A. (2006). Wnt signal pathways and neural stem cell differentiation. *Neurodegener Dis 3*, 76-86.

Laurenti, E., Wilson, A. and Trumpp, A. (2009). Myc's other life: stem cells and beyond. *Curr Opin Cell Biol 21*, 844-54.

Li, B., Ma, Y., Wang, S. and Moran, P. M. (2005). Influence of carboxyl group density on neuron cell attachment and differentiation behavior: gradient-guided neurite outgrowth. *Biomaterials 26*, 4956-63.

Li, H., Babiarz, J., Woodbury, J., Kane-Goldsmith, N. and Grumet, M. (2004). Spatiotemporal heterogeneity of CNS radial glial cells and their transition to restricted precursors. *Dev Biol 271*, 225-38.

Li, H., Chang, Y. W., Mohan, K., Su, H. W., Ricupero, C. L., Baridi, A., Hart, R. P. and Grumet, M. (2008a). Activated Notch1 maintains the phenotype of radial glial cells and promotes their adhesion to laminin by upregulating nidogen. *Glia 56*, 646-58.

Li, H. and Grumet, M. (2007). BMP and LIF signaling coordinately regulate lineage restriction of radial glia in the developing forebrain. *Glia 55*, 24-35.

Li, H., Hader, A. T., Han, Y. R., Wong, J. A., Babiarz, J., Ricupero, C. L., Godfrey, S. B., Corradi, J. P., Fennell, M., Hart, R. P., Plummer, M. R. & Grumet, M. (2011). Isolation of a novel rat neural progenitor clone that expresses Dlx family transcription factors and gives rise to functional GABAergic neurons in culture. *Dev Neurobiol* (in press)

Li, H. and Shi, W. (2010). Neural Progenitor Diversity and their Therapeutic Potential for Spinal Cord Repair. *Front. Biol. 5*, 386-395.

Li, Q. J., Tang, Y. M., Liu, J., Zhou, D. Y., Li, X. P., Xiao, S. H., Jian, D. X. and Xing, Y. G. (2007). Treatment of Parkinson disease with C17.2 neural stem cells overexpressing NURR1 with a recombined republic-deficit adenovirus containing the NURR1 gene. *Synapse* 61, 971-7.

Lie, D. C., Song, H., Colamarino, S. A., Ming, G. L. and Gage, F. H. (2004). Neurogenesis in the adult brain: new strategies for central nervous system diseases. *Annu Rev Pharmacol Toxicol* 44, 399-421.

Liu, W. G., Lu, G. Q., Li, B. and Chen, S. D. (2007). Dopaminergic neuroprotection by neurturin-expressing c17.2 neural stem cells in a rat model of Parkinson's disease. *Parkinsonism Relat Disord* 13, 77-88.

Lu, P., Jones, L. L., Snyder, E. Y. and Tuszynski, M. H. (2003). Neural stem cells constitutively secrete neurotrophic factors and promote extensive host axonal growth after spinal cord injury. *Exp Neurol* 181, 115-29.

Lundberg, C. and Bjorklund, A. (1996). Host regulation of glial markers in intrastriatal grafts of conditionally immortalized neural stem cell lines. *Neuroreport* 7, 847-52.

Lundberg, C., Englund, U., Trono, D., Bjorklund, A. and Wictorin, K. (2002). Differentiation of the RN33B cell line into forebrain projection neurons after transplantation into the neonatal rat brain. *Exp Neurol* 175, 370-87.

Lundberg, C., Winkler, C., Whittemore, S. R. and Bjorklund, A. (1996). Conditionally immortalized neural progenitor cells grafted to the striatum exhibit site-specific neuronal differentiation and establish connections with the host globus pallidus. *Neurobiol Dis* 3, 33-50.

Macias, M. Y., Syring, M. B., Pizzi, M. A., Crowe, M. J., Alexanian, A. R. and Kurpad, S. N. (2006). Pain with no gain: allodynia following neural stem cell transplantation in spinal cord injury. *Exp Neurol* 201, 335-48.

Martinez-Serrano, A. and Bjorklund, A. (1997). Immortalized neural progenitor cells for CNS gene transfer and repair. *Trends Neurosci* 20, 530-8.

Mayer-Proschel, M., Kalyani, A. J., Mujtaba, T. and Rao, M. S. (1997). Isolation of lineage-restricted neuronal precursors from multipotent neuroepithelial stem cells. *Neuron* 19, 773-85.

McKay, R. (1997). Stem cells in the central nervous system. *Science* 276, 66-71.

Min, S., Mascarenhas, N. T. and Taparowsky, E. J. (1993). Functional analysis of the carboxy-terminal transforming region of v-Myc: binding to Max is necessary, but not sufficient, for cellular transformation. *Oncogene* 8, 2691-701.

Min, S. and Taparowsky, E. J. (1992). v-Myc, but not Max, possesses domains that function in both transcription activation and cellular transformation. *Oncogene* 7, 1531-40.

Nakagawa, M., Takizawa, N., Narita, M., Ichisaka, T. and Yamanaka, S. (2010). Promotion of direct reprogramming by transformation-deficient Myc. *Proc Natl Acad Sci U S A* 107, 14152-7.

Nevins, J. R. (1992). E2F: a link between the Rb tumor suppressor protein and viral oncoproteins. *Science* 258, 424-9.

Noble, M., Arhin, A., Gass, D. and Mayer-Proschel, M. (2003). The cortical ancestry of oligodendrocytes: common principles and novel features. *Dev Neurosci* 25, 217-33.

Noctor, S. C., Flint, A. C., Weissman, T. A., Wong, W. S., Clinton, B. K. and Kriegstein, A. R. (2002). Dividing precursor cells of the embryonic cortical ventricular zone have morphological and molecular characteristics of radial glia. *J Neurosci* 22, 3161-73.

Obradovic, D., Gronemeyer, H., Lutz, B. and Rein, T. (2006). Cross-talk of vitamin D and glucocorticoids in hippocampal cells. *J Neurochem* 96, 500-9.

Onifer, S. M., Cannon, A. B. and Whittemore, S. R. (1997). Altered differentiation of CNS neural progenitor cells after transplantation into the injured adult rat spinal cord. *Cell Transplant* 6, 327-38.

Ossato, G., Digman, M. A., Aiken, C., Lukacsovich, T., Marsh, J. L. and Gratton, E. (2010). A two-step path to inclusion formation of huntingtin peptides revealed by number and brightness analysis. *Biophys J* 98, 3078-85.

Pahnke, J., Mix, E., Knoblich, R., Muller, J., Zschiesche, M., Schubert, B., Koczan, D., Bauer, P., Bottcher, T., Thiesen, H. J. et al. (2004). Overexpression of glial cell line-derived neurotrophic factor induces genes regulating migration and differentiation of neuronal progenitor cells. *Exp Cell Res* 297, 484-94.

Park, J. Y., Hwang, E. M., Park, N., Kim, E., Kim, D. G., Kang, D., Han, J., Choi, W. S., Ryu, P. D. and Hong, S. G. (2007). Gateway RFP-fusion vectors for high throughput functional analysis of genes. *Mol Cells* 23, 357-62.

Philips, M. F., Mattiasson, G., Wieloch, T., Bjorklund, A., Johansson, B. B., Tomasevic, G., Martinez-Serrano, A., Lenzlinger, P. M., Sinson, G., Grady, M. S. et al. (2001). Neuroprotective and behavioral efficacy of nerve growth factor-transfected hippocampal progenitor cell transplants after experimental traumatic brain injury. *J Neurosurg* 94, 765-74.

Pollock, K., Stroemer, P., Patel, S., Stevanato, L., Hope, A., Miljan, E., Dong, Z., Hodges, H., Price, J. and Sinden, J. D. (2006). A conditionally immortal clonal stem cell line from human cortical neuroepithelium for the treatment of ischemic stroke. *Exp Neurol* 199, 143-55.

Reddy, E. P., Reynolds, R. K., Watson, D. K., Schultz, R. A., Lautenberger, J. and Papas, T. S. (1983). Nucleotide sequence analysis of the proviral genome of avian myelocytomatosis virus (MC29). *Proc Natl Acad Sci U S A* 80, 2500-4.

Renfranz, P. J., Cunningham, M. G. and McKay, R. D. (1991). Region-specific differentiation of the hippocampal stem cell line HiB5 upon implantation into the developing mammalian brain. *Cell* 66, 713-29.

Riess, P., Zhang, C., Saatman, K. E., Laurer, H. L., Longhi, L. G., Raghupathi, R., Lenzlinger, P. M., Lifshitz, J., Boockvar, J., Neugebauer, E. et al. (2002). Transplanted neural stem cells survive, differentiate, and improve neurological motor function after experimental traumatic brain injury. *Neurosurgery* 51, 1043-52; discussion 1052-4.

Roy, N. S., Nakano, T., Keyoung, H. M., Windrem, M., Rashbaum, W. K., Alonso, M. L., Kang, J., Peng, W., Carpenter, M. K., Lin, J. et al. (2004). Telomerase immortalization of neuronally restricted progenitor cells derived from the human fetal spinal cord. *Nat Biotechnol* 22, 297-305.

Ryu, M. Y., Lee, M. A., Ahn, Y. H., Kim, K. S., Yoon, S. H., Snyder, E. Y., Cho, K. G. and Kim, S. U. (2005). Brain transplantation of neural stem cells cotransduced with tyrosine hydroxylase and GTP cyclohydrolase 1 in Parkinsonian rats. *Cell Transplant* 14, 193-202.

Sadri-Vakili, G., Bouzou, B., Benn, C. L., Kim, M. O., Chawla, P., Overland, R. P., Glajch, K. E., Xia, E., Qiu, Z., Hersch, S. M. et al. (2007). Histones associated with downregulated genes are hypo-acetylated in Huntington's disease models. *Hum Mol Genet* 16, 1293-306.

Sah, D. W., Ray, J. and Gage, F. H. (1997). Bipotent progenitor cell lines from the human CNS. *Nat Biotechnol* 15, 574-80.

Salto, C., Saindon, E., Bolin, M., Kanciurzewska, A., Fahlman, M., Jager, E. W., Tengvall, P., Arenas, E. and Berggren, M. (2008). Control of neural stem cell adhesion and density by an electronic polymer surface switch. *Langmuir* 24, 14133-8.

Schwob, A. E., Nguyen, L. J. and Meiri, K. F. (2008). Immortalization of neural precursors when telomerase is overexpressed in embryonal carcinomas and stem cells. *Mol Biol Cell* 19, 1548-60.

Sharma, R., McMillan, C. R. and Niles, L. P. (2007). Neural stem cell transplantation and melatonin treatment in a 6-hydroxydopamine model of Parkinson's disease. *J Pineal Res* 43, 245-54.

Shaw, J., Hayman, M. J. and Enrietto, P. J. (1985). Analysis of a deleted MC29 provirus: gag sequences are not required for fibroblast transformation. *J Virol* 56, 943-50.

Sherman, L., Sleeman, J. P., Hennigan, R. F., Herrlich, P. and Ratner, N. (1999). Overexpression of activated neu/erbB2 initiates immortalization and malignant transformation of immature Schwann cells in vitro. *Oncogene* 18, 6692-9.

Shihabuddin, L. S., Hertz, J. A., Holets, V. R. and Whittemore, S. R. (1995). The adult CNS retains the potential to direct region-specific differentiation of a transplanted neuronal precursor cell line. *J Neurosci* 15, 6666-78.

Siddall, P. J., Taylor, D. A., McClelland, J. M., Rutkowski, S. B. and Cousins, M. J. (1999). Pain report and the relationship of pain to physical factors in the first 6 months following spinal cord injury. *Pain* 81, 187-97.

Soldati, C., Biagioni, S., Poiana, G. and Augusti-Tocco, G. (2008). beta-Catenin and actin reorganization in HGF/SF response of ST14A cells. *J Neurosci Res* 86, 1044-52.

Son, G. H., Geum, D., Chung, S., Park, E., Lee, K. H., Choi, S. and Kim, K. (2005). A protective role of 27-kDa heat shock protein in glucocorticoid-evoked apoptotic cell death of hippocampal progenitor cells. *Biochem Biophys Res Commun* 338, 1751-8.

Staflin, K., Honeth, G., Kalliomaki, S., Kjellman, C., Edvardsen, K. and Lindvall, M. (2004). Neural progenitor cell lines inhibit rat tumor growth in vivo. *Cancer Res* 64, 5347-54.

Thomas, R. J., Hope, A. D., Hourd, P., Baradez, M., Miljan, E. A., Sinden, J. D. and Williams, D. J. (2009). Automated, serum-free production of CTX0E03: a therapeutic clinical grade human neural stem cell line. *Biotechnol Lett* 31, 1167-72.

Tominaga, M., Honda, S., Okada, A., Ikeda, A., Kinoshita, S. and Tomooka, Y. (2005). A bipotent neural progenitor cell line cloned from a cerebellum of an adult p53-deficient mouse generates both neurons and oligodendrocytes. *Eur J Neurosci* 21, 2903-11.

Truckenmiller, M. E., Vawter, M. P., Zhang, P., Conejero-Goldberg, C., Dillon-Carter, O., Morales, N., Cheadle, C., Becker, K. G. and Freed, W. J. (2002). AF5, a CNS cell line immortalized with an N-terminal fragment of SV40 large T: growth, differentiation, genetic stability, and gene expression. *Exp Neurol* 175, 318-37.

Valenza, M., Rigamonti, D., Goffredo, D., Zuccato, C., Fenu, S., Jamot, L., Strand, A., Tarditi, A., Woodman, B., Racchi, M. et al. (2005). Dysfunction of the cholesterol biosynthetic pathway in Huntington's disease. *J Neurosci* 25, 9932-9.

Vescovi, A. L. and Snyder, E. Y. (1999). Establishment and properties of neural stem cell clones: plasticity in vitro and in vivo. *Brain Pathol* 9, 569-98.

Villa, A., Liste, I., Courtois, E. T., Seiz, E. G., Ramos, M., Meyer, M., Juliusson, B., Kusk, P. and Martinez-Serrano, A. (2009). Generation and properties of a new human ventral mesencephalic neural stem cell line. *Exp Cell Res* 315, 1860-74.

Villa, A., Navarro-Galve, B., Bueno, C., Franco, S., Blasco, M. A. and Martinez-Serrano, A. (2004). Long-term molecular and cellular stability of human neural stem cell lines. *Exp Cell Res* 294, 559-70.

Villa, A., Snyder, E. Y., Vescovi, A. and Martinez-Serrano, A. (2000). Establishment and properties of a growth factor-dependent, perpetual neural stem cell line from the human CNS. *Exp Neurol* 161, 67-84.

Wang, X. J., Liu, W. G., Zhang, Y. H., Lu, G. Q. and Chen, S. D. (2007). Effect of transplantation of c17.2 cells transfected with interleukin-10 gene on intracerebral immune response in rat model of Parkinson's disease. *Neurosci Lett* 423, 95-9.

Warfvinge, K., Kamme, C., Englund, U. and Wictorin, K. (2001). Retinal integration of grafts of brain-derived precursor cell lines implanted subretinally into adult, normal rats. *Exp Neurol* 169, 1-12.

Watson, D. K., Psallidopoulos, M. C., Samuel, K. P., Dalla-Favera, R. and Papas, T. S. (1983). Nucleotide sequence analysis of human c-myc locus, chicken homologue, and myelocytomatosis virus MC29 transforming gene reveals a highly conserved gene product. *Proc Natl Acad Sci U S A* 80, 3642-5.

Weidong, L., Shen, C. and Jankovic, J. (2009). Etiopathogenesis of Parkinson disease: a new beginning? *Neuroscientist* 15, 28-35.

Weinelt, S., Peters, S., Bauer, P., Mix, E., Haas, S. J., Dittmann, A., Petrov, S., Wree, A., Cattaneo, E., Knoblich, R. et al. (2003). Ciliary neurotrophic factor overexpression in neural progenitor cells (ST14A) increases proliferation, metabolic activity, and resistance to stress during differentiation. *J Neurosci Res* 71, 228-36.

Whittemore, S. R. (1999). Neuronal replacement strategies for spinal cord injury. *J Neurotrauma* 16, 667-73.

Whittemore, S. R. and Snyder, E. Y. (1996). Physiological relevance and functional potential of central nervous system-derived cell lines. *Mol Neurobiol* 12, 13-38.

Whittemore, S. R. and White, L. A. (1993). Target regulation of neuronal differentiation in a temperature-sensitive cell line derived from medullary raphe. *Brain Res* 615, 27-40.

Wierod, L., Rosseland, C. M., Lindeman, B., Oksvold, M. P., Grosvik, H., Skarpen, E. and Huitfeldt, H. S. (2008). Activation of the p53-p21(Cip1) pathway is required for CDK2 activation and S-phase entry in primary rat hepatocytes. *Oncogene* 27, 2763-71.

Yamada, K., Hisatsune, T., Uchino, S., Nakamura, T., Kudo, Y. and Kaminogawa, S. (1999). NMDA receptor mediated Ca2+ responses in neurons differentiated from p53-/- immortalized Murine neural stem cells. *Neurosci Lett* 264, 165-7.

Yan, J., Welsh, A. M., Bora, S. H., Snyder, E. Y. and Koliatsos, V. E. (2004). Differentiation and tropic/trophic effects of exogenous neural precursors in the adult spinal cord. *J Comp Neurol* 480, 101-14.

Yang, M., Stull, N. D., Berk, M. A., Snyder, E. Y. and Iacovitti, L. (2002). Neural stem cells spontaneously express dopaminergic traits after transplantation into the intact or 6-hydroxydopamine-lesioned rat. *Exp Neurol* 177, 50-60.

Zhang, L., Gu, S., Zhao, C. and Wen, T. (2007). Combined treatment of neurotrophin-3 gene and neural stem cells is propitious to functional recovery after spinal cord injury. *Cell Transplant* 16, 475-81.

3

Neural Stem Cells: Exogenous and Endogenous Promising Therapies for Stroke

M. Guerra-Crespo[1,2], A.K. De la Herrán-Arita[1],
A. Boronat-García[1], G. Maya-Espinosa[1],
J.R. García-Montes[1], J.H. Fallon[3] and R. Drucker-Colín[1,2]
[1]*Departamento de Neuropatología Molecular, Instituto de Fisiología Celular*
[2] *Grupo Células Troncales Adultas, Regeneración Neuronal y Enfermedad de Parkinson*
Universidad Nacional Autónoma de México
[3]*Department of Psychiatry and Human Behavior, University of California, Irvine*
[1,2]*México*
[3]*USA*

1. Introduction

In the last three decades, neuroscience has been profoundly involved in stem cell research that focuses in attempting to develop mechanisms and strategies for secure therapy for different types of brain injury. The limited capacity for cellular regeneration in the highly specialized adult brain makes it particularly vulnerable to cellular damage produced by injuries, such as stroke, which results in a permanent loss of function. Stroke is a a vascular accident characterized by dramatic neuronal loss following a sudden cease of blood flow.

According to the World Health Organization, 15 million people worldwide suffer a stroke event each year. Of those 5 million pass away and another 5 million are permanently disabled (World Health Organization, 2007). Chronic stroke can have a devastating impact on the patient, family, and caregivers; but it also incurs in high economic costs to society. In the United States, stroke is the leading cause of adult disability with an estimated annual medical cost of approximately $40 billion.

High blood pressure contributes to the majority of stroke events, accounting for 12.7 million strokes over the world (World Health Organization, 2007). In developed countries, the incidence of stroke is declining, largely due to efforts in attempting to lower blood pressure and reduce smoking. However, the overall rate of stroke remains high due to the aging of the population.

There are two main types of stroke. One is ischemic stroke, which is caused by a blockage of an artery; the other is hemorrhagic stroke, which is the result of a tear in an artery's wall that produces a blood outflow into the brain. Ischemic stroke is the most common type, it accounts for about 85 percent of all stroke events (Foulkes *et al.*, 1988). In both cases, prompt treatment could mean the difference between life and death. Early treatment can also minimize damage to the brain and potential disability. The consequences of stroke on bodily functions and the severity of stroke depend on the affected area of the brain and the extent of the damage.

1.1 Current treatments for stroke

In general terms, a stroke event can be divided in acute, sub-acute and chronic phase, by taking in consideration the time course of the injury. The therapeutic strategies to each relative time point are different and centered to ameliorate different sorts of damage.

In the acute phase, the use of thrombolytic agents may dissolve the blood clot in order to slow down or prevent the cascading process that destroys nerve cells after a few hours of ischemic stroke. A currently available and successful intervention to reduce the size of the infarct is the employment of recombinant tissue plasminogen activator (t-PA). T-PA allows the dissolution of a blood clot occluding a cerebral vessel by converting plasminogen into plasmin, an important enzyme present in blood that degrades many blood plasma proteins, most notably, fibrin clots.

Administration of t-PA is approved only within 3 hours of the onset of ischemia, although optimal results are observed if given within 90 minutes (Hacke et al., 2004). Unfortunately, due to this narrow time window as well as a number of contraindications, t-PA therapy is only available to about 5% of stroke patients evaluated in the emergency room. Of these, t-PA may be expected to yield an approximate of 30% increase in the number of patients avoiding long-term neurologic deficits (Ropper & Brown, 2005).

Surgical interventions have enhanced over time and proved to be effective in some cases; however, their success is still below a desired echelon. Although surgical decompression after a stroke event has proved to lessen mortality in severe cases, doubling the probability to survive in a favorable condition, the odds of surviving in a condition requiring assistance from others increases around 10 times (Vahedi et al., 2007). Advances in endovascular techniques may improve recanalization sufficiently to improve patient or cell survival, but these have yet to be substantiated by randomized clinical trials (Burns et al., 2008).

Given the narrow window of time in which thrombolytic drugs and surgical procedures are effective, current research is focused in developing neuroprotective agents that maintain the cellular viability of threatened neuronal tissue (ischemic penumbra) and reduce the secondary damage after ischemic stroke. Many drugs currently undergoing investigation target the excitatory amino acids, such as glycine and glutamate, released by dying neural cells, which are known to lead to downstream changes that destroy nerve cells several hours to several days after a stroke. Dejectedly, although a plethora of neuroprotective compounds have shown promise in animal models, currently their employment has not shown any effectiveness in clinical trials (Dirnagl, 2006).

This fact implicates that nowadays, not a single treatment has been successful in reversing the effects of the chronic stroke. Physical therapy is used to promote functional recovery in long-term stroke patients, but recovery is often incomplete. Therefore, reversal of symptoms after a chronic stroke is a daunting problem that requires the improvement of the patient's lost function achieved by the replacement of lost neurons and glia in the injured region, as well as the establishment of new functional connections. These requirements call for bold new treatments that induce new neural cells to differentiate and integrate into the circuitry that was damaged by the stroke, the cell replacement therapy.

Considering the large amount of data acquired over the past four decades, it has been confirmed that neural stem cells (NSCs) are present throughout life and that thousands of neurons are born on a daily basis in two specific zones of the brain, the subventricular zone (SVZ) and the hippocampus (For extensive review see Zhao *et al.*, 2008).

NSCs are endowed with a self-renewal capacity and are specified to give rise only to nervous tissue-specific cell types, including neurons, glia and oligodendroglia (Reynolds and Weiss, 1996). These features together with the recent finding of the NSCs endogenous response to certain types of insults, such as stroke, lead to the persistent pursue to replace the cellular loss that takes place in the central nervous system (CNS) after injury or neurodegenerative diseases. With the advent of neuroregeneration discipline, new insights have come to the management of stroke. In general, two broad approaches are currently in development for cell replacement therapy in stroke: the recruitment of endogenous neural stem cells and exogenous stem cells transplanted into the affected area.

For a successful therapy, both approaches require to follow a highly regulated process known as neurogenesis, defined as the birth or generation of new neurons from NSCs (Zhao *et al.*, 2008). Neurogenesis follows a course where important cellular steps such as proliferation, migration and differentiation (PMD reponse), as well as cell survival are taking place. However, without a doubt, in order to develop a successful cell therapy, more understanding about how the neurogenesis process is occurring is of foremost relevance.

To achieve this goal, some important questions emerge: what are the characteristics required from the microenvironment that allow the neurogenic process to persist throughout life in the adult brain? What are the underlying mechanisms of neurogenesis regulation? And what is the cellular and molecular process regulating neurogenesis under pathological conditions?

In this chapter we will describe the current knowledge about the cellular organization and the molecular regulation that takes place in the SVZ, mechanisms that could provide the basis for the development of cell therapy in stroke and other neurodegenerative diseases. Afterward, the chapter will depict the effects of several growth factors with towering therapeutic potential for their capacity to induce endogenous cell replacement. Finally, this chapter will depict the therapeutic potential of NSCs and other cell types that are suitable for transplantation and ergo, for regeneration therapy in human patients afflicted with cerebral ischemia.

2. Cellular and molecular regulation of adult NSCs in the SVZ

2.1 The SVZ and rostral migratory stream (RMS): A general view

The study of adult neurogenesis in mammalian CNS began in the 1960's with the pioneering observations made by Joseph Altman, who managed to observe cell proliferation in the adult brain with ^{3}H-thymidine, a recognized cell division marker (Altman 1963, 1965, 1969). In spite of the controversy, further studies corroborated the existence of brain areas with the potential to generate new neurons from NSCs and defined as neurogenic niches. Nowadays, it is well accepted that the main neurogenic areas in the adult mammalian brain are the SVZ located in the walls of the lateral ventricles and the subgranular layer of the dentate gyrus (DG) of the hippocampus (Figure 1).

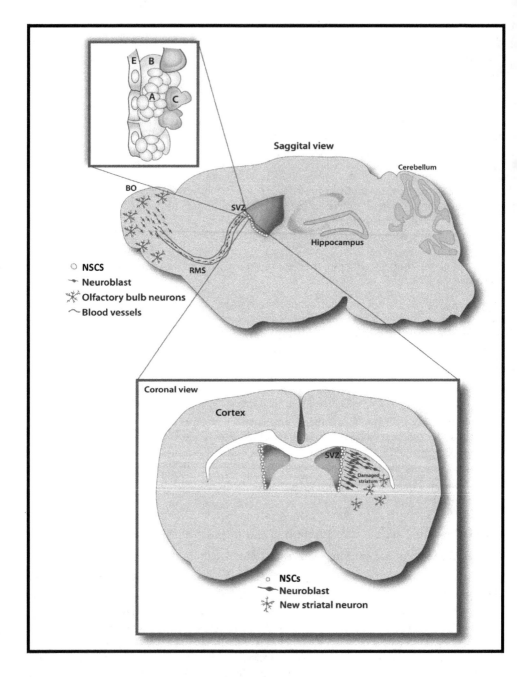

Fig. 1. Stroke and neurogenesis in the subventricular zone .

The SVZ contains many cell types, in addition to chemical and physical factors that create a special microenvironment, conducive to accurately regulate the self-renewal and multipotentiality properties of NSCs (Fuchs *et al.*, 2004). It also regulates the neurogenic processes of PMD as well as the less characterized cell integration.

The cellular composition and cytoarchitecture of the SVZ is remarkable peculiar and complex (Figure 1). There are at least five main different cell types integrating the SVZ: Astrocytes, also called B cells, divided in B1 (apical B) and B2 (tangential B); transit amplifying cells (C cells, the putative precursor); neuroblasts (A cells); tanycytes (D cells) and ependymal cells, divided in E1 and E2 (E cells) (Doetsch *et al.*, 1997; Mirzadeh *et al.*, 2008; Shen *et al.*, 2008). To give rise to new neuron, B cells generate C cells and their subsequent division generates A cells that migrate tangentially in clusters via the RMS pathway towards the OB (Figure 1) (Doetsch & Alvarez-Buylla, 1996; Lois *et al.*, 1996). In the OB, neuroblasts migrate radially to the granular and glomerular layers, where they differentiate as local interneurons and integrate into functional circuits (Belluzzi *et al.*, 2003; Carleton *et al.*, 2003; Kosaka *et al.*, 1995; Whitman *et al.*, 2007). Although uncertain, the functional relevance of the cell replacement that occurs in the OB throughout the lifespan of rodents is attributed to the olfactory adjustment to odor changes in the environment.

Without a doubt, the features shared by the many cellular types of the SVZ contributed to the debate about the true identity of NSCs (for review, Chojnacki *et al.*, 2009). Mitotic cells (astrocytes or B cells) have been generally considered to be the true NSCs, owing to their self-renew capacity and their ability to indefinitely produce neuronal and glial progeny (García-Verdugo *et al.*, 1998; Doetsch *et al.*, 1999). Nevertheless, *in vivo* observations suggest that ependymal cells function as NSCs (Johansson *et al.*, 1999). Nowadays, astrocytes are the current accepted NSCs in the adult SVZ. Nonetheless, it is well accepted that the combined stimuli of injury and a growth factor (e.g. transforming growth factor alpha,TGFα) induces a PMD response by NSCs in the ependymal layer and in the SVZ (Gleason *et al.*, 2008; Guerra *et al.*, 2009).

More recently, the presence of NSCs has been determined in the RMS (Gritti *et al.*, 2002), which was considered solely as a migratory pathway for neuroblasts that were migrating rostrally from the SVZ to their final destination, the OB (Lledo *et al.*, 2008). This cellular movement within the RMS is called "chain migration", a term established by Lois and coworkers in 1996; they showed that neuroblasts migrated in clusters without axonal guidance or radial glia regulation and instead, used a network of astrocytes that form "glial tubes" (Lois *et al.*, 1996). This unique type of migration is thought to enable cells to draw on neighboring cells as their scaffold for migration (Murase & Horwitz, 2002).

The close proximity to the striatum, shared by the SVZ and the RMS raised interest as a cellular replacement option for focal stroke occurring at the basal ganglia. Several molecules have been implicated in the highly regulated neurogenesis processes taking place in both areas. Some of them play multiple essential roles by regulating different levels of the PMD response. For the development of a thriving cell therapy, it is essential to control the processes of proliferation and migration, by means of increasing the number of proliferating cells and redirecting them to the injured area. Therefore, the mechanisms that will allow us to control neuronal fate are of great interest in the neurorepair field and represent a promising subject for the development of a factual clinical treatment.

In the following fraction, we describe the main molecules and cellular events that have been involved in the NSCs differentiation route. Table 1 summarizes the main findings.

2.2 Regulation of the NSCs development in the OB pathway

The tangential homotypic traverse of the cells that depart from the SVZ through the RMS is finely controlled by several molecules at different levels. Growth factors are the main mitogenic signals received by NSCs that trigger cell division. A subsequent generation of neuroblasts takes place after such signals; these neuroblasts are confined within the RMS via the combined effect of diffusible chemoattractants and chemorepellents that are flowing at a concentration gradient from the SVZ to the RMS. Noteworthy, the precise migration route is determined by cell-cell interaction mechanisms to ascertain their oriented organization into a continuous alignment. This migration configuration requires individual morphology arrangements in the wanderer neuroblasts, in order to make them suitable for migration.

2.2.1 Growth factors: Regulating multiple effects

Growth factors and neurotrophins have been implicated in the regulation of neurogenesis at early and postnatal development by controlling proliferation, migration and differentiation. Here, we describe some of these factors, including epidermal growth factor (EGF), fibroblast growth factor-2 (FGF-2), TGFα, brain derived neurotrophic factor (BDNF) and vascular endothelial growth factor (VEGF) for their critical role in these processes.

2.2.1.1 EGF, TGFα and FGF-2: Mitogenic signals

EGF and TGFα, two members of the EGF family, were the first growth factors to be associated to regulate SVZ proliferation through its binding to EGF receptor (EGFR). This tyrosine kynase receptor has been immunodetected in C cells (Doetsch et al., 2002) and in astrocytes of the SVZ (Höglinger et al., 2004). In vitro, studies have demonstrated that NSCs derived from the SVZ proliferate in the presence of EGF or FGF-2, as free-floating neurospheres that have the potential to differentiate into neurons and glia under appropriate conditions (Doetsch et al., 1999; Gritti et al., 1999; Reynolds & Weiss, 1992). In vivo, intraventricular infusion of EGF and TFGα resulted in an increase of NSCs proliferation in the SVZ (Craig et al., 1996; Khun et al., 1997; Morshead et al., 2003). Grippingly, only TGFα-knockout mice presented a significant reduction in proliferation and neuroblast migration in the SVZ and RMS (Tropepe et al., 1997), pointing out its direct role in these two cellular processes.

Alternatively, FGF is a large family that is widely expressed in the central nervous system. Twenty-two members of the FGF family have been identified in humans (Itoh & Orniz, 2011) and have been related to several neuronal processes, for instance, development, adult neurogenesis and repair mechanisms (Reuss & von Bohlen, 2003). To accomplish its mentioned functions, FGF binds with different affinity to each one of the FGF receptor (FGFR) family, integrated by four different members (FGFR 1 to 4) (Ornitz et al., 1996, Johnson & Williams, 1993).

From all the integrants of the FGF family, FGF-2 is the one commonly related to regulate adult neurogenesis. FGF-2 and its receptor, FGFR-1, have been described in the SVZ (Mudó et al.,

2007). *In vitro*, FGF-2 stimulates the proliferation of NSCs located in the SVZ and that these progenitors expressing nestin (neural progenitor marker) are able to differentiate into several brain cell types including neurons (Gritti *el al.*, 1996, 1999). *In vivo* studies demonstrated that a subcutaneous injection of FGF-2 increases mitotic activity in the adult SVZ (Wagner *et al.*, 1999) and restores the proliferative rates in aging rats (Fluxe *et al.*, 2008; Jin *et al.*, 2003). Nevertheless, the expression levels of FGF-2 and FGFR-1 in the SVZ do not change during aging, suggesting that although FGF-2/FGFR-1 interaction is involved in cell proliferation, it does not regulate the age-dependent declining of NSCs proliferation (Frinchi *et al.*, 2010).

2.2.1.2 BDNF: A multitask molecule

A neurotrophin recognized to undertake multiple roles in SVZ neurogenesis is BDNF. BDNF and its receptors of high and low affinity, TrkB and p75[NTR], respectively, are expressed all over the SVZ-RMS in a mutually exclusive pattern; with higher expression of BDNF and TrkB in the RMS when compared to the SVZ (Bath *et al.*, 2008; Chiaramello *et al.*, 2007; Galvão *et al.*, 2008; Gascon *et al.*, 2007; Giuliani *et al.*, 2004; Maisonpierre *et al.*, 1990; Snapyan *et al.*, 2009; Young *et al.*, 2007). In the adult RMS, BDNF mRNA expression was identified in endothelial cells of blood vessels, and absent in astrocytes as well as neuroblasts (Snapyan *et al.* 2009), whereas TrkB was found predominantly in astrocytes (Snapyan *et al.* 2009). Conversely, active TrkB (phosphorylated form) as well as the low affinity receptor p75[NTR] have been observed in migrating neuroblasts (Bath *et al.*, 2008, Galvão *et al.*, 2008; Snapyan *et al.*, 2009). P75[NTR] is also present in a small subset of GFAP-immunopositive cells and transit amplifying cells (C-cells) in the RMS (Bath *et al.*, 2008, Galvão *et al.*, 2008; Snapyan *et al.*, 2009). The BDNF-TrkB-p75 interaction is correlated to multiple cellular processes in the SVZ-RMS, in particular, those regarding survival, proliferation, migration and cell differentiation.

Luskin and Goldman's groups, who were working independently in a parallel fashion, were the firsts studying the effect of BDNF on adult neurogenesis. They both demonstrated that infusion or overexpression of BDNF into the lateral ventricles increased cell proliferation in the SVZ and migration through the default migratory pathway towards the OB (Benraiss *et al.*, 2001; Pencea *et al.*, 2001; Zigova *et al.*, 1998). Of equal relevance, was their discovery that a higher number of newborn neurons occur in the OB, highlighting its role in differentiation. Simultaneously, new heterotopic spiny neurons were found in the striatum; this finding raises the possibility to redirect the migration of neuroblasts after BDNF infusion, an astonishing breakthrough for endogenous replacement therapy (Benraiss *et al.*, 2001; Pencea *et al.*, 2001).

More recently, an additional function has been attributed to BDNF, the chemoattraction; defined as the movement of cells towards a chemical concentration gradient. Chiaramello *et al.*, tested the hypothesis that the lower expression pattern of BDNF in the RMS and a higher expression pattern in the OB is consistent with the chemoattraction property.

In explants cell cultures, the addition of this neurotrophin resulted essential for survival in addition to, a dose-dependent increase of migrating newly dividing cells. Interestingly, BDNF-induced motility on SVZ neuroblast explants was suppressed by blocking TrkB receptor autophosphorylation and by blocking BDNF action with neutralizing antibodies (Chiaramello *et al.*, 2007). Together, these results prove that BDNF has a chemoattractive function through an autocrine and/or paracrine signaling.

Despite the conclusive data concerning BDNF, the mechanisms responsible for maintaining the cells in proper formation while navigating towards the OB core still are unclear. New relevant information comes out from an interesting study from Snapyan and coworkers. They identified BDNF as a molecular signal released from endothelial cells of blood vessels (not from astrocytes or neuroblasts) in the SVZ-RMS, and demonstrated that it promotes neuronal migration via p57^{NTR} activation on neuroblasts (Snapyan et al., 2009). They proposed a vasculature-guided migration model in which migrating neuroblasts in the RMS are retained and migrate along this pathway, secondary to the presence of blood vessels that are oriented in a parallel fashion to the RMS (Snapyan et al., 2009). This newly proposed model however, does not exclude the previously stated chemoatraction model, since the possibility that both mechanisms are operating is plausible (Snapyan et al., 2009).

2.2.1.3 VEGF: Regulator of proliferation and a probable chemoattractive molecule in the SVZ

Another growth factor regulating cellular proliferation in the SVZ is VEGF, a glycoprotein known to be involved in angiogenesis and vasculogenesis. Intraventricular infusion of VEGF leads to an increase in cell proliferation of the SVZ (Jin et al., 2002; Sun et al., 2006). This finding has been confirmed by inducing the overexpression of VEGF in an ischemic model, where an increase in SVZ proliferation and migration of new cells into the ischemic injury was observed (Wang et al., 2007a, 2007b).

The VEGF family ranges from VEGF-A to VEGF-D factors, which have an affinity to several tyrosine kinase receptors: VEGF receptor (VEGFR) 1 (Flt1), VEGFR2 (KDR/Flk1), VEGFR3 (Flt4) and neuropilin receptors (NP1/2) (Matsumoto & Claesson-Welsh, 2001). One of these receptors, VGFR2, has been demonstrated to mediate a chemotactic activity for VEGF in cell cultures (Zhang et al., 2003). Its role as a chemoattractive guidance molecule for migrating neural progenitors arising from the SVZ only takes place when these cells are maintained under FGF-2 administration. These in vitro essays show that FGF-2 stimulates neural progenitors to express VGFR2, which confers them the capacity to respond to VEGF (Zhang et al., 2003).

The chemoattractant function of VEGF in adult brain is still not clear. In vivo, intraventricular VEGF administration revealed that VEGFR2/Flk-1 receptors predominate in neurogenic niches such as the SVZ and co-localize with migrating neuroblasts as well as astroglial, endothelial and neuronal cells (Jin et al., 2002; Schänzer et al., 2004). VEGF expression is observed in astrocytes, being higher in astrocytes of the SVZ and RMS than in astrocytes from non-permissive regions (Balenci et al., 2007). This expression represents an endogenous source of VEGF that can be related to neurogenesis and might have a direct effect on the migration of neural progenitors within neurogenic regions (Balenci et al., 2007).

2.2.2 Chain migration: Molecules implicated

Neuroblast chain formation requires a myriad of specific and regulated interactions to constrain the migrating cells into a precisely organized shape of the RMS. Here, we are describing the main molecules orchestrating the cellular processes involved in chain formation.

2.2.2.1 Ephrin family: Driving proliferation and proper cell positioning in migrating chains

Ephrins are transmembrane-associated proteins that exert their actions through its binding to Ephrin (Eph) receptors; the largest family of tyrosine kynase receptors. Ligands and receptors are divided in two subclasses (A and B), based on their binding properties and structural homologies (Mosch *et al.*, 2010). In general, ephrin-A ligands (ephrin-A1 to A6) bind preferentially to EphA receptor (EphA1 to A9), whereas ephrin-B (ephrin-B1 to B3) ligands bind to EphB receptor (EphB1 to B6). The interaction triggers a bidirectional cascade signal, where ephrins mediate a "reverse" signal and receptors mediate a "forward" signal (Cowan & Henkemeyer, 2002).

Ephrins-Eph interaction during development has been implicated in multiple roles, including axonal growth and cell guidance (For review see Wilkinson, 2001). In the adult brain, this interaction has also been related to several roles during neurogenesis (Conover *et al.*, 2000; Holmberg *et al.*, 2005; Theus *et al.*, 2010).

The SVZ and RMS express Eph-B1-3 and EphA4 receptors (Conover *et al.*, 2000; Theus *et al.*, 2010). In the RMS, EphB2 receptor seems to be surrounding chains of migrating neuroblasts, whereas cells expressing EphB2 in the SVZ are yet still to be determined (astrocytes, neuroblasts or ependymal cells) (Conover *et al.*, 2000). On the other hand, ephrin-B ligands are expressed in astrocytes that envelop chains of migrating neuroblast along the RMS pathway. This ephrin/Eph complementary expression pattern seems to regulate the classic ephrin contact-mediated repulsive response to give a position to the cells in specific sites.

Interestingly, blocking Ephrin-B/EphB interactions originates an increase in astrocyte proliferation in the SVZ and promotes a disorganization of the chain network (Conover *et al.*, 2000). Therefore, ephrin-B/EphB interaction is a negative regulator of cell proliferation and controls spatial organization in the SVZ. Additionally, this result suggests that inhibition of cell proliferation is required to maintain the germinative niches homeostasis.

Recently, Theus and collaborators revealed the anti-proliferative effect of EphB3, another EphB receptor in the SVZ. EphB3 is expressed in neuronal stem progenitor cells and in neuroblasts. In the traumatic brain injury (TBI) model, where an increase in neurogenesis in the SVZ is induced, Theus's group observed a significant reduction of EphB3 expression, coincidently with enhanced NSCs precursors survival and proliferation post-injury. These findings were corroborated in both ephrin-B3 and EphB3 knockout mice. The two models showed a significant augmentation in SVZ proliferation. Interestingly, in ephrinB3$^{-/-}$ mice, cell division can be reverted by infusion of a soluble form of ephrinB3 (ephrinB3-Fc) in the lateral ventricle. Furthermore, its infusion also prevents TBI-induced neural stem progenitor cell proliferation (Theus *et al.*, 2010).

Studies made in ephrin subclass A receptors gave similar results to the ones observed on ephrin-B. The use of ephrin-A2 and ephA7 knockout mice showed that this ligand-receptor interaction is a key inhibitor of cell proliferation in adult brains (Holmberg *et al.*, 2005). Ephrin-A2$^{-/-}$ and EphA7$^{-/-}$ mice show an increase in SVZ proliferation concomitant to an increase in the number of new cells in the OB; suggesting that these cells migrate in a regular fashion to the OB. In this study, it was observed that Ephrin-A2 is expressed in neural progenitor cells and neuroblasts of the lateral ventricles, whereas EphA7 receptor was expressed in ependymal cells and astrocytes of the SVZ. Interestingly, once again it seems that they are localized in a mutually exclusive manner, proper to promote ligand-receptor interactions (Holmberg *et al.*, 2005).

Altogether, these findings indicate that ephrin signaling is involved in the regulation of at least two processes of adult neurogenesis, the proliferation and neuroblast guidance into migrating chains, although, the mechanisms controlling these events still have to be determined.

2.2.2.2 ErbB receptors and neuregulins: Chemoattractive implications in proliferation and migration

The ErbB family, also called EGFR family, is integrated by four related tyrosine kinase receptors (ErbB1-ErbB4); one of them involved in cell migration signaling. Anton and coworkers determined that ErbB4 is expressed in neuronal precursor cells (type A cells) residing in the SVZ and the RMS. Additionally, in a small subset of type B cells and type C cells (Anton *et al.*, 2004). Ghashghaei and collaborators detected the presence of ErbB4 in a subgroup of CD24+ ependymal cells (Ghashghaei *et al.*, 2006).

Experiments in mice lacking ErbB4 receptor, determined its role in the organization of the SVZ-RMS pathway (Anton *et al.*, 2004). ErbB4-null mice had a disorganized structure of the SVZ, whereas the neuronal precursors, typically organized in clusters of chains along the SVZ and RMS, were instead forming fragmented chains that migrated as individual cells with an altered orientation. Moreover, impaired placement of interneurons in the OB was observed. *In vitro*, explants from these mutant mice were also unable to form compact neuronal chains, suggesting that loss of ErbB4 disrupts the characteristic "glial" tubular organization in the RMS (Anton *et al.*, 2004).

In the SVZ, ErbB4 receptors can be activated by neuroregulins (NRGs), proteins belonging to the EGF family and directly involved in the migration process as chemoattractants (Anton *et al.*, 2004). NRGs are a family of four signaling proteins that mediate cell-cell interactions in different organs, including the brain. They have been related to the activation of intracellular signaling pathways that lead to specific cellular responses, including stimulation or inhibition of proliferation, apoptosis, migration, differentiation and adhesion (Yarden *et al.*, 2001).

Two NRG types, NRG1 and NRG2, are controlling adult neurogenesis, in particular, cell proliferation and migration. NRG1 type III isoform is highly expressed in the RMS and the OB in the early postnatal development period (Anton *et al.*, 2004). *In vitro*, NRG1 type III has been characterized as the preferred chemoattractive protein (compared to NRG1 type I), aiding the migration of neuronal precursor cells from the SVZ (Anton *et al.*, 2004).

NRG2 is expressed by immature neuroblasts and in a subset of astrocytes that are lining the ventricles of the SVZ (Ghashghaei *et al.*, 2006). Ghashghaei and collaborators demonstrated that NRG1 and NRG2 have different functions in the same niche. Intraventricular infusion of NRG1 induces the aggregation of proliferating precursors into clusters in the SVZ. This aggregation is fundamental for their proper migration, probably by a chemoattractive property. On the other hand, intraventricular infusion of NRG2 promotes astrocyte proliferation and a subsequent increase of neuroblast and GABAergic interneurons in the olfactory bulb (Ghashghaei *et al.*, 2006).

2.2.2.3 βI integrins: Receptors regulating chain formation and migration through laminin binding

Integrins are heterodimeric cell surface glycoproteins that regulate proliferation and cell adhesion. Their mechanism of action is mediated through the binding to ECM proteins (fibronectin, laminin), other proteins such as ADAMs (a desintegrin and metalloprotease) and Ig-superfamily cell surface counter-receptors (such as VCAM-1). Two different subunits have been identified, α (18) and β (8), which assemble at least into 24 distinct types of integrins (Hynes, 2002).

Integrins play an important role directing the migration of neuronal precursors demonstrated in both *in vivo* and *in vitro* experiments. At least 11 integrin subunits have been identified in the SVZ-RMS pathway (α1, α2, α3, α6, α7, αv, β1, β3, β5, β6 and β8) with modifications in the temporal expression pattern during development (Belvindrah *et al.*, 2007; Murase & Horwitz, 2002). The expression of α1, α6, and α7 integrin subunits in neuroblast of the RMS seems to be higher than the one observed in the SVZ (Belvindrah *et al.*, 2007) and grippingly, all of them are able to heterodimerize with a β1 subunit (Hynes, 2002). A model for NSCs-vascular niche adhesion in the SVZ proposes integrins as a receptor for laminin, a protein deposited between neuroblasts and mainly expressed by endothelial cells that surround the SVZ. Laminin is a chemoattractant molecule for SVZ-RMS neuronal precursors that has been proposed to promote cell-cell interactions for chain formation via binding to β1-integrin (Belvindrah *et al.*, 2007). As a counterpart, β5 integrin is dispensable for chain migration.

Another integrin, α6β1, is expressed in chain migrating cells along the rodent SVZ-OB pathway, mainly in cell-cell junctions (Belvindrah *et al.*, 2007; Emsley & Hagg, 2003; Jacques *et al.*, 1998). Laminin is the only known ligand for α6β1 integrin. It has been observed that laminin is recruited to the cell surface of migrating neuroblasts, where it induces chain formation in SVZ explants and the aggregation of neuronal precursors *in vivo*. In addition, it also induces chain migration *in vitro* and *in vivo* (Belvindrah *et al.*, 2007; Emsley & Hagg, 2003). Worthy of notice, laminin infusion, in regions where precursor cells are not normally seen, redirects neural precursors toward these locations, as it has been observed in the neostriatum (Emsley& Hagg, 2003). The evidence, strongly supports the idea that laminin-α6β1 interaction is involved in the directional guidance of neuronal precursors, and promotes the formation of cell chains in the adult RMS, as well as maintaining the integrity of glial tubes in the RMS (Belvindrah *et al.*, 2007; Emsley & Hagg, 2003).

2.2.2.4 Poly-sialated neural-cell adhesion (PSA-NCAM) molecule: Forming the chain migration process and controlling differentiation

NCAM is a cell surface glycoprotein, member of the immunoglobulin superfamily that mediates cell-cell homotypic interactions, while PSA is a polymer of neuroaminic acid residues added to the NCAM molecule that is highly expressed during development and persists in the adult nervous system. Interestingly, in the adult brain, its expression is particularly confined to neurogenic niches (Seki & Arai, 1993). Specifically, neuroblasts conforming the chain migration in the RMS express PSA-NCAM (Rousselot *et al.*, 1995).

In explants cultures, it has been observed, the absence of PSA produced by endoneuraminidase-N (endoN) treatment incites the dispersion of migrating chains, although neuroblasts are still able to migrate as single cells (Hu, 2000). Furthermore, *in vivo* essays demonstrate that these cells do not easily disperse, probably because the tubular glial structures that are ensheating the neuroblasts are confining the migrating cells (Hu, 2000). This clearly indicated that lack of PSA causes a decrease in cell-cell interactions in neural progenitor chains. Therefore, PSA is an important element for neuroblast chain formation (Hu, 2000).

Other studies have demonstrated that PSA is additionally controlling neuroblast differentiation (Battista *et al.*, 2010; Petridis *et al.*, 2004). Removal of PSA moieties secondary to endoN administration inhibits cell contact dependent differentiation *in vivo*. Furthermore, it promotes a minimal and ectopic dopaminergic differentiation of neural progenitors in the SVZ (Petridis *et al.*, 2004). PSA elimination can also result in a dispersal of progenitor cells from the SVZ to the surrounding regions such as cortex and striatum, where neuroblasts differentiate into a calretinin and GABAergic phenotypes (Battista *et al.*, 2010).

The effects of NCAM mutations are quite different compared to the ones observed after PSA depletion. NCAM mutations produce a dramatic size reduction of the OB (~30%), while disruption of PSA increases this effect (Cremer *et al.*, 1994). PSA-NCAM deficient mice have an altered RMS, where the normal borders are exceeded as a result of an altered accumulation of migrating cells (Chazal *et al.*, 2000).

Altogether, it seems that PSA-NCAM mutations lead neural precursors to fail in the tangential migration to the OB. On the other hand, the ability to migrate radially into the same structure remains unaltered under PSA removal. This was demonstrated after transplanting SVZ cells in the OB of normal and PSA depleted mice OBs (by endoN), in both cases, no differences in radial migration distance or cell morphology were detected, which indicate that PSA does not regulate radial migration (Hu, 1996).

2.2.2.5 Doublecortin (DCX): Cytoskeletal dynamics for cell translocation

DCX is a neuron-specific phosphoprotein associated with microtubules that is localized in cell bodies and leading processes. It is involved in the regulation of cytoskeletal dynamics. It is expressed in neuroblasts (type A cells) and immature neurons wherein induces polymerization, in addition to promote the stabilization of microtubules that contribute to cell locomotion (Francis *et al.*, 1999, Gleeson *et al.*, 1999).

DCX expression is downregulated in postmigratory neurons in the OB. Its co-distribution with PSA-NCAM characterizes early committed neurons within the RMS; therefore, DCX is selectively expressed in migratory cell populations within the SVZ, RMS and proximal OB (Moores *et al.*, 2004; Ocbina *et al.*, 2006).

This factor promotes and maintains a bipolar cell morphology, which allows nuclear translocation and therefore cellular migration. DCX deletion results in alterations of the RMS, instigating a thickening of the RMS by the double of its size; it also results in a multipolar neuroblast morphology that correlates to a pause in migration. Furthermore, the migratory cells suffer from an unpaired nuclear translocation towards the centrosome and undergo some defects in the length of leading processes, which suggests a failure in neurite stabilization (Koizumi *et al.*, 2006).

2.2.2.6 A Desintegrin And Metalloproteinase (ADAM) protein: Propelling migration

ADAM proteins are transmembrane proteins formed by metalloprotease and desintegrin domains. These molecules appear to be related to neuroblast migration, given the fact that other proteins involved in this process require cleavage-dependent activation promoted by ADAMs. The possible mechanism of regulation might be the high capacity of ADAMs to bind to integrins, which, as previously mentioned, are fundamental to this process (Yang *et al.*, 2006). ADAMs are widely expressed in the CNS and approximately 17 different ADAMs have been detected in the CNS, however, so far, only ADAM2 and ADAM21 are directly related to SVZ-RMS cell dynamics (Murase *et al.*, 2008; Yang *et al.*, 2005).

ADAM2 is a protein expressed in the RMS neuroblasts. Lack of ADAM2 results in defects in migration and morphological alterations of the RMS, which is caudally thicker and rostrally thinner, as seen in ADAM2-null mice. ADAM2 probably regulates migration by promoting polarized cell morphology that enables migration, since ADAM2-knockout mice present short leading cell processes and a slow cell migration rate compared with neuroblasts in wild type mice (Murase *et al.*, 2008).

ADAM21 is a protein expressed in ependymal and SVZ cells. The cell processes extending from the SVZ that express ADAM21 are surrounded by glial cells and project to blood vessels that course along the RMS. They are associated with integrin α6β1 in neuroblasts and its location among neural progenitors and neuroblasts suggest that ADAM21 is involved in both cell proliferation and migration (Yang *et al.*, 2005).

2.2.2.7 Chondroitin Sulphate Proteoglycans (CSPGs): Confinement of neuroblast migration

Chondroitin sulfate is a sulfated glycosaminoglycan (GAG), composed of repeated disaccharide units of glucoronic acid (GlcA) and N-acetylgalactosamine (GalNAc). It is commonly attached to proteins as part of a proteoglycan and is a major component of the ECM that interacts with other proteins due to its negative charges (Viapiano & Matthews, 2006).

The adult brain is composed of a type of glia hallmarked by the expression of chondroitin sulfate proteoglycan NG2; which are called NG2 cells. These glial cells are widely distributed in the CNS, are present in multiple branched processes and have the capacity to differentiate into oligodendrocytes (Dawson *et al.*, 2003).

NG2 cells are aligned along the border of the SVZ and are more abundant as they are further distal to the RMS, being higher in the OB. This spatial pattern suggests a correlation between neuroblast maturity and the presence of NG2 cells. Furthermore, in the glomerular cell layer of the OB, these cells are in direct contact to cells expressing immature and mature neuronal markers (DCX, PSA-NCAM and the neuronal nuclear antigen, NeuN). The spatial organization of NG2 in SVZ-RMS raises the possibility that these cells confine the migration of neuroblasts within the RMS and prevents its dispersion (Komitova *et al.*, 2009) However, to make this assumption further research is required.

2.2.2.8 Slit and Robo proteins, chemorepulsive interactions for appropriate migration

Slit and Roundabout (Robo), ligand and receptor respectively, are evolutionarily conserved proteins in *Drosophila* and vertebrates. In mammals, Slit1-3 and Robo1-3 have been identified and implicated in axonal repulsion and cell guidance (Brose and Tessier-Lavigne 2000). Slit is a secreted protein that binds directly to Robo and functions as a chemorepellent for OB axons (Li *et al.*, 1999).

Slit and Robo function on the migratory pathway just started to be unraveled through *in vitro* experiments. Brain explants show that Slit 1 and Slit2 are expressed in the septum, where it repels progenitor cells rising from the SVZ and maintained along the RMS (Wu *et al.*, 1999). Moreover, Slit2 is expressed in the choroid plexus where it repels neural progenitors (Hu, 1999). Given the fact that Robo2 and Robo3 receptor expression has been determined in the SVZ and RMS (Marillat *et al.*, 2002), it is presumable that a Slit-Robo interaction is occurring in the migratory stream.

Slit1 deficient mice contributed to clarify the role of Slit1 in SVZ migration. Neuroblasts raised from the SVZ of knockout Slit1 mice migrate caudally to the corpus callosum, rather than to the RMS, which supports the idea that Slit1 plays an important role in directing migration. Moreover, Slit1 is also expressed in type A and type C cells within the SVZ and RMS, indicating that Slit presence is not limited to chemorepulsion activity, but possibly in parallel way, act as a individual cell migration inhibitor and might maintain chain migration integrity because Slit-mutant neurospheres migrate farther and in a disperse manner (Nguyen-Ba-Charvet *et al.*, 2004). Therefore, the evidence suggests that Slit1 and Slit2 are involved at least, in the beginning of the cell migration pathway from the SVZ towards the OB, orchestrating migration through a concentration gradient (Wu *et al.*, 1999).

2.2.2.9 Semaphorin-Neuropilin complex: Does it regulate SVZ-RMS migration?

Semaphorins are axonal guidance molecules with attractant or repellent activity that participate in early development, angiogenesis and cell migration (Tamagone & Comoglio, 2000). In vertebrates, semaphorins are divided in two groups; class 3 for secreted semaphorins and classes 4 to 7, which include transmembrane semaphorins (Raper, 2000). There is one receptor family manly involved in the regulation of semaphorin responses in the CNS: The neuropilins, NP1 and NP2 (De Wit & Verhaagen, 2003; Raper, 2000). Neuropilins are preserved throughout the entire adulthood (Giger *et al.*, 1998) and it is well known that these receptors maintain and stabilize neuronal connections and prevent axonal sprouting (Giger *et al.*, 2000; Wit & Verhaagen 2003).

Semaphorin 3A and its homodimer receptor NP1 are present along the entire RMS in the adult brain; they appear to be related to the regulation of neuroblast migration. NP1 is located in endothelial cells and binds to VEGF, an important angiogenic factor (Soker *et al.*, 1998). Therefore, it has been suggested that semaphorin 3A modulates angiogenesis. This might support the notion that the guidance of migrant neuroblasts chains could be regulated by semaphorin 3A through the indirect action of remodeling blood vessels (Melendez-Herrera *et al.*, 2008).

Complex/Molecule		Migration /Participate in proliferation(*)	Cell type expression		Reference
			Receptors	Ligands	
Growth Factors	EGF-EGFR	Negative effect on neuroblast migration (*+)		Neuronal precursor cells	Craig et al., 1996; Doetsch et al., 1999;
	EGF-TGFα	Neuroblast migration (*+)	EGFR:C cells, neuroblasts, and astrocytes	TGFα:Astrocytes	Doetsch et al., 2002; Gritti et al., 1999; Kim et al. 2009; Morshead et al., 2003; Reynolds & Weiss, 1992; Tropepe et al., 1997
	BDNF-TrkB	Autophosphorylation induces motility on SVZ neuroblasts (*+)	TrkB:migrating neuroblasts TrkB-T1: astrocytes and ependymal cells	BDNF:Endothelial cells	Maisonpierre et al., 1990; Giuliani et al., 2004; Chiaramello et al., 2007; Gascon et al., 2007; Young et al., 2007; Galvão et al., 2008; Snapyan et al., 2009
	BDNF-P75NTR	Promotes neuroblast migration	P75NTR: Neuroblasts, astrocytes and C-cells		
	FGF-2	Cell guidance with VEGF interaction (*+)	FGFR: Neural precursors (Nestin+)	FGF-2:Glial cells	Mudó et al., 2007; Frinchi et al., 2010
	VEGFR-VEGF	Neuroblasts guidance (*+)	VEGFR: Neuroblasts	VEGF:Astrocytes, endothelial cells	Jin et al., 2002; Zhang et al., 2003; Schänzer et al., 2004; Schmidt el al., 2009
Tyrosine kinase receptors	Ephrins	Chain organization (*-)	EphB3:C cells and neuroblasts EphA7:Ependymal cells and astrocytes	Ephrin B:Astrocytes Ephrin A2:Neuroblasts	Conover et al., 2000; Holmberg et al., 2005
	Erb	ErbB4:Chain organization NRG1:Neuroblast aggregation NRG2:SVZ-cell organization (*+)	ErbB4:Neuroblasts, C cells, ependymal cells	NRG1:Neuroblasts NRG2:Neuroblasts and astrocytes	Anton et al., 2004; Ghashghaei et al., 2006
Integrins	Integrins	Neuroblast aggregation and chain formation (*+)	α6β1-integrin: Neuroblasts and NSCs	Laminin:Recruited to the cell surface of neuroblasts Highly abundant around blood vessels in endothelial cells	Jacques et al., 1998; Emsley & Hagg, 2003; Belvindrah et al., 2007; Shen et al., 2008

Complex/Molecule		Migration /Participate in proliferation(*)	Cell type expression		Reference
			Receptors	Ligands	
Immunoglobulin superfamily	PSA-NCAM	Chain formation. Cell adhesion for translocation	-	Neuroblasts and non-migrating glial progenitors	Seki and Arai 1993; Hu et al., 1996; Chazal et al., 2000; Petridis et al., 2004
Microtubule-associated proteins	DCX	Stabilization of microtubules. Bipolar morphology for nuclear translocation	-	Neuroblasts	Francis et al., 1999; Gleeson et al., 1999; Moores et al., 2004; Ocbina et al., 2006
Extracelular matrix molecules	ADAMs	Chain formation. Maintains cell morphology	Integrins	ADAM2:Neuroblasts (RMS) ADAM21:Ependymal and SVZ cells	Komitova et al., 2009; Murase et al., 2008 Viapiano et al., 2006; Yang et al., 2006
	CSPGs	Neuroblast migration	Integrins	NG2 glial cells	Viapiano et al., 2006; Komitova et al., 2009
	Tenascin-R	Radial migration in OB	Not determined	Granular layer of the OB	Saghatelyan et al., 2004
Slit-Robo	Slit-Robo	Chemorepulsion	Robo1:OB Robo2 and Robo3: SVZ-RMS neuroblasts	Slit1 and Slit2:Septum Slit1:Type A and C cells	Li et al., 1999; Wu et al., 1999; Marillat et al., 2002; Nguyen-Ba-Charvet et al., 2004
Semaphorin-NP	Semaphorin-NP	Suggested that modulates neuroblast migration	NP1:Endotelial cells (RMS)	Semaphorin 3A: Endothelial cells (RMS)	Tamagone & Comoglio 2000; Meléndez-Herrera et al., 2008
Reelin/ApoER2-VLDLR	Reelin/ApoER2-VLDLR	Radial migration in the OB by cell detachment	ApoER2-VLDLR: Neuroblasts	Reelin:Mitral cells of the OB	D´Arcangelo et al., 1999; Hack et al., 2002; Simó et al., 2007
Prokineticin2	PK2/Prokr2	Cell detachment, radial migration in OB	Prokr2: OB Glomerular layer	PK2: OB Glomerular layer	Ng et al., 2004; Prosser et al., 2007

(*+) Increase cell proliferation, (*-) Decrease cell proliferation

Table 1. Regulation of NSCs proliferation and neuroblast migration in the SVZ-RMS pathway.

2.2.2.10 Radial migration in the OB: Reelin, Tenascin-R and Prokineticin2 as detachment signals

After completing chain migration through the RMS, neuroblasts finally arrive to the OB, where a shift in migration occurs, from a tangential to radial direction. To accomplish this cellular step, a neuroblast detachment signal is required. The most described ligand-receptor complex involved in this process is reelin/ApoER2-VLDLR. Reelin is an ECM secreted glycoprotein expressed in mitral cells of the OB. The surface receptors for reelin are the apolipoprotein E receptor 2 (ApoER2) and the very low-density lipoprotein receptor (VLDLR), both expressed in migrating neuroblasts. To allow the migratory switch, binding of reelin to its receptors induces phosphorylation of the intracellular adaptor protein disabled-1 (Dab1) and Src family kinases (SFK) (D´Arcangelo *et al.*, 1999, Hiesberger *et al.*, 1999).

In vitro, SVZ explants supplemented with reelin exhibit a loss of neuroblast chain formation, which gives raise to individual cell migration. Furthermore, *in vivo* observations of reeling-null mice reveal that neuroblasts fail to migrate radially in the OB and remain in clusters (Hack *et al.*, 2002). Additionally, the experimental overexpression of reelin by grafting reelin-expressing cells in the SVZ produces a dispersion of neuroblasts around the ventricular structures by chemokinetic activity and detachment (Courtes *et al.*, 2011).

Recently, another function of reelin has been hypothesized. It was demonstrated that reelin expression is reactivated after brain injury (focal demyelinization of corpus callosum) in mature neurons at the proximal damaged area. It is suggested that reelin enhances chemoattraction exerted by lesion-derived cytokines that contribute to neuroblast recruitment in the boundary of the damaged area. All together, these results support reelin's performance as a detachment and migration key factor (Courtes *et al.*, 2011).

There are other molecules involved in radial migration in the OB; one of these molecules is tenascin-R, an ECM glycoprotein expressed in the granular layer of the OB, where it initiates neuroblast chain detachment and radial migration. Tenascin-R-null mutant mice show a cell reduction in the granular layer, whereas neuroblasts remain in clusters in the OB (Saghatelyan *et al.*, 2004).

Finally, other molecule involved in OB migration is Prokineticin2 (PK2), which is expressed in the granular and periglomerular layers of the OB and acts as detachment signal and chemoattractant. PK2 receptor-null mice (Prokr2) exhibit a decrease in the volume of the OB and have an abnormal accumulation of neuroblasts around the olfactory ventricle. This suggests a deficiency in neuroblast migration and defects in chain migration detachment (Prosser *et al.*, 2007). Furthermore, *in vitro*, SVZ explants co-cultured with cells obtained from the glomerular layer of the OB, begin cell migration toward the glomerular layer of the explants; whereas cells from the glomerular layer of PK2-null mice do not exhibit chemotactic activity (Ng *et al.*, 2005).

3. Growth factors as an endogenous approach for neurorepair therapy

3.1 Endogenous response after stroke

We just described in the previous section the existence of a substantial number of molecules and its complex signaling regulating PMD response at the SVZ under basal conditions.

However, studies also reveal that neurogenesis could be triggered secondary to specific injury conditions, including stroke. Focal cerebral ischemia promotes neurogenesis in the DG of the hippocampus and in the SVZ (Arvidsson et al., 2002; Jin et al., 2001; Liu et al., 1998; Parent et al., 2002; Zhang et al., 2001); both being a feature shared by rodent and the human brain (Jin et al., 2006; Martí-Fabregas et al., 2010). Moreover, these studies demonstrate that the default migratory pathway, followed by neuron precursors from the SVZ that supply the OB region, can be partially diverted to other destinations including the striatum and cortex after stroke injury. Recently, it was demonstrated that stroke enhances long-term neurogenesis, although, decreased in magnitude when compared to the acute phase (Thored et al., 2006). These findings are of paramount relevance for their therapeutic potential in the field of neuronal damage reestablishment, by taking advantage of an endogenous cell source. However, Ardvisson et al., in their seminal work, determined that within 6 weeks of transient focal stroke uniquely 0.2% of newborn neurons from the SVZ were integrated in the damaged striatum. Thus, neurogenesis occurring after cerebral ischemia represents an insufficient cell source for the purpose of neuronal replacement therapy (Ardvisson et al., 2002).

3.2 Self-renewal induced by growth factors: The endogenous neuronal repair

The rationale for self-renewal induced by growth factors relies on the existence of neurogenic niches in the brain with the potential to modulate the proliferative response by either injury or growth factors. The purpose of this approach has been to determine whether growth factors are able to amplify the endogenous response of NSCs in a meaningful level that can account an increase of neuronal differentiation. The concept however, was not new in the field of stroke studies. One of us, Dr. James Fallon (Fallon et al., 2000) employed the 6-hydroxydopamine lesion rodent model of Parkinson's disease, where he and collaborators demonstrated that proliferating cells significantly increased in the striatal SVZ ipsilateral to the injured side, however, this increase was exclusive in animals that also received an striatal infusion of TGF-α; neuroblasts then migrated in mass into the striatum to become neurons.

There is a long and increasing list of growth factors that has the potential to be implemented as a therapeutic tool in the recovery process after a stroke event, exploiting their neuroprotection and neurogenesis features. Here, we are focusing on studies that unveil that growth factors are modifying neurogenesis subsequent to the onset of focal cerebral ischemia, specifically in the SVZ-RMS. Table 2 represents a chronological compendium of such studies. The hematopoietic factors known to compel neurogenesis were omitted in our chapter, nonetheless, they are extensively reviewed by others (Greenberg & Jin, 2006).

The majority of the research described in this section of the chapter employs the most common method to study focal stroke, the middle cerebral artery occlusion (MCAO) model, which affects the striatum and/or cortex, resembling the injury that commonly occurs in stroke patients (Figure 1). To induce this kind of ischemia, an incision in the neck is made and after exposition of the common, external and internal carotid arteries, a monofilament suture is then carefully introduced via the external carotid artery through the lumen of the internal carotid artery until it reaches and occludes the middle cerebral artery (MCA).

3.2.1 EGF family of growth factors

It is important to highlight that in practically all the protocols regarding neurogenesis, the quintessential strategy to identify newborn cells is the administration of bromodeoxyuridine (BrdU), a marker of cell division, which intercalates into the DNA of cells that are undergoing proliferation. The neuronal (or glial) lineage of BrdU-labeled cells is determined by the co-staining with specific markers of immature or mature phenotypes, which may differs depending on the goal of the study.

3.2.1.1 EGF

Teramoto and collaborators reported in 2003 the first study about the effect of a growth factor on neurogenesis in the SVZ after an ischemic insult (Teramoto *et al.*, 2003). The antecedents implicating EGF as a factor that promotes NSCs proliferation and migration from the SVZ to the striatum lead them to test if EGF could induce a PMD response in the damaged brain after an ischemic event. They administered an intraventricular dose of EGF two days after stroke for a period of one week that allow a noteworthy neuronal replacement increase after week 13th post MCAO. Interestingly, Teramoto determined that the BrdU+/NeuN+ cells observed at the boundary zone of the stroke lesion were not DARPP-32 (dopamine and adenosine 3′,5′-monophosphate–regulated phosphoprotein of 32KD) positive, the prevailing neuronal population in the striatum. Rather than, they found 65% of the new cells matured into aspiny parvalbumin-containing (PV) interneurons. This effect is intriguing, given the fact that *in vitro*, EGF stimulates the DARPP-32 phenotype (Reynolds & Weiss, 1992). Therefore, albeit EGF is probably directing the mechanisms related to neuronal commitment and fate specification, such claims need further study.

3.2.1.2 Heparin-binding epidermal growth factor-like growth factor (HB-EGF)

Another member of this family is the HB-EGF that also has a clear effect in increasing proliferation of NSCs in the SVZ. However, its effect on migration and differentiation is not fully disclosed. In one study, Jin and coworkers analyzed such effect 4 weeks after stroke and observed an increase in the number of BrdU cells (approximately 40%) and the number of BrdU cells co-localizing with the immature neuronal marker TUC-4 in the SVZ. Nonetheless, a concomitant decrease of approximately 60% of neuroblasts (DCX+) migrating towards the striatum was also observed. The authors suggested that this effect is probably due to its chemoattractant properties. In spite of the decrease in migration, a significant improvement in neurological outcome was accounted, probably due to a reduction in infarct size promoted by the growth factor (Jin *et al.*, 2004). Later on, another study conducted by Sugiura and coworkers determined that recombinant adenovirus-expressing HB-EGF promotes neurogenesis and angiogenesis in the SVZ. Nonetheless, opposite to the study developed by Jin *et al.*, no effect limiting migration of newborn cells toward the striatum was reported. Therefore, also in contrast, an increase of neuronal cells was observed in the ischemic striatum, going from 2 BrdU+/NeuN+ cells to 23 cells per mm^2 (Sugiura *et al.*, 2005) Additionally, a functional recovery was observed. The discrepancy in both results still remains to be discerned, however, it could be due to the different methods employed to deliver the growth factor, which impose differences in concentration and availability.

3.2.1.3 TGF-α

The first report of TGFα's effect on neurogenesis in rats that were subjected to transient MCAO, was made by our group (Guerra-Crespo *et al.*, 2009). The majority of stroke studies analyze the effect of growth factors in the acute phase of ischemia. However, we were interested in the delayed administration of the growth factor, since it resembles the typical situation in humans with preexisting stroke injuries, who might benefit from this type of therapy. Therefore, we infused TGFα directly in the striatum four weeks after injury, when the infarction area was no longer expanding and the cellular deterioration had stabilized, indicating that the acute phase was completed and the chronic phase had begun.

Eight weeks after MCAO, and four weeks after the onset of TGFα administration, we found a 4-fold increase of BrdU labeled cells arising from the ependymal layer and the SVZ. Many of the BrdU-labeled cells of the SVZ and others under migration were expressing the immature neuronal marker Meis2, a transcription factor that is strongly expressed in striatal precursors. Additionally, we found around the site of the infarction about a 7-fold increase of BrdU cells that were co-labeled with the neuronal-fate marker NeuN, whereas, several of the newborn cells co-labeled with DARPP-32, indicating that they differentiate into striatal neurons, which are typical for this brain region. These results indicate that TGFα treatment significantly increased the yield of neurons produced in the injury response. Although we did not examine the long-term survival of these neurons, an approximately 90% of behavioral recovery (corner and cylinder test) in the chronic animal suggests that many of them became functionally and integrated in the host's CNS (Guerra-Crespo *et al.*, 2009).

In the same year, another group (Leker *et al.*, 2009) reported an increase in neurogenesis as well as angiogenesis induced by TGFα. Leker *et al.*, administered an intraparenchymal dose of the growth factor 1 day after ischemia, for a consecutive period of 14 days and analyzed the long-term response. TGFα increased the number of BrdU cells and allow a 2-fold increase of neuroblasts in the ischemic hemisphere. Nonetheless, only a slight number of newborn neurons in proximity to the infarct border were observed, suggesting that under these specific experimental conditions, TGFα leads to a moderate but significant neuronal differentiation. Concomitant to neurogenesis, TGFα expanded (2.4-fold) the area covered by blood vessels in the ischemic border zone. The mechanism involved the recruitment of endothelial bone marrow-derived cells into newly formed cerebral blood vessels.

3.2.1.4 Intranasal infusion of TGFα

The employment of growth factors in patients is impeded by the facts that intracranial infusion is impractical and that many growth factors intravenously administrated are not able to cross the blood-brain barrier (BBB). Even though there are methods for bypassing the BBB, they typically consist of invasive neurosurgeries that would restrict clinical application to the most severe cases. Noninvasive techniques that are capable of delivering growth factors to the CNS represent a therapeutic alternative to surgery. A pioneer work was the intranasal administration of neurotrophic growth factor (NGF), which demonstrated that delivered growth factors could bypass the BBB. Since then, the prevalence of the intranasal administration technique for CNS treatment has grown considerably (Capsoni *et al.*, 2002; De Rosa *et al.*, 2005; Frey *et al.*, 1997; Liu *et al.*, 2004; Ma *et al.*, 2008). With this approach of administration, therapeutic molecules traverse the BBB through the olfactory pathway and the less-studied trigeminal neural pathway (Thorne *et al.*, 2004). The advantage of this method is that factors are delivered directly into the brain and thereby avoid adverse systemic effects. The simplicity of the intranasal administration of growth factors makes it an outstanding strategy. This non-surgical approach represents a potential therapeutic strategy for human patients.

Based in this knowledge, we delivered an intranasal dose of a pegylated form of TGFα (PEG-TGFα) to make it more stable for the nasal route. We found that intranasal delivery is a viable alternative because PEG-TGFα was able to induce the proliferation and migration of neural progenitors to the damaged striatum (in terms of BrdU incorporation and nestin expression), although of less magnitude compared to intracranial TGFα administration. This finding is associated with significant behavioral improvement in the MCAO model, measured by the corner and cylinder test. Therefore, intranasal delivery of PEG-TGFα holds great therapeutic potential.

3.2.2 FGF-2

From the FGF family, FGF-2 is the member which neurogenic properties have been demonstrated. The first study, performed in 2003, reported that, regardless of a 30% increase of BrdU+/DCX+ cells, no BrdU+/NeuN+ cells were observed (Wada *et al.*, 2003). In the same year, Matsuoka and collaborators also reported an increase (2.1 fold) of BrdU+ cells in the SVZ of a global ischemia rodent model, through FGF-2 gene delivery by an adenoviral vector. Although neuronal differentiation in the striatum was not analyzed, a small number of newborn cells (3%) were labeled positive for NeuN amongst the different layers of the cortex and by the proximity to the SVZ suggesting that such cells were derived from the SVZ (Matsuoka *et al.*, 2003). Matsuoka's research set a precedent on gene therapy field, since was the first time that a growth factor was administered through viral vector in a stroke model

Both former works were focused on the study of acute phase of stroke, where a short infusion period of the growth factor or a short time analysis after the growth factor-adenovirus transduction was made. More recently, Leker and coworkers employed an ischemia model with predominant cortical damage and an adenovirus delivery system that allowed overexpression of FGF-2 for a long time period. They were able to observe that FGF-2 increased proliferation and migration from the SVZ and that the immature neurons were localized in the border of damaged cortex when analyzed at 30 and 90 days after stroke. Additionally, the results shown that the group treated with FGF-2 presented a 2-fold increase of newborn cells expressing NeuN and even a higher increase (22 *versus* 1.6%) of cells labeled with the immature neuronal marker Hu. In either Matsuoka *et al.*, or Leker *et al.*, studies, no lineage analyses was performed to asseverate without a doubt, that such cells were originated in the SVZ, since they could be also produced in the cortex. Nevertheless, the evidence suggests that the majority of the cells arose from the SVZ (Leker *et al.*, 2007).

The previous studies disclose the enhancement achieved on endogenous neurogenesis in the SVZ when EGF or FGF-2 are administered independently. However, a more interesting fact would be to analyze the simultaneous effect of both growth factors in order to increase neurogenesis. Nakatomi *et al.*, in a breakthrough work addressed that question in a transient ischemia model with specific pyramidal hippocampal damage. The results demonstrated that endogenous proliferation and migration are enhanced by intraventricular co-administration of growth factors after stroke. However, that the growth factor induced neuronal regeneration of approximately 40% of the CA1 pyramidal layer, one month after stroke, was a remarkable finding (Nakatomi *et al.*, 2002). This study was centered in the analysis of the hippocampus; however, only a few years later, Baldauf and Reymann examined the combined effect of EGF/FGF-2 on the SVZ. They observed an increase (almost double) in the number of BrdU+/DCX+ cells in the ipsilateral striatum, in spite of a concomitant increase in the infarct volume. Unfortunately, neuronal fate and behavior were not analyzed; therefore, further analyses are required to conclusively discern the effect of the synchronic administration of EGF and FGF-2 for striatum neuronal replacement (Baldauf and Reymann 2005).

3.2.3 Neurotrophic factors: BDNF

The neuroprotective effects of the intraventricular infusion of BDNF after global ischemia were reported for the first time in 1994 (Beck *et al.*, 1994). However, the role of BDNF in neurogenesis was recently demonstrated. In one report (Gustafsson *et al.*, 2003), BDNF expression was successfully attained in the substantia nigra by means of an adenovirus; the objective was to transport BDNF anterogradely to the striatum and avoid damage in its cytoarchitecture. The transduction of the viral vector took place 4 to 5 weeks prior to the MCAO. With this strategy, they found a significant increase of neuroblast migration towards the striatum at 2 weeks after ischemia. Additionally, a higher number of BrdU cells co-laballed with early neuronal marker Hu and striatal neuronal marker Meis2 were observed. The significant relevance for replacement therapy cannot be established with these findings, because the transduction of the viral vector generated anomalous behavior patterns and therefore, the behavioral outcome cannot be correctly analyzed. Moreover, the high expression levels of BDNF aggravated the cellular death of cholinergic, PV and neuropeptide Y interneurons in the striatum, which could override the neuroprotective effects observed in former studies performed by the same research group (Andsberg *et al.*, 2002).

Some years later, in another attempt to determine the effect of BDNF on neurogenesis, Schavitz and coworkers induced a parietal cortical lesion, and after an intravenous injection of BDNF on the following 5 days, were able to observe precursor cells rising from the SVZ that were migrating toward the ipsilateral striatum. A substantial number of neuroblasts were recruited to the ischemic hemisphere 37 days after the last injection; still, neuronal replacement was not observed with this paradigm of cortical injury, since no BrdU+/NeuN+ cells were observed. Additionally, the authors were unable to detect cortical neurogenesis (Schavitz *et al.*, 2007).

In summary, a variety of growth factors have been tested in experimental stroke models and irrespective of their nature, practically all of them can induce proliferation on NSCs that reside in the SVZ. Most of them, enhance in a parallel fashion the recruitment of neuroblasts toward the peri-infarcted area, either striatum or cortex. However, extensive differences in neuronal differentiation have been observed in the damaged area (even when employing the same growth factor), ranging from a highly significant increase to a decrease in differentiation levels. The behavioral outcome, measured as an indirect index of functional integration, has been analyzed only in the minority of the studies, finding an important level of recovery in some of them.

The potential of growth factors for endogenous cell replacement is evident; however, clinical studies are not currently being undertaken, given the fact that growth factors encompass a strong and dangerous mitogenic effect.

Growth factor	Stroke Model	Delivery Method	Time period of infusion	Effect on Neurogenesis	Behavioral outcome	Reference
EGF Family						
EGF	Mouse Left MCAO	Minipump in lateral ventricle	21 days after ischemia for 7 days	- 65% of new PV interneurons 13 weeks after stroke - 100 fold of neuronal replacement	NA	Teramoto et al., 2003
HB-EGF	Rat Right MCAO	Minipump in lateral ventricle	24 hours after ischemia for 3 days	- Increase of BrdU+ cells expressing TUC-4 -60% decrease in migrating neuroblasts 4 weeks after stroke	Improvement in neurological score	Jin et al., 2004
HB-EGF	Rat Left MCAO	Adenoviral vector in lateral ventricle	3 days after ischemia	- 2-fold increase of vascular density (angiogenesis) - Increase of BrdU+/NeuN+ cells (2 vs 23 cells per mm²) 28 days after ischemia	Improvement in rotarod test	Sugiura et al., 2005
TGFα	Rat Left MCAO	Minipump in striatum	1 month after ischemia for 28 days (chronic treatment)	- 4-fold increase of BrdU+ cells - 7-fold increase of BrdU+/NeuN+ cells and several BrdU+/DARPP-32+ two months after stroke	90% of improvement in corner and cylinder test	Guerra-Crespo et al., 2009
TGFα	Mouse Left MCAO	Minipump intra-parenchyma	1 day after ischemia for 14 days	- 2.4 fold increase in blood vessel cover area in the infarct border - Small number of newborn neurons in the infarct border 90 days post-infusion	NA	Leker et al., 2009
TGFα	Rat Left MCAO	Intranasal delivery	4 intranasal doses per month (1 per week)	- Increased BrdU+ cells in SVZ and ischemic striatum - Increased neurogenesis (BrdU+/Nestin+ cells) in the peri-infarcted striatum	50% of improvement in corner and cylinder test	Guerra-Crespo et al., 2010

Growth factor	Stroke Model	Delivery Method	Time period of infusion	Effect on Neurogenesis	Behavioral outcome	Reference
EGF Family						
FGF-2 (bFGF)	Rat Right MCAO (cortex)	Intracisternal injection	Injections 24 and 48 hrs after stroke	- 30% increase of BrdU+/DCX+ cells at day 7 and 2% at day 21 - No BrdU+/NeuN+ cells	NA	Wada et al., 2003
FGF-2	Gerbil Global ischemia	Adenoviral vector in lateral ventricle	Transduction 3 hrs after stroke	- 2.1 fold increase of BrdU+ cells in the SVZ 7 days after ischemia - 3% of BrdU+/NeuN+ in cortex 30 days post-stroke	NA	Matsuoka et al., 2003
FGF-2	Hypertensive Rat MCAO (cerebral cortex)	Adenoviral vector in the infarct border	Transduction starting the same day of ischemia (chronic treatment)	- Increase of BrdU+ cells expressing neural transcription factors MASH1 and Pax6 in the peri-infarcted area 30 days after stroke - Increase of BrdU+/Hu+ cells (22% vs 1.6%)	Improvement in motor disability score	Leker et al., 2007
FGF-2+ EGF	Rat Left MCAO	Minipump in lateral ventricle	10 min after ischemia for 14 days	- Increased proliferation in the striatum - 2 fold increase of BrdU+/DCX+ cells in striatum 14 days after stroke	NA	Baldauf et al., 2005
Neurotrophin						
BDNF	Rat MCAO	Adenoviral vector in SN transported anterogradely towards striatum	5 weeks previously to MCAO	- Increased neuroblasts (DCX+) - Increased neuronal death in the striatum - Increased BrdU+/Meis2+ cells 2 weeks post-ischemia	Vector-induced abnormal motor behavior	Gustafsson et al., 2003
BDNF	Rat Photothrombotic ischemia (cortical stroke)	Intravenous injection	1 hour post-ischemia 2nd to 5th day	- Highly significant increase of neuroblasts in striatum 37 days after last injection - No BrdU+/NeuN+ cells	Improvement in neurological score and adhesive tape removal test	Schavitz et al., 2007

Table 2. Growth factors induce SVZ neurogenesis in ischemic stroke.

4. NSCs transplant therapy: A new expectation

Neural transplantation is a promising strategy for treatment of several CNS pathologies that offers long-lasting improvement and the prospect of permanent cure. The most obvious possibility is to use neural transplantation as a technique for cell replacement therapy whereby the cells would occupy the place or the function of dead or degenerated cells. Potential advantages to this approach may include greater control over cell fate, the ability to deliver any desired number of cells, and reduced risks associated with mitogen infusion. A number of different cell types have been considered for cell transplantation with goals ranging from replacement of host circuitry to delivery of neuroprotective or immunomodulatory compounds.

The majority of studies to date have shown relatively limited cell replacement from endogenous NSCs. Further, the technology for mobilizing endogenous NSCs is relatively new. In contrast, work has been in progress for decades to replace lost neural cells by transplantation of either fetal brain tissue or more recently, NSCs.

Recent studies have highlighted the enormous potential of cell transplantation therapy for stroke. In this branch of the chapter, we will describe the experimental trials that utilized NSCs in the MCAO model, which placed the stepping stone for the first human trials of NSCs transplant therapy.

Fetal brain tissue transplants have been shown to produce some recovery in animal models of stroke (Mattsson et al., 1999; Nishino et al., 2000; Riolobos et al., 2001), but ethical considerations and a short supply of human fetal tissue limited this approach. As a result, a variety of cell types have been tested in stroke models, they include human bone marrow cells, human umbilical cord blood cells (Chen et al., 2001a; Chen et al., 2001b; Savitz et al., 2002; Zhao et al., 2002), rat trophic factor-secreting kidney cells (Mattsson et al., 1999; Nishino et al., 2000; Riolobos et al., 2001; Savitz et al., 2002), and immortalized cell lines such as the human neuron-like NT2N (hNT) cells (Borlongan et al., 1998; Saporta et al., 1999) and MHP36, an embryonic murine immortalized neuroepithelial cell line (Modo et al., 2002; Veizovic et al., 2001). In spite of the vast types of transplanted cells employed, they yet need to demonstrate a significant behavioral recovery in animal models of stroke and a long-lasting survival of the grafted tissue (Table 3).

From the previously mentioned cell types employed for transplant, human cells that have been used in these studies fall into 3 categories: A) Neural stem/progenitor cells (NPCs) cultured from fetal tissue; B) immortalized neural cell lines, hematopoietic/endothelial progenitors and stromal cells isolated from bone marrow, umbilical cord blood, peripheral blood or C) adipose tissue. Even though transplanted human cells have shown promise, other sorts of cells have arisen to address the need for a quintessential cell source for transplant therapy.

Amongst them, NSCs have been proposed as a potential source of new cells to replace those lost due to central nervous system injury such as stroke, as well as a source of trophic molecules to minimize damage and promote recovery in clinical trials.

In the background of this imperative clinical need, hundreds of studies have recently published the therapeutic potential of either endogenous or transplanted NSCs in laboratory models of stroke. To their advantage, NSCs have the capacity to respond actively to their environment, migrate to areas of injury, and secrete neuroprotective compounds. Such properties may afford them therapeutic potential both in the acute phase and at later time points when the employment of conventional medical therapies would no longer be effective.

NSCs can be isolated from many regions of the CNS of embryonic as well as adult mammals. As mentioned in other section of the chapter, they can be propagated in culture in the presence of EGF and/or FGF-2 as proliferative clusters of cells termed neurospheres. Recent studies have demonstrated that rather than being homogeneous aggregates of stem cells, neurospheres actually represent a heterogeneous collection of cells including true stem cells, committed progenitors, and differentiated progeny. This is in contrast to embryonic stem cells (ESCs), which in the presence of appropriate signaling molecules can be maintained as a relatively homogeneous population of stem cells. NSCs also differ from ESCs in terms of the variety of neurons they can generate. Profiles of NSCs gene expression tend to point to NSCs expanded as neurospheres in EGF and FGF-2 as adopting a forebrain profile.

Consistent with this, attempts to differentiate NSCs into cells from other regions of the CNS, such as dopaminergic neurons, cerebellar Purkinje cells, or motoneurons have in most cases been unsuccessful. Nevertheless, NSCs can be successfully differentiated into representative cell types in parts of the brain most commonly affected by stroke, such as cortical projection neurons (Englund et al., 2002), interneurons (Scheffler et al., 2005) and hippocampal pyramidal neurons (Corti et al., 2005). Retrograde labeling, synaptic integration, and action potential generation from NSCs-derived neurons has been demonstrated in vivo (Englund et al., 2002).

Given the fact that NSCs have the capability to differentiate into neurons (Kelly et al., 2004; Song et al., 2002a; Song et al., 2002b), astrocytes (Eriksson et al., 2003; Herrera et al., 1999; Winkler et al., 1998), oligodendrocytes (Pluchino et al., 2003; Yandava et al., 1999), and perhaps endothelium (Wurmser et al., 2004), advocates that conception that NSCs should be capable of replacing most of the cell types affected by an ischemic injury.

4.1 From theory to practice: NSCs transplant in rodent models of stroke

Actual results in preclinical studies, however, have been quite varied. NSCs, including human, can clearly survive after transplantation, have a tendency to migrate toward areas of infarct (Kelly et al., 2004), and can generate functional neurons (Englund et al., 2002) that may form connections with host cells (Park et al., 2002). Although several studies have found NSCs to predominantly differentiate into glia after transplantation into normally non-neurogenic regions (Eriksson et al., 2003; Herrera et al., 1999; Winkler et al., 1998), robust neural differentiation has been observed after transplantation of cells cultured on laminin (Wu et al., 2002; Yan et al., 2007).

Most studies have not observed substantial changes in infarct size after NSCs transplantation (Kelly et al., 2004; Pollock et al., 2006); however, neuroprotective (Lee et al., 2007; Ourednik et al., 2002) and immunomodulatory (Fujiwara et al., 2004; Pluchino et al., 2005) effects of NSCs in addition to their potential for at least some cell replacement (Sinden et al., 1997), have collectively yielded beneficial effects in multiple animal models of neurodegeneration and brain injury, including stroke (Chu et al., 2004; Pollock et al., 2006; Sinden et al., 1997).

NSCs transplantation enhances endogenous cell proliferation in the SVZ and promotes angiogenesis in the peri-infarct zone of adult rats, even if it is performed in the acute phase of ischemic injury. In addition, this transplanted NSCs managed to survive, migrate, differentiate, and also induce improvement in neurological functions (Zhang et al., 2009a, 2009b; Zhang et al., 2010). Grafted NSCs enhanced the number of BrdU-positive cells in ischemic ipsilateral SVZ at 7 days after transplantation, an effect that persisted to at least 14 days post-transplantation. These results revealed that NSCs transplantation increases cell proliferation in the SVZ and promotes angiogenesis in the peri-infarct zone after focal cerebral ischemia in adult rats. The reason that grafted NSCs increase endogenous NSPCs proliferation may be due to the production of certain growth factors or repression of inflammation and apoptosis.

In addition to promote proliferation, it has been shown that human fetal striatum derived NSCs, transplanted as neurospheres, survive in stroke-damaged rat striatum, migrate toward the site of the injury, and differentiate into mature neurons in the absence of tumor formation (Darsalia et al., 2007).

Evidence of cell migration to the site of ischemic injury from administration by various routes has been seen, including intravenous, intraarterial, and intraparenchymal brain injection. Migration potential may differ according to cell type and route, but this has not been systematically explored for most cell lines. Animal studies with a number of NSCs lines have shown evidence of cell survival and in some studies improvement in behavioral outcomes after focal ischemic injury (Bacigaluppi et al., 2008; Borlongan et al., 1998; Chu et al., 2004; Ishibashi et al., 2004; Jiang et al., 2006; Modo et al., 2002; Pollock et al., 2006; Wei et al., 2005).

In a follow-up work, Darsalia et al. showed that transplantation shortly after stroke (48 hours) resulted in better cell survival than did transplantation 6 weeks after stroke, but the delayed transplantation did not influence the magnitude of migration, neuronal differentiation, and cell proliferation in the grafts. Additionally, transplanting greater numbers of grafted NSCs did not result in a greater number of surviving cells or increased neuronal differentiation. They observed a substantial number of activated microglia 48 hours after the insult in the injured striatum, but reached maximum levels 1 to 6 weeks after stroke (Darsalia et al., 2011). Their findings show that the best survival of grafted human NSCs in stroke-damaged brain requires optimum numbers of cells to be transplanted in the early post stroke phase, before the inflammatory response is established.

In an attempt to improve transplant survival and behavioral outcome, Jin et al. found that intralesional transplantation of nestin/Sox2-immunopositive neuronal precursor cells (NPCs) derived from BG01 human embryonic stem cells 3 weeks after distal MCAO in rats reduced infarct volume and improved behavioral outcome 4–9 weeks post-transplant (Jin et al., 2010a). In another study, they found that the beneficial effects of transplantation occurred in both young adult (3-month-old) and aged (24-month-old) rats (Jin et al., 2010b).

NPCs express many factors known to influence neurite plasticity and thus have the potential to enhance structural plasticity after stroke. With that notion in mind, Andres et al. decided to analyze the effects of transplanted NPCs on structural plasticity and axonal transport in the ischemic rat brain. They found that NPCs transplant one week after the ischemic event enhanced dendritic plasticity in both the ipsi- and contralesional cortex. Moreover, stem cell-grafted rats demonstrated increased corticocortical, corticostriatal, corticothalamic and corticospinal axonal rewiring from the contralesional side; with the transcallosal and corticospinal axonal sprouting correlating with functional recovery (Andres et al., 2011).

With the advent and enhancement of molecular biology technology, tumor-derived neuronal tissues, including immortal teratocarcinoma-derived cells such as NT2N and hNT cells have been tested in stroke models (Bacigaluppi et al., 2008; Borlongan et al., 1998). Human fetal cortex cells have been immortalized by genetic modification (e.g. insertion of transcription factor genes including v-myc (Cacci et al., 2007) and c-myc (Pollock et al., 2006).

Irrespective of cell type or route of administration, cell survival has been limited. Quantification of cell survival is poorly reported. Reports, from the few studies that have attempted to quantify cell survival, range from 1% (Hicks et al., 2009) to 30% (Darsalia et al., 2007). Site of transplantation may be relevant to cell survival, with pathological evidence of $33.4 \pm 6.1\%$ viable cells when human fetal neural stem cells (hNSCs) were transplanted in non-ischemic tissue medial to the ischemic lesion (Kelly et al., 2004). In contrast 30–50% of hNT cells have been suggested to survive in and around the ischemic tissue (Bliss et al., 2006). Inflammation following ischemic stroke may aid cell migration (Belmadani et al., 2006), but a negative correlation between cell survival and inflammatory response has also been observed (Kelly et al., 2004), and may be a factor to consider when timing cell administration.

Although transplanted NSCs can recover some of the function lost after stroke, recovery has shown to be incomplete and restoration of lost tissue is minimal in most of the cases. The challenge set was to provide transplanted cells with matrix support in order to optimize their ability to engraft the damaged tissue. Bible et al. demonstrated that plasma polymerised allylamine (ppAAm)-treated poly(D,L-lactic acid-co-glycolic acid) (PLGA) scaffold particles can act as a structural support for neural stem cells injected directly through a needle into the lesion cavity using magnetic resonance imaging-derived coordinates. Upon implantation, the neuro-scaffolds integrated efficiently within the rat host tissue forming a primitive neural tissue. These work demonstrated that neuro-scaffolds could be a more advanced method to enhance brain repair. This study provides a substantial step in the technology development required for the translation of this approach.

Other cell sources employed for this purpose are the induced pluripotent stem (iPS) cell and mesenchymal stem cells (MSCs). iPS cells can be produced with high reproduction ability and pluripotency to differentiate into various types of cells, making them a feasible resource for transplantation, with the additional benefit of obtaining these cells from the same patient. On the other hand, MSC are multipotent stem cells that can differentiate into a variety of cell types.

In one study, undifferentiated iPS cells were transplanted into the ipsilateral striatum of a MCAO model of stroke; the transplanted iPS cells expanded and formed larger tumors in the post-ischemic brain compared with the control condition. iPS cells formed a tridermal teratoma (Kawai et al., 2010). Despite this finding, iPS cells are still a hopeful alternative to provide neural cells for ischemic brain injury; however, tumor formation still needs to be prevented and controlled.

In another study that employed human bone marrow-derived MSCs (hBMSCs) found a significant recovery of behavior in the hBMSCs-treated rats beginning at 14 days after MCAO compared with the control animals. High levels of BDNF, neurotrophin-3 (NT-3), and VEGF were detected in the hBMSCs-treated brain, as well as an increased proliferation of neuronal progenitor cells in the SVZ (Bao et al., 2011). This indicates that it is unlikely that

MSCs replaced the damaged tissue and more likely that they secreted trophic factors that promoted functional recovery after stroke.

Altogether, these findings, therefore, placed the stepping stone for direct clinical implications. However, evidence indicates that NSCs transplantation may protect the CNS from inflammatory damage via a "bystander" mechanism rather than by direct cell replacement (Martino & Pluchino, 2006).

4.2 Human trials with stem cells

Results of NSCs transplantation in ischemic stroke patients have not been reported, although in 2010 ReNeuron, a company in the United Kingdom received an approval to start a clinical trial using expanded NSCs. Therefore, we will witness the first clinical results of NSCs transplants. Nonetheless, the potential of precursor cells as an exogenous source for transplant therapy has been already assessed in some clinical trials (summarized in table 3).

Neural cells derived from an immortalized human teratocarcinoma cell line (NT2N cells) underwent two small clinical studies after showing improved behavioral outcomes in rats (Borlongan et al., 1998). In the first human safety study (Stilley et al., 2004), twelve patients who had suffered ischemic stroke on average 27 months earlier, received doses of between 2 and 6 million cells by direct injection into the basal ganglia. No cell related adverse events were reported. Some motor improvement was reported in around half the subjects at 6 months based on one clinical stroke scale and an increase in 18F-flurodeoxyglucose uptake on brain positron emission tomography (PET) scans was also reported, although of unclear significance. Subsequently Kondziolka and colleagues (Kondziolka et al., 2005) reported on an open-label randomized phase II efficacy trial of 5–10 million NT2N cells including 14 actively treated subjects with stroke between 1 and 6 years earlier. Patients were randomized to receive cells with rehabilitation or rehabilitation alone in a 7:2 ratio and two ascending dose arms. Ischemic and hemorrhagic stroke formed half of the subjects each. No cell related adverse events were noted, and the major adverse events reported (seizure and subdural hematoma) were considered to be procedure-related. Neurological motor scores that were stable 6 months prior to surgery were reported to improve in 6/14 subjects by 6 months while in 4/14 subjects the scores deteriorated. There was no indication of any dose-related effects.

Savitz and colleagues used the intra-parenchymal route for delivery of fetal porcine derived cells in five patients, who suffered stroke 3–10 months prior (Savitz et al., 2005). The study was halted after the fourth and fifth patients had worsening motor deficits and seizures. Whether cell or procedure related complications were the cause, it still remains unclear.

Mesenchymal stem cells have been administered intravenous in a controlled trial (Bang et al., 2005) and autologous cells have been transplanted intraparenchymally in an open study (Suárez-Monteagudo et al., 2009). Neither trial reported any cell or procedure related adverse events up to one year follow-up. In the latter study, clinical scores showed minimal and insignificant changes. Bang and colleagues reported improvement in one functional score of activities of daily living (Barthel index scores measured at 3, 6 and 12 months after cell therapy) but not in other clinical measures of outcome (modified-Rankin scale and National Institutes of Health Stroke Scale scores) and the number of subjects was small (5 actively treated and 25 controls).

Cell Source	Stroke Area	Time period (after transplant)	Behavioral outcome	N° of surviving cells	Reference
NSCs transplant therapy in rodent models of stroke					
Human Neuron-Like NT2N	MCAO	24 weeks	3-fold improvement of Passive Avoidance Test	NA	Borlongan et al., 1998
Rat Trophic Factor-Secreting Kidney Cells	MCAO	20 weeks	1 point augmentation in Prehensile Traction Test	NA	Mattsson et al., 1999
Human NT Neurons	MCAO	12 weeks	50% of behavioral improvement in functional tests	24,217 ± 9,260	Saporta et al., 1999
Human Umbilical Cord Blood Cells	MCAO	5 weeks	Two points reduction of Modified Neurological Severity Score	32 600 ± 1689	Chen et al., 2001a
Rat Bone Marrow Cells	MCAO	2 weeks	50% of behavioral improvement in functional tests	∼14% (Total of $4×10^5$)	Chen et al., 2001b
MHP36 Human Immortalized Cell Line	MCAO	8 weeks	2-Fold improvement in Water Maze Acquisition Test	∼7500	Veizovic et al., 2001
MHP36 Human Immortalized Cell Line	MCAO	4 weeks	30% of behavioral improvement in functional tests	∼7500	Modo et al., 2002
Human Bone Marrow Cells	MCAO	2-6 weeks	33.5 ± 8.7% of somatosensory asymmetries	NA	Zhao et al., 2002
Human NSCs neurospheres	Distal MCAO	4 weeks	NA	100,147 ± 28,944	Kelly et al., 2004
CTX0E03 Human Neural Stem Cells	MCAO	6-12 weeks	50% of behavioral improvement in functional tests	NA	Pollock et al., 2006
iPS cells	MCAO	7 weeks	None	Tumor of $50mm^3$	Kawai et al., 2010
Human Bone Marrow-Derived Mesenchymal	MCAO	4 weeks	Decrease of 4 points in the Modified Neurological Severity Scores	NA	Bao et al., 2011
NSCs transplant therapy in stroke patients					
Cell Source	Stroke Area	Time period (after transplant)	Behavioral outcome	N° of surviving cells	Reference
Neural MSCs derived	MCA	48 weeks	Significant improvement for 12 weeks in Barthel Index (30 points augmentation)	NA	Bang et al., 2005
Human Neuronal Cells	NA	96 weeks	Improvement of 6.9 points in the European Stroke Scale at 24 weeks	NA	Kondziolka et al., 2005

Cell Source	Stroke Area	Time period (after transplant)	Behavioral outcome	N° of surviving cells	Reference
Neural Fetal Porcine Cells	Basal Ganglia	192 weeks	Improvement in speech, language and/or motor impairments in 40% of the patients	NA	Savitz *et al.*, 2005
Bone Marrow Stem Cells	NA	48 weeks	None	NA	Suárez-Monteagudo *et al.*, 2009

Table 3. Experimental and clinical NSCs transplant therapy in stroke.

4.3 The prospect of NSCs transplant therapy for stroke

NSCs transplantation therapy for stroke holds great promise. However, the mechanisms of recovery are not completely understood. It is very likely that more than one mechanism is involved in the processes of recovery, and it still remains to be answered.

To this end, some standardization of the basic research, especially for behavior, is needed so that direct comparisons can be made between studies. Furthermore, longer-term studies are required to determine whether the cell-enhanced recovery is sustained and also to determine the tumorigenic potential of the cells. Other challenges include ensuring appropriate characterization, manufacturing, and quality control of transplanted cells and rigorous testing of viral and adventitious agents. Clearly, more research is needed to understand the bidirectional interaction between the transplanted cells and the host to optimize the chances of success before proceeding to the clinic.

Although reconstructing normal brain circuitry following stroke via NSCs is not likely in the foreseeable future, and although great care must be taken to ensure safety before considering clinical trials, preliminary evidence supports the therapeutic potential of NSCs for treatment of ischemic brain injury in animal models.

Understanding the mechanism of action of human NPCs in the post-ischemic brain will be important for the successful translation of cell transplantation strategies to the clinic. For example, if modulation of host brain plasticity is a major human NPCs mechanism of action, this could dictate the best time to transplant cells after stroke; "network relearning" occurs within weeks of stroke and continues for several months, making it a good therapeutic target with a large time window of intervention. Furthermore, knowing what changes the human NPCs elicit in the brain offers useful surrogate indicators of transplanted cell activity.

5. Conclusions

Under normal and pathological conditions, the adult brain is able to preserve regions with regenerative potential. Current research of neurogenic niches is revealing their complex homeostatic process, but at the same time, is bestowing with expectation that unraveling the characteristics of the unique molecular environment of the SVZ and the understanding of the underlying mechanisms that regulate the creation of new neurons in the adult brain will allow us to manipulate NSCs to yield a significant number of neurons capable of integration into human functional brain circuitries that were damaged and improve the motor deficits secondary to stroke or neurodegenerative diseases.

Long-term studies reviewed here support the persistence of an attenuate plasticity process residing within the neurogenic SVZ and RMS throughout life, which can be modulated in major extent by the action of some growth factors. The employment of growth factors could circumvent the technical and ethical constraints by using stem cells for transplant therapy. In addition, autologous transplantation of NSCs expanded *in vitro* could also avoid these concerns, and for this reason, it can be considered as a promising alternative. The first transplant of NSCs in stroke patients is currently in progress.

Altogheter, the large body of evidence supports the manipulation of endogenous NSCs and employment of grafted stem cells as future treatments for acute and chronic stroke. In spite of current efforts, the effectiveness and safety of both approaches are still being developed. It is clear that further investigation is necessary before such methods can be applied for human treatment and in our opinion, successful cell therapy for stroke patients, is still in a distant future.

6. Acknowledgments

We thank to Diana Millán-Aldaco and Marcela Palomero-Rivero for their relevant critical input on the manuscript. This work was supported by IMPULSA of the Universidad Nacional Autónoma de México (UNAM); by the Iniciativa de Apoyo complementario a la realización de las obras determinadas (IACOD), UNAM Grant No. I1201911 and by Programa de Apoyo a Proyectos de Investigación e Innovación Tecnológica (PAPIIT), UNAM Grant No. IN225209-3.

7. References

Altman, J. (1963) Autoradiographic investigation of cell proliferation in the brains of rats and cats. *The Anatomical record*, 145: 573–91.

Altman, J., Das, G.D. (1965) Autoradiographic and histological evidence of postnatal hippocampal neurogenesis in rats. *J Comp Neurol.*, 124:319–335.

Altman, J. (1969) Autoradiographic and histological studies of postnatal neurogenesis IV. Cell proliferation and migration in the anterior forebrain, with special reference to persisting neurogenesis in the olfactory bulb. *J Comp Neurol.*, l137:433–458.

American Heart Association. (2007) International Cardiovascular Disease Statistics; www.americanheart.org.

Andres, R.H., Horie, N., Slikker, W., Keren-Gill, H., Zhan, K., Sun, G., Manley, N.C., Pereira, M.P., Sheikh, L.A., McMillan, E.L., Schaar, B.T., Svendsen, C.N., Bliss, T.M., Steinberg, G.K. (2011) Human neural stem cells enhance structural plasticity and axonal transport in the ischaemic brain. *Brain*, 134:1777-1789.

Andsberg, G., Kokaia, Z., Klein, R.L., Muzyczka, N., Lindvall, O., Mandel, R.J. (2002) Neuropathological and behavioral consequences of adeno-associated viral vector-mediated continuous intrastriatal neurotrophin delivery in a focal ischemia model in rats. *Neurobiol Dis.*, 9:187-204.

Anton, E.S., Ghashghaei, H.T., Weber, J.L., McCann, C., Fischer, T.M., Cheung, I.D., Gassmann, M., Messing, A., Klein, R., Loyd, K.C.K., Lai, C. (2004) Receptor tyrosine kinase ErbB4 modulates neuroblast migration and placement in the adult forebrain. *Nat Neurosci.*, 7:1319-1328.

Arvidsson, A., Collin, T., Kirik, D., Kokaia, Z., Lindvall, O. (2002) Neuronal replacement from endogenous precursors in the adult brain after stroke. *Nat Med.*, 8:963-70.

Bacigaluppi, M., Pluchino, S., Martino, G., Kilic, E., Hermann, D.M. (2008) Neural stem/precursor cells for the treatment of ischemic stroke. *J Neurol Sci.*, 265:73-77.

Baldauf, K., Reymann, K.G. (2005) Influence of EGF/bFGF treatment on proliferation, early neurogenesis and infarct volume after transient focal ischemia. *Brain Res.*, 1056:158-167.

Balenci, L., Saoudi, Y., Grunwald, D., Deloulme, J.C., Bouron, A., Bernards, A., Baudier, J. (2007) IAGAP1 regulates adult neural progenitors in vivo and vascular endothelial growth factor-triggered neural progenitor migration in vitro. J Neurosci., 27:4716-4724.

Bang, O.Y., Lee, J.S., Lee, P.H, Lee, G. (2005) Autologous mesenchymal stem cell transplantation in stroke patients. Ann Neurol., 57:874-882.

Bao, X., Wei, J., Feng, M., Lu, S., Li, G., Dou, W., Ma, W., Ma, S., An, Y., Qin, C., Zhao, R.C., Wang, R. (2011) Transplantation of human bone marrow-derived mesenchymal stem cells promotes behavioral recovery and endogenous neurogenesis after cerebral ischemia in rats. Brain Res., 1367:103-113.

Bath, K.G., Mandairon, N., Jing, D., Rajagopal, R., Kapoor, R., Chen, Z.Y., Khan, T., Proenca, C.C., Kraemer, R., Cleland, T.A., Hempstead, B.L., Chao, M.V., Lee, F.S. (2008) Variant brain-derived neurotrophic factor (Val66Met) alters adult olfactory bulb neurogenesis and spontaneous olfactory discrimination. J Neurosci., 28:2383-2393.

Battista, D., Rutishauser, U. (2010) removal of polysialic acid triggers dispersion of subventricularly derived neuroblasts into surrounding CNS tissues. J Neurosci., 11:3995- 4003.

Belluardo, N., Mudó, G., Bonomo, A., Di Liberto, V., Frinchi, M., Fluxe, K. (2008). Nicotine induced fibroblast growth factor-2 restores the age-related decline of precursor cell proliferation in the subventricular zone of rat brain. Brain Res., 1193:12-24.

Belluzzi, O., Benedusi, M., Ackman, J., LoTurco, J.J. (2003) Electrophysiological differentiation of new neurons in the olfactory bulb. *J Neurosci.*, 23, 10411-10418.

Belmadani, A., Tran, P.B., Ren, D., Miller, R.J. (2006) Chemokines regulate the migration of neural progenitors to sites of neuroinflammation. *J Neurosci.*, 26:3182-3191.

Belvindrah, R., Hankel, S., Walker, J., Patton, B.L., Müller, U. (2007) Integrins Control the Formation of Cell Chains in the Adult Rostral Migratory Stream. *J Neurosci.*, 27:2704-2717.

Benraiss, A., Chmielnicki, E., Lerner, K., Roh, D., Goldman, S.A. (2001) Adenoviral brain-derived neurotrophic factor induces both neostriatal and olfactory neuronal recruitment from endogenous progenitor cells in the adult forebrain. *J Neurosci.*, 21, 6718-6731.

Bible, E., Chau, D.Y., Alexander, M.R., Price, J., Shakesheff, K.M., Modo, M. (2009) The support of neural stem cells transplanted into stroke-induced brain cavities by PLGA particles. *Biomaterials.*, 30:2985-9294.

Bliss, T.M., Kelly, S., Shah, A.K., Foo, W.C., Kohli, P., Stokes, C., Sun, G.H., Ma, M., Masel, J., Kleppner, S.R., Schallert, T., Palmer, T., Steinberg, G.K. (2006) Transplantation of hNT neurons into the ischemic cortex: cell survival and effect on sensorimotor behavior. *J Neurosci Res.*, 83:1004-1014.

Borlongan, C.V., Tajima, Y., Trojanowski, J.Q., Lee, V.M., Sanberg, P.R. (1998) Transplantation of cryopreserved human embryonal carcinoma-derived neurons (NT2N cells) promotes functional recovery in ischemic rats *Exp. Neurol.* 149:310-321.

Brose, K., Tessier-Lavigne, M. (2000) Slit proteins: key regulators of axon guidance, axonal branching, and cell migration. *Curr Opin Neurobiol.,* 10:95-102.

Burns, T.C., Rodriguez, G.J., Patel, S., Hussein, H.M., Georgiadis, A.L., Lakshminarayan, K., Qureshi, A.I. (2008) Endovascular interventions following intravenous thrombolysis may improve survival and recovery in patients with acute ischemic stroke: a case control study. *Am J Neuroradiol.,* 29:1918-1924.

Cacci, E., Villa, A., Parmar, M., Cavallaro, M., Mandahl, N., Lindvall, O., Martinez-Serrano, A., Kokaia, Z. (2007) Generation of human cortical neurons from a new immortal fetal neural stem cell line. *Exp Cell Res.,* 313:588-601.

Capsoni, S., Giannotta, S., Cattaneo, A. (2002) Nerve growth factor and galantamine ameliorate early signs of neurodegeneration in anti-nerve growth factor mice. *Proc Natl Acad Sci USA,* 99:12432-7.

Carleton, A., Petreanu, L.T., Lansford, R., Alvarez-Buylla, A., Lledo, P.M. (2003) Becoming a new neuron in the adult olfactory bulb. *Nat Neurosci.,* 6:507-518.

Chazal, G., Durbec, P., Jankovski, A., Rougon, G., Cremer, H. (2000) Consequences of neural cell adhesion molecule deficiency on cell migration in the rostral migratory stream of the mouse. *J Neurosci.,* 20:1446-1457.

Chen, J., Li, Y., Wang, L., Lu, M., Zhang, X., Chopp, M. (2001b) Therapeutic benefit of intracerebral transplantation of bone marrow stromal cells after cerebral ischemia in rats. *J. Neurol. Sci.,* 189:49-57.

Chen, J., Sanberg, P.R., Li, Y., Wang, L., Lu, M., Willing, A.E., Sanchez-Ramos, J., Chopp, M. (2001a) Intravenous administration of human umbilical cord blood reduces behavioral deficits after stroke in rats. *Stroke,* 32:2682-2688.

Chiaramello, S., Dalmasso, G., Bezin, L., Marcel, D., Jourdan, F., Peretto, P., Fasolo, A., De Marchis, S. (2007) BDNF/TrkB interaction regulates migration of SVZ precursor cells via PI3-K and MAP-K signalling pathways. *Eur J Neurosci.,* 26:1780-1790.

Chojnacki, A.K., Mak, G.K., Weiss, S. (2009) Identity crisis for adult periventricular neural stem cells: subventricular zone astrocytes, ependymal cells or both?. *Nat Rev Neurosci.,* 10:153-63.Chu, K., Kim, M., Park, K.I., Jeong, S.W., Park, H.K., Jung, K.H., Lee, S.T., Kang, L., Lee, K., Park, D.K., Kim, S.U., Roh, J.K. (2004) Human neural stem cells improve sensorimotor deficits in the adult rat brain with experimental focal ischemia. *Brain Res.,* 1016:145-153.

Conover, J.C., Doetsch, F., Garcia-Verdugo, J.M., Gale, N.W., Yancopoulos, G.D., Alvarez-Buylla, A. (2000) Disruption of Eph/ephrin signaling affects migration and proliferation in the adult subventricular zone. *Nat Neurosci.,* 3:1091-1097.

Corti, S., Locatelli, F., Papadimitriou, D., Donadoni, C., Del Bo, R., Fortunato, F., Strazzer, S., Salani, S., Bresolin, N., Comi, G.P. (2005) Multipotentiality, homing properties, and pyramidal neurogenesis of CNS-derived LeX(ssea-1)_/CXCR4_ stem cells. *FASEB J.,* 19:1860 -1862.

Courtès, S., Vernerey, J., Pujadas, L., Magalon, K., Cremer, H., Soriano, E., Durbec, P., Cayre, M. (2011) reelin controls progenitor cell migration in the healthy and pathological adult mouse brain. *PLoS ONE,* 6:e20430.

Cowan, C.A., Henkemeyer, M. (2002). Ephrins in reverse, park and drive. *Trends Cell Biol.*, 12: 339–346.

Craig, C.G., Tropepe, V., Morshead, C.M., Reynolds, B.A., Weiss, S., van der Kooy, D. (1996) In vivo growth factor expansion of endogenous subependymal neural precursor cell populations in the adult mouse brain. *J Neurosci.*, 16:2694-2658.

Cremer, H., Lange, R., Christoph, A., Plomann, M., Vopper, G., Roes, J., Brown, R., Baldwin, S., Kraemer, P., Scheff, S., Barthels, D., Rajewsky, K., Wille, W. (1994) Inactivation of the N-CAM gene in mice results in size reduction of the olfactory bulb and deficits in spatial learning. *Nature*, 367:455–459.

D'Arcangelo, G., Miao, G.G., Chen, S.C., Soares, H.D., Morgan, J.I., Curran, T. (1995) A protein related to extracelular matrix proteins deleted in the mouse mutant reeler. *Nature*, 374:719–723.

Darsalia, V., Kallur, T., Kokaia, Z. (2007) Survival, migration and neuronal differentiation of human fetal striatal and cortical neural stem cells grafted in stroke-damaged rat striatum. *Eur J Neurosci.*, 26:605–14.

Darsalia, V., Allison, S.J., Cusulin, C., Monni, E., Kuzdas, D., Kallur, T., Lindvall, O., Kokaia, Z. (2011) Cell number and timing of transplantation determine survival of human neural stem cell grafts in stroke-damaged rat brain. *J Cereb Blood Flow Metab.*, 31:235-42.

Dawson, M.R., Polito, A., Levine, J.M., Reynolds, R. (2003) NG2-expressing glial progenitor cells: an abundant and widespread population of cycling cells in the adult rat CNS. *Mol Cell Neurosci.*, 24:476–488.

De Rosa, R., Garcia, A.A., Braschi, C., Capsoni, S., Maffei, L., Berardi, N., Cattaneo, A. (2005) Intranasal administration of nerve growth factor (NGF) rescues recognition memory deficits in AD11 anti-NGF transgenic mice. *Proc Natl Acad Sci USA*, 102:3811-6.

De Wit, J., Verhaagen, J. (2003) Role of semaphorins in the adult nervous system. *Prog Neurobiol.*, 71:249-67.

Dirnagl U. (2006) Bench to bedside: the quest for quality in experimental stroke research. *J Cereb Blood Flow Metab.*, 26:1465–1478.

Doetsch, F., Alvarez-Buylla, A. (1996) Network of tangentially phatways for neuronal migration in adult mammalian brain. *Proc Natl Acad Sci USA.*, 93:14895–14900.

Doetsch, F., Garcia-Verdugo, J. M., Alvarez-Buylla, A. (1997) Cellular composition and three-dimensional organization of the subventricular germinal zone in the adult mammalian brain. *J Neurosci.*, 17:5046–5061.

Doetsch, F., Caille, I., Lim, D. A., Garcia-Verdugo, J. M., Alvarez-Buylla, A. (1999) Subventricular zone astrocytes are neural stem cells in the adult mammalian brain. *Cell*, 97:703–716.

Doetsch, F., Petreanu, L., Caille, I., Garcia-Verdugo, J.M., Alvarez-Buylla, A. (2002) EGF converts transit-amplifying neurogenic precursors in the adult brain into multipotent stem cells. *Neuron.*, 36:1021-1034.

Drescher, U. (1997) The Eph family in the patterning of neural development. *Curr Biol.*, 7:799–807.

Emsley, J.G., Hagg, T. (2003) alpha6beta1 integrin directs migration of neuronal precursors in adult mouse forebrain. *Exp. Neurol.*, 183:273–285.

Englund, U., Bjorklund, A., Wictorin, K., Lindvall, O., Kokaia, M. (2002) Grafted neural stem cells develop into functional pyramidal neurons and integrate into host cortical circuitry. *Proc Natl Acad Sci USA*, 99:17089–17094.

Eriksson, P.S., Perfilieva, E., Bjork-Eriksson, T., Alborn, A.M., Nordborg, C., Peterson, D.A., Gage, F.H. (1998) Neurogenesis in the adult human hippocampus. *Nat Med.*, 4:1313–1317.

Fallon, J., Reid, S., Kinyamu, R., Opole, I.., Opole, R., Baratta, J., Korc, M., Endo, T.L., Duong, A., Nguyen, G., Karkehabadhi, M., Twardzik, D., Patel, S., Loughlin, S. (2000) *In vivo* induction of massive proliferation, directed migration, and differentiation of neural cells in the adult mammalian brain. *Proc Natl Acad Sci USA*, 97:14686-91.

Foulkes, M.A., Wolf, P.A., Price, T.R., Mohr, J.P., Hier, D.B. (1988) The Stroke Data Bank: design, methods, and baseline characteristics. *Stroke*, 19:547-54.

Francis, F., Koulakoff, A., Boucher, D., Chafey, P., Schaar, B., Vinet, M.C., Friocourt, G., McDonnell, N., Reiner, O., Kahn, A., McConnell, S.K., Berwald-Netter, Y., Denoulet, P., Chelly, J. (1999) Doublecortin is a developmentally regulated, microtubule-associated protein expressed in migrating and differentiating neurons. *Neuron*, 23:247-56.

Frey, W.H. 2nd, Liu, J., Chen, X., Thorne, R.G., Fawcett, J.R., Ala, T.A., Rahman, Y.E. (1997) Delivery of 125I-NGF to the brain via the olfactory route. *Drug Delivery*, 4:87-92.

Frinchi, M., Di Liberto, V., Olivieri, M., Fuxe, K., Belluardo, N., Mudò, G. (2010) FGF-2/FGFR1 neurotrophic system expressionlevel and its basal activation do not account for the age-dependent decline of precursor cell proliferation in the subventricular zone of rat brain. *Brain Res.*, 1358:39–45.

Fuchs, E., Tumbar, T., Guasch, G. (2004) Socializing with the neighbors: stem cells and their niche. *Cell*, 116:769–778.

Fujiwara, Y., Tanaka, N., Ishida, O., Fujimoto, Y., Murakami, T., Kajihara, H., Yasunaga, Y., Ochi, M. (2004) Intravenously injected neural progenitor cells of transgenic rats can migrate to the injured spinal cord and differentiate into neurons, astrocytes and oligodendrocytes. *Neurosci Lett.*, 366:287–291.

Galvão, R.P., Garcia-Verdugo, J.M., Alvarez-Buylla, A. (2008) Brain-derived neurotrophic factor signaling does not stimulate subventricular zone neurogenesis in adult mice and rats. *J Neurosci.*, 28: 13368-13383.

García-Verdugo, J.M., Doetsch, F., Wichterle, H., Lim, D.A., Alvarez-Buylla, A. (1998) Architecture and cell types of the adult subventricular zone: in search of the stem cells. *J Neurobiol.*, 36:234-248.

Gascon, E., Vutskits, L., Jenny, B., Durbec, P., Kiss, J.Z. (2007) PSA-NCAM in postnatally generated immature neurons of the olfactory bulb: a crucial role in regulating p75 expression and cell survival. *Development*, 134:1181–1190.

Ghashghaei, H.T., Weber, J., Pevny, L., Schmid, R., Schwab, M.H., Lloyd, K.C.K., Eisenstat, D.D., Lai, C., Anton, E.S. (2006) The role of neuregulin–ErbB4 interactions on the proliferation and organization of cells in the subventricular zone. *Proc Natl Acad Sci USA*, 103:1930–1935.

Giger, R.J., Pasterkamp, R.J., Heijnen, S., Holtmaat, A.J., Verhaagen, J. (1998) Anatomical distribution of the chemorepellent semaphorin III/collapsin-1 in the adult rat and human brain: predominant expression in structures of the olfactory-hippocampal pathway and the motor system. *J Neurosci Res.*, 52:27–42.

Giger, R.J., Cloutier, J.F., Sahay, A., Prinjha, R.K., Levengood, D.V., Moore, S.E., Pickering, S., Simmons, D., Rastan, S., Walsh, F.S., Kolodkin, A.L., Ginty, D.D., Geppert, M. (2000) Neuropilin-2 is required in vivo for selective axon guidance responses to secreted semaphorins. *Neuron*, 25:29–41.

Giuliani, A., D'Intino, G., Paradisi, M., Giardino, L., Calza, L. (2004) p75(NTR)-immunoreactivity in the subventricular zone of adult male rats: expression by cycling cells. *J Mol Histol.*, 35:749–758

Gleason, D., Fallon, J.H., Guerra, M., Liu, J.C., Bryant, P.J. (2008) Ependymal stem cells divide asymmetrically and transfer progeny into the subventricular zone when activated by injury. *Neuroscience*, 156:81-8.

Gleeson, J.G., Lin, P.T., Flanagan, L.A., Walsh, C.A. (1999) Doublecortin is a microtubule-associated protein and is expressed widely by migrating neurons. *Neuron*, 23:257-71.

Greenberg, D.A., Jin, K. (2006) Growth factors and stroke. *NeuroRx*, 3:458-65.

Gritti, A., Parati, E.A., Cova, L., Frolichsthal, P., Galli, R., Wanke, E., Faravelli, L., Morassutti, D.J., Roisen, F., Nickel, D.D., Vescovi, A.L. (1996) Multipotential stem cells from the adult mouse brain proliferate and self-renew in response to basic fibroblast growth factor. *J Neurosci.*, 16:1091–1100.

Gritti, A., Frölichsthal-Schoeller, P., Galli, R., Parati, E.A., Cova, L., Pagano, S.F., Bjornson, C.R., Vescovi, A.L. (1999) Epidermal and fibroblast growth factors behave as mitogenic regulators for a single multipotent stem cell-like population from the subventricular region of the adult mouseforebrain. *J Neurosci.*, 19:3287-3297.

Gritti, A., Bonfanti, L., Doetsch, F., Caille, I., Alvarez-Buylla, A., Lim D., Galli R., Garcia-Verdugo J.M., Herrera, D.G., Vescovi, A.L. (2002) multipotent neural stem cells reside into the rostral extension and olfactory bulb of adult rodents. *J Neurosci.*, 22:437-445.

Guerra-Crespo, M., Gleason, D., Sistos, A., Toosky, T., Solaroglu, I., Zhang, J.H., Bryant, P.J., Fallon, J.H. (2009) Transforming growth factor-alpha induces neurogenesis and behavioral improvement in a chronic stroke model. *Neuroscience*, 160:470-83.

Guerra-Crespo, M., Sistos, A., Gleason, D., Fallon, J.H. (2010) Intranasal administration of PEGylated transforming growth factor-alpha improves behavioral deficits in a chronic stroke model. *J Stroke Cerebrovasc Dis.*, 19:3-9.

Gustafsson, E., Andsberg, G., Darsalia, V., Mohapel, P., Mandel, R.J., Kirik, D., Lindvall, O., Kokaia, Z. (2003) Anterograde delivery of brain-derived neurotrophic factor to striatum via nigral transduction of recombinant adeno-associated virus increases neuronal death but promotes neurogenic response following stroke. *Eur J Neurosci*, 17:2667-2678.

Hack, I., Bancila, M., Loulier, K., Carroll, P., Cremer, H. (2002) Reelin is a detachment signal in tangential chain-migration during postnatal neurogenesis. *Nat Neurosci.*, 5: 939-945.

Hacke, W., Donnan, G., Fieschi, C., Kaste, M., von Kummer, R., Broderick, J.P., Brott T, Frankel M, Grotta JC, Haley EC Jr, Kwiatkowski T, Levine SR, Lewandowski C, Lu M, Lyden P, Marler JR, Patel S, Tilley BC, Albers G, Bluhmski E, Wilhelm M, Hamilton S, ATLANTIS Trials Investigators, ECASS Trials Investigators, NINDS rt-PA Study Group Investigators. (2004) Association of outcome with early stroke treatment: pooled analysis of ATLANTIS, ECASS, and NINDS rt-PA stroke trials. *Lancet*, 363:768–774.

Herrera, D.G., Garcia-Verdugo, J.M., Alvarez-Buylla, A. (1999) Adult-derived neural precursors transplanted into multiple regions in the adult brain. *Ann Neurol.*, 46:867–877.

Hicks, A.U., Lappalainen, R.S., Narkilahti, S., Suuronen, R., Corbett, D., Sivenius, J., Hovatta, O., Jolkkonen, J. (2009) Transplantation of human embryonic stem cell-derived neural precursor cells and enriched environment after cortical stroke in rats: cell survival and functional recovery. *Eur J Neurosci.*, 29:562-574.

Hiesberger, T., Trommsdorff, M., Howell, B.W., Goffinet, A., Mumby, M.C., Cooper, J.A., Herz, J. (1999) Direct binding of Reelin to VLDL receptor ApoE receptor 2 induces tyrosine phosphorylation of disabled-1 and modulates tau phosphorylation. *Neuron*, 24:481--489.

Höglinger, G.U., Rizk, P., Muriel, M.P., Duyckaerts, C., Oertel, W.H., Caille, I., Hirsch, E.C. (2004) Dopamine depletion impairs precursor cell proliferation in Parkinson disease. *Nat Neurosci.*, 7:726-7235.

Holmberg, J., Armulik, A., Senti, K.A., Edoff, K., Spalding, K., Momma, S., Cassidy, R., Flanagan, J.G., Frisén, J. (2005) Ephrin-A2 reverse signaling negatively regulates neural progenitor proliferation and neurogenesis *Genes Dev.*, 19:462-471.

Hu, H., Tomasiewicz, H., Magnuson, T., Rutishauser, U. (1996) The role of polysialic acid in migration of olfactory bulb interneuron precursors in the subventricular zone. *Neuron*, 16:735–743.

Hu, H. (1999) Chemorepulsion of neuronal migration by Slit2 in the developing mammalian forebrain. *Neuron*, 23:703–711.

Hu, H. (2000) Polysialic acid regulates chain formation by migrating olfactory interneuron precursors. *J Neurosci Res.*, 61:480–492.

Hynes, R.O. (2002) Integrins: Bidirectional, Allosteric Signaling Machines. *Cell*, 110:673–687.

Ishibashi, S., Sakaguchi, M., Kuroiwa, T., Yamasaki, M., Kanemura, Y., Shizuko, I., Shimazaki, T., Onodera, M., Okano, H., Mizusawa, H. (2004) Human neural stem/progenitor cells, expanded in long-term neurosphere culture, promote functional recovery after focal ischemia in Mongolian gerbils. *J Neurosci Res.*, 78:215-223.

Itoh, N., Ornitz, D.M. (2011) Fibroblast growth factors: from molecular evolution to roles in development, metabolism and disease. *J Biochem.*, 149:121–130.

Jacques, T.S., Relvas, J.B., Nishimura, S., Pytela, R., Edwards, G.M., Streuli, C.H., ffrench-Constant, C. (1998) Neural precursor cell chain migration and division are regulated through different beta1 integrins. *Development*, 125:3167-3177.

Jiang, Q., Zhang, Z.G., Ding, G.L., Silver, B., Zhang, L., Meng, H., Lu, M., Pourabdillah-Nejed-D, S., Wang, L., Savant-Bhonsale, S., Li, L., Bagher-Ebadian, H., Hu, J., Arbab, A.S., Vanguri, P., Ewing, J.R., Ledbetter, K.A., Chopp, M. (2006) MRI detects white matter reorganization after neural progenitor cell treatment of stroke. Neuroimage, 32:1080-1089.

Jin, K., Minami, M., Lan, J.Q., Mao, X.O., Batteur, S., Simon, R.P., Greenberg, D.A. (2001) Neurogenesis in dentate subgranular zone and rostral subventricular zone after focal cerebral ischemia in the rat. *Proc Natl Acad Sci USA*, 98:4710-5.

Jin, K., Zhu, Y., Sun, Y., Mao, X.O., Xie, L., Greenberg, D.A. (2002) Vascular endothelial growth factor (VEGF) stimulates neurogenesis in vitro and in vivo. *Proc Natl Acad Sci USA*, 99:11946–11950.

Jin, K., Sun, Y., Xie, L., Batteur, S., Mao, X.O., Smelick, C., Logvinova, A., Greenberg, D.A. (2003) Neurogenesis and aging: FGF-2 and HB-EGF restore neurogenesis in hippocampus and subventricular zone of aged mice. *Aging Cell*, 2:175-183.

Jin, K., Sun, Y., Xie, L., Childs, J., Mao, X.O., Greenberg, D.A. (2004) Post-ischemic administration of heparin-binding epidermal growth factor-like growth factor (HB-EGF) reduces infarct size and modifies neurogenesis after focal cerebral ischemia in the rat. *J Cereb Blood Flow Metab.*, 24:399-408.

Jin, K., Wang, X., Xie, L., Mao, X.O., Zhu, W., Wang, Y., Shen, J., Mao, Y., Banwait, S., Greenberg, D.A. (2006) Evidence for stroke-induced neurogenesis in the human brain. *Proc Natl Acad Sci USA*, 103:13198-202.

Jin, K., Mao, X., Xie, L., Galvan, V., Lai, B., Wang, Y., Gorostiza, O., Wang, X., Greenberg, D.A. (2010a) Transplantation of human neural precursor cells in Matrigel scaffolding improves outcome from focal cerebral ischemia after delayed postischemic treatment in rats. *J. Cereb. Blood Flow Metab.*, 30:534-544.

Jin, K., Mao, X., Xie, L., Greenberg, R.B., Peng, B., Moore, A., Greenberg, M.B., Greenberg, D.A. (2010b) Delayed transplantation of human neural precursor cells improves outcome from focal cerebral ischemia in aged rats. *Aging Cell*, 9:1076–108.

Johansson, C.B., Momma, S., Clarke, D.L., Risling, M., Lendahl, U., Frisén, J. (1999) Identification of a neural stem cell in the adult mammalian central nervous system. *Cell*, 96: 25-34.

Johnson, D.E., Williams, L.T. (1993) Structural and functional diversity in the FGF receptor multigene family. *Adv. Cancer Res.*, 60:1-41.

Kawai, H., Yamashita, T., Ohta, Y., Deguchi, K., Nagotani, S., Zhang, X., Ikeda, Y., Matsuura, T., Abe, K. (2010) Tridermal tumorigenesis of induced pluripotent stem cells transplanted in ischemic brain. *J Cereb Blood Flow Metab.*, 30:1487-1493.

Kelly, S., Bliss, T.M., Shah, A.K., Sun, G.H., Ma, M., Foo, W.C., Masel, J., Yenari, M.A., Weissman, I.L., Uchida, N., Palmer, T., Steinberg, G.K. (2004) Transplanted human fetal neural stem cells survive, migrate, and differentiate in ischemic rat cerebral cortex. *Proc Natl Acad Sci., U S A*, 101:11839–11844.

Koizumi, H., Higginbotham, H., Poon, T., Tanaka, T., Brinkman, B.C., Gleeson, J.G. (2006) Doublecortin maintains bipolar shape and nuclear translocation during migration in the adult forebrain. *Nat Neurosci.*, 9:779–786.

Komitova, M., Zhu, X., Serwanski, D.R., Nishiyama, A. (2009) NG2 cells are distinct from neurogenic cells in the postnatal mouse subventricular zone. *J Comp Neurol.*, 512:702-16.

Kondziolka, D., Steinberg, G.K., Wechsler, L., Meltzer, C.C., Elder, E., Gebel, J., Decesare, S., Jovin, T., Zafonte, R., Lebowitz, J., Flickinger, J.C., Tong, D., Marks, M.P., Jamieson, C., Luu, D., Bell-Stephens, T., Teraoka, J. (2005) Neurotransplantation for patients with subcortical motor stroke: a phase 2 randomized trial. *J Neurosurg.*, 103:38-45.

Kuhn, H.G., Winkler, J., Kempermann, G., Thal, L.J., Gage, F.H. (1997) Epidermal growth factor and fibroblast growth factor-2 have differenteffects on neural progenitors in the adult rat brain. *J Neurosci.*, 17:5820-5828.

Lee, J.P., Jeyakumar, M., Gonzalez, R., Takahashi, H., Lee, P.J., Baek, R.C., Clark, D., Rose, H., Fu, G., Clarke, J., McKercher, S., Meerloo, J., Muller, F.J., Park, K.I., Butters, T.D., Dwek, R.A., Schwartz, P., Tong, G., Wenger, D., Lipton, S.A., Seyfriend, T.N., Platt, F.M., Snyder, E.Y. (2007) Stem cells act through multiple mechanisms to benefit mice with neurodegenerative metabolic disease. *Nat Med.*, 13:439–447.

Leker, R.R., Soldner, F., Velasco, I., Gavin, D.K., Androutsellis-Theotokis, A., McKay, R.D. (2007) Long-lasting regeneration after ischemia in the cerebral cortex. *Stroke*, 38:153-161.

Leker, R.R., Toth, Z.E., Shahar, T., Cassiani-Ingoni, R., Szalayova, I., Key, S., Bratincsák, A., Mezey, E. (2009) Transforming growth factor alpha induces angiogenesis and neurogenesis following stroke. *Neuroscience*, 163:233-43.

Li, H.S., Chen, J.H., Wu, W., Fagaly, T., Zhou, L., Yuan, W., Dupuis, S., Jiang, Z.H., Nash, W., Gick, C. (1999) Vertebrate slit, a secreted ligand for the transmembrane protein roundabout, is a repellent for olfactory bulb axons. *Cell*, 96:807-818.

Liu, J., Solway, K., Messing, R.O., Sharp, F.R. (1998) Increased neurogenesis in the dentate gyrus after transient global ischemia in gerbils. *J Neurosci.*, 18:7768-78.

Liu, X.F., Fawcett, J.R., Hanson, L.R., Frey, W.H. 2nd. (2004) The window of opportunity for treatment of focal cerebral ischemic damage with noninvasive intranasal insulin-like growth factor-I in rats. *J Stroke Cerebrovasc Dis.*, 13:16-23.

Lledo, P.M., Merkle, F.T., Alvarez-Buylla, A. (2008) Origin and function of olfactory bulb interneuron diversity. *Trends Neurosci.*, 31:392-400.

Lois, C., Alvarez-Buylla, A. (1994), Long distance neuronal migration in the adult mammalian brain. *Science*, 264:1145–1148.

Lois, C., Garcia-Verdugo, J.M., Alvarez-Buylla, A. (1996) Chain migration of neuronal precursors. *Science*, 271:978–981.

Ma, M., Ma, Y., Yi, X., Guo, R., Zhu, W., Fan, X., Xu, G., Frey, W.H. 2nd, Liu, X. (2008) Intranasal delivery of transforming growth factor-beta1 in mice after stroke reduces infarct volume and increases neurogenesis in the subventricular zone. *BMC Neurosci.*, 9:117.

Maisonpierre, P.C., Belluscio, L., Friedman, B., Alderson, R.F., Wiegand, S.J., Furth, M.E., Lindsay, R.M., Yancopoulos, G.D. (1990) NT-3, BDNF, and NGF in the developing rat nervous system: parallel as well as reciprocal patterns of expression. *Neuron*, 5:501-509.

Marillat, V., Cases, O., Nguyen-Ba-Charvet, K.T., Tessier-Lavigne, M., Sotelo, C., Chedotal, A. (2002) Spatiotemporal expression patterns of slit and robo genes in the rat brain. *J Comp Neurol.*, 442:130-155.

Martí-Fàbregas, J., Romaguera-Ros, M., Gómez-Pinedo, U., Martínez-Ramírez, S., Jiménez-Xarrié, E., Marín, R., Martí-Vilalta, J.L., García-Verdugo, J.M. (2010) Proliferation in the human ipsilateral subventricular zone after ischemic stroke. *Neurology*, 74:357-65.

Martino,. G, Pluchino, S. (2006) The therapeutic potential of neural stem cells. *Nat Rev Neurosci.*, 7:395–406.

Matsumoto, T., Claesson-Welsh, L. (2001) VEGF receptor signal transduction. *Sci. STKE*, 2001:Re21.

Matsuoka, N., Nozaki, K., Takagi, Y., Nishimura, M., Hayashi, J., Miyatake, S., Hashimoto, N. (2003) Adenovirus-mediated gene transfer of fibroblast growth factor-2 increases BrdU-positive cells after forebrain ischemia in gerbils. *Stroke*, 34:1519-25.

Mattsson, B., Sorensen, J.C., Zimmer, J., Johansson, B.B. (1997) Neural grafting to experimental neocortical infarcts improves behavioral outcome and reduces thalamic atrophy in rats housed in enriched but not in standard environments. *Stroke*, 28:1225–1231.

Meléndez-Herrera, E., Colín-Castelán, D., Varela-Echavarría, A., Gutiérrez-Ospina, G. (2008) Semaphorin-3A and its receptor neuropilin-1 are predominantly expressed in endothelial cells along the rostral migratory stream of young and adult mice. *Cell Tissue Res.*, 333:175-84.

Mirzadeh, Z., Merkle, F. T., Soriano-Navarro, M., Garcia-Verdugo, J. M., Alvarez-Buylla, A. (2008) Neural stem cells confer unique pinwheel architecture to the ventricular surface in neurogenic regions of the adult brain. *Cell Stem Cell*, 3:265–278.

Modo, M., Stroemer, R.P., Tang, E., Patel, S., Hodges, H. (2002) Effects of implantation site of stem cell grafts on behavioral recovery from stroke damage. *Stroke*, 33:2270–2278.

Moores, C.A., Perderiset, M., Francis, F., Chelly, J., Houdusse, A., Milligan, R.A. (2004) Mechanism of microtubule stabilization by doublecortin. *Mol Cell*, 14:833-9.

Morshead, C.M., Garcia, A.D., Sofroniew, M.V., van Der Kooy, D. (2003) The ablation of glial fibrillary acidic proteinpositive cells from the adult central nervous system results in the loss of forebrain neural stem cells but not retinal stem cells. *Eur J Neurosci.*, 18:76–84.

Mosch, B., Reissenweber, B., Neuber, C., Pietzsch, J. (2010) Eph receptors and ephrin ligands: Important players in angiogenesis and tumor angiogenesis. *J Onc.*, 2010:1-12.

Mudó, G., Belluardo, N., Fuxe, K. (2007) Acute intermittent nicotine treatment induces fibroblast growth factor-2 in the subventricular zone of the adult rat brain and enhances neuronal precursor cell proliferation. *Neuroscience*, 145:470-83.

Murase, S., Horwitz, A. F. (2002) deleted in colorectal carcinoma and differentially expressed integrins mediate the directional migration of neural precursors in the rostral migratory stream. *J Neurosci.*, 22:3568–3579.

Murase, S., Cho, C., White, J.M., Horwitz, A.F. (2008) ADAM2 promotes migration of neuroblasts in the rostral migratory stream to the olfactory bulb. *Eur J Neurosci.*, 27:1585-95.

Nakatomi, H., Kuriu, T., Okabe, S., Yamamoto, S., Hatano, O., Kawahara, N., Tamura, A., Kirino, T., Nakafuku, M. (2002) Regeneration of hippocampal pyramidal neurons after ischemic brain injury by recruitment of endogenous neural progenitors. *Cell*, 110:429-41.

Ng, K.L., Li, J.D., Cheng, M.Y., Leslie, F.M., Lee, A.G., Zhou, Q.Y. (2005) Dependence of olfactory bulb neurogenesis on prokineticin 2 signaling. *Science*, 308:1923–1927.

Nguyen-Ba-Charvet, K.T., Picard-Riera, N., Tessier-Lavigne, M., Baron-Van, Evercooren, A., Sotelo, C., Chedotal, A. (2004) Multiple roles for slits in the control of cell migration in the rostral migratory stream. *J Neurosci.*, 24:1497–1506.

Nishino, H., Borlongan, C.V. (2000) Restoration of function by neural transplantation in the ischemic brain. *Prog. Brain Res.*, 127:461–476.

Ocbina, P.J., Dizon, M.L., Shin, L., Szele, F.G. (2006) Doublecortin is necessary for the migration of adult subventricular zone cells from neurospheres. *Mol Cell Neurosci.,* 33:126-35.

Ornitz, D.M., Xu, J., Colvin, J.S., McEwen, D.G., MacArthur, C.A., Coulier, F., Gao, G., Goldfarb, M. (1996) Receptor specificity of the fibroblast growth factor family. *J Biol Chem.,* 271:15292-15297.

Ourednik, J., Ourednik, V., Lynch, W.P., Schachner, M., Snyder, E.Y. (2002) Neural stem cells display an inherent mechanism for rescuing dysfunctional neurons. *Nat Biotechnol.,* 20:1103-1110.

Parent, J.M., Vexler, Z.S., Gong, C., Derugin, N., Ferriero, D.M. (2002) Rat forebrain neurogenesis and striatal neuron replacement after focal stroke. *Ann Neurol.,* 52:802-13.

Park, K.I., Lachyankar, M., Nissim, S., Snyder, E.Y. (2002) Neural stem cells for CNS repair: state of the art and future directions. *Adv Exp Med Biol.,* 506:1291-1296.

Pencea, V., Bingaman, K.D., Wiegand, S.J., Luskin, M.B. (2001) Infusion of brain-derived neurotrophic factor into the lateral ventricle of the adult rat leads to new neurons in the parenchyma of the striatum, septum, thalamus, and hypothalamus. *J Neurosci.,* 21:6706-6717.

Petridis, A.K., El-Maarouf, A., Rutishauser, U. (2004) Polysialic acid regulates cell contact-dependent neuronal differentiation of progenitor cells from the subventricular zone. *Dev Dyn.,* 230:675-684.

Pluchino, S., Quattrini, A., Brambilla, E., Gritti, A., Salani, G., Dina, G., Galli, R., Del Carro, U., Amadio, S., Bergami, A., Furlan, R., Comi, G., Vescovi, A.L., Martino, G. (2003) Injection of adult neurospheres induces recovery in a chronic model of multiple sclerosis. *Nature,* 422:688-694.

Pollock, K., Stroemer, P., Patel, S., Stevanato, L., Hope, A., Miljan, E., Dong, Z., Hodges, H., Price, J., Sinden, J.D. (2006) A conditional immortal clonal stem line from human cortical neuroepithelium for the treatment of ischemic stroke. *Exp Neurol.,* 199:143-155.

Prosser, H.M., Bradley, A., Caldwell, M.A. (2007) Olfactory bulb hypoplasia in Prokr2 null mice stems from defective neuronal progenitor migration and differentiation. *Eur J Neurosci.,* 12: 3339-3344.

Raper, J.A. (2000) Semaphorins and their receptors in vertebrates and invertebrates. *Curr Op Neurobiol.,* 10:88-94.

Reuss, B., Von, Bohlen., Halbach, O. (2003) Fibroblast growth factors and their receptors in the central nervous system. *Cell Tissue Res.,* 313:139-157

Reynolds, B.A., Weiss, S. (1992) Generation of neurons and astrocytes from isolated cells of the adult mammalian central nervous system. *Science,* 255:1707-1710.

Reynolds, B.A., Weiss, S. (1996) Clonal and population analyses demonstrate that an EGF-responsive mammalian embryonic CNS precursor is a stem cell. *Dev Biol.,* 175:1-13.

Riolobos, A. S., Heredia, M., de la Fuente, J.A., Criado, J.M., Yajeya, J., Campos, J., Santacana, M. (2001) Functional recovery of skilled forelimb use in rats obliged to use the impaired limb after grafting of the frontal cortex lesion with homotopic fetal cortex. *Neurobiol Learn Mem.,* 75:274-292.

Ropper, A.H., Brown, R.H. (2009) Adams and Victor's principles of neurology, 9th Ed. New York: McGraw-Hill.

Rousselot, P., Lois, C., Alvarez-Buylla, A. (1995) Embryonic (PSA) N-CAM reveals chains of migrating neuroblasts between the lateral ventricle and the olfactory bulb of adult mice. *J Comp Neurol.*, 351:51-61.

Saghatelyan, A., de Chevigny, A., Schachner, M., Lledo, P.M. (2004). Tenascin-R mediates activity-dependent recruitment of neuroblasts in the adult mouse forebrain. *Nat Neurosci.*, 7:347-356.

Saporta, S., Borlongan, C.V., Sanberg, P.R. (1999) Neural transplantation of human neuroteratocarcinoma (hNT) neurons into ischemic rats. A quantitative dose-response analysis of cell survival and behavioral recovery. *Neuroscience*, 91:519-525.

Savitz, S.I., Rosenbaum, D.M., Dinsmore, J.H., Weschler, L.R., Caplan, L.R. (2002) Cell transplantation for stroke *Ann. Neurol.*, 53:266-275.

Savitz, S.I., Dinsmore, J., Wu, J., Henderson, G.V., Stieg, P., Caplan, L.R. (2005) Neurotransplantation of fetal porcine cells in patients with basal ganglia infarcts: a preliminary safety and feasibility study. *Cerebrovasc Dis.*, 20:101-107.

Schabitz, W.R., Steigleder, T., Cooper-Kuhn, C.M., Schwab, S., Sommer, C., Schneider, A., Kuhn, H.G. (2007) Intravenous brain-derived neurotrophic factor enhances poststroke sensorimotor recovery and stimulates neurogenesis. *Stroke*, 38:2165-2172.

Schänzer, A., Wachs, F.P., Wilhelm, D., Acker, T., Cooper-Kuhn, C., Beck, H., Winkler, J., Aigner, L., Plate, KH., Kuhn, H.G. (2004) Direct stimulation of adult neural stem cells in vitro and neurogenesis in vivo by vascular endothelial growth factor. *Brain Pathol.*, 14:237-48.

Scheffler, B., Walton, N.M., Lin, D.D., Goetz, A.K., Enikolopov, G., Roper, S.N., Steindler, D.A. (2005) Phenotypic and functional characterization of adult brain neuropoiesis. *Proc Natl Acad Sci., U S A*, 102:9355-9358.

Seki, T., Arai, Y. (1993) Highly polysialylated neural cell adhesion molecule (NCAM-H) is expressed by newly generated granule cells in the dentate gyrus of the adult rat. *J Neurosci.*, 13:2351-2358.

Shen, Q., Wang, Y., Kokovay, E., Lin, G., Chuang, S.M., Goderie, S.K., Roysam, B., Temple, S. (2008) Adult SVZ stem cells lie in a vascular niche: a quantitative analysis of niche cell-cell interactions. *Cell Stem Cell*, 3:289-300.

Sinden, J.D., Rashid-Doubell, F., Kershaw, T.R., Nelson, A., Chadwick, A., Jat, P.S., Noble, M.D., Hodges, H., Gray, J.A. (1997) Recovery of spatial learning by grafts of a conditionally immortalized hippocampal neuroepithelial cell line into the ischaemia-lesioned hippocampus. *Neuroscience*, 81:599-608.

Snapyan, M., Lemasson, M., Brill, M.S., Blais, M., Massouh, M., Ninkovic, J., Gravel, C., Berthod, F., Götz, M., Barker, P.A., Parent, A.,Saghatelyan, A. (2009) Vasculature guides migrating neuronal precursors in the adult mammalian forebrain via brain-derived neurotrophic factor signaling. *J Neurosci.*, 29:4172-4188.

Soker, S., Takashima, S., Miao, H.Q., Neufeld, G., Klagsbrun, M. (1998) Neuropilin-1 is expressed by endothelial and tumor cells as an isoformspecific receptor for vascular endothelial growth factor. *Cell*, 92:735-745.

Song, H.J., Stevens, C.F., Gage, F.H. (2002a) Astroglia induce neurogenesis from adult neural stem cells. *Nature*, 417:39-44.

Song, H.J., Stevens, C.F., Gage, F.H. (2002b) Neural stem cells from adult hippocampus develop essential properties of functional CNS neurons. *Nat Neurosci.*, 5:438-445.

Stilley, C.S., Ryan, C.M., Kondziolka, D., Bender, A., DeCesare, S., Wechsler, L. (2004) Changes in cognitive function after neuronal cell transplantation for basal ganglia stroke. *Neurology*, 63:1320-1322.

Suárez-Monteagudo, C., Hernández-Ramírez, P., Alvarez-González, L., García-Maeso, I., de la Cuétara-Bernal, K., Castillo-Díaz, L., Bringas-Vega, M.L., Martínez-Aching, G., Morales-Chacón, L.M., Báez-Martín, M.M., Sánchez-Catasús, C., Carballo-Barreda, M., Rodríguez-Rojas, R., Gómez-Fernández, L., Alberti-Amador, E., Macías-Abraham, C., Balea, E.D., Rosales, L.C., Del Valle Pérez, L., Ferrer, B.B., González, R.M., Bergado, J.A. (2009) Autologous bone marrow stem cell neurotransplantation in stroke patients. An open study. *Restor Neurol Neurosci.*, 27:151-161.

Sugiura, S., Kitagawa, K., Tanaka, S., Todo, K., Omura-Matsuoka, E., Sasaki, T., Mabuchi, T., Matsushita, K., Yagita, Y., Hori, M. (2005) Adenovirus-mediated gene transfer of heparin-binding epidermal growth factor-like growth factor enhances neurogenesis and angiogenesis after focal cerebral ischemia in rats. *Stroke*, 36:859-864.

Sun, Y., Jin, K., Childs, J.T., Xie, L., Mao, X.O., Greenberg, D.A. (2006) Vascular endothelial growth factor-B (VEGFB) stimulates neurogenesis: Evidence from knockout mice and growth factor administration. *Dev Biol.*, 289:329-33.

Tamagnone, L., Comoglio, P.M. (2000) Signaling by semaphorin receptors: cell guidance and beyond. *Trends Cell Biol.*, 10, 377-383.

Teramoto, T., Qiu, J., Plumier, J.C., Moskowitz, M.A. (2003) EGF amplifies the replacement of parvalbumin-expressing striatal interneurons after ischemia. *J Clin Invest.*, 111:1125-1132.

Theus, M.G., Ricard, J., Bethea, J.R., Liebl, D.J. (2010) EphB3 limits the expansion of neural progenitor cells in the subventricular zone by regulatinf p53 during homeostasis and following traumatic brain injury. *Stem Cells*, 28:1231-1242.

Thored, P., Arvidsson, A., Cacci, E., Ahlenius, H., Kallur, T., Darsalia, V., Ekdahl, C.T., Kokaia, Z., Lindvall, O. (2006) Persistent production of neurons from adult brain stem cells during recovery after stroke. *Stem Cells*, 24:739-47.

Thorne, R.G., Pronk, G.J., Padmanabhan, V., Frey, W.H. 2nd. (2004) Delivery of insulin-like growth factor-I to the rat brain and spinal cord along olfactory and trigeminal pathways following intranasal administration. *Neuroscience*, 127:481-96.

Tropepe, V., Craig, C.G., Morshead, C.M., van der Kooy, D. (1997) Transforming growth factor-alpha null and senescent mice show decreased neural progenitor cell proliferation in the forebrain subependyma. *J Neurosci.*, 17:7850-7859.

Vahedi, K., Hofmeijer, J., Juettler, E., Vicaut, E., George, B., Algra, A., Amelink, G.J., Schmiedeck, P., Schwab, S., Rothwell, P.M., Bousser, M.G., van der Worp, H.B., Hacke, W., DECIMAL, DESTINY, and HAMLET investigators. (2007) Early decompressive surgery in malignant infarction of the middle cerebral artery: a pooled analysis of three randomised controlled trials. *Lancet Neuro.*, 6:215-222.

Veizovic, T., Beech, J.S., Stroemer, R.P., Watson, W.P., Hodges, H. (2001) Resolution of stroke deficits following contralateral grafts of conditionally immortal neuroepithelial stem cells. *Stroke*, 32:1012-1019.

Viapiano, M.S., Matthews, R.T. (2006) From barriers to bridges: chondroitin sulfate proteoglycans in neuropathology. *Trends Mol Med.*, 12:488-496.

Wada, K., Sugimori, H., Bhide, P.G., Moskowitz, M.A., Finklestein, S.P. (2003) Effect of basic fibroblast growth factor treatment on brain progenitor cells after permanent focal ischemia in rats. *Stroke*, 34:2722-2728.

Wagner, J.P., Black, I.B., DiCicco-Bloom, E. (1999) Stimulation of neonatal and adult brain neurogenesis by subcutaneous injection of basic fibroblast growth factor. *J Neurosci.*, 19:6006–6016.

Wang, Y.Q., Jin, K., Mao, X.O., Xie, L., Banwait, S., Marti, H.H., Greenberg, D.A. (2007a) VEGF-overexpressing transgenic mice show enhanced post-ischemic neurogenesis and neuromigration. *J Neurosci Res.*, 85:740–747.

Wang, Y.Q., Guo, X., Qiu, M.H., Feng, X.Y., Sun, F.Y. (2007b) VEGF overexpression enhances striatal neurogenesis in brain of adult rat after a transient middle cerebral artery occlusion. *J Neurosci Res.*, 85:73–82.

Wei, L., Cui, L., Snider, B.J., Rivkin, M., Yu, S.S., Lee, C.S., Adams, L.D., Gottlieb, D.I., Johnson, E.M. Jr Yu, S.P., Choi, D.W. (2005) Transplantation of embryonic stem cells overexpressing Bcl-2 promotes functional recovery after transient cerebral ischemia. *Neurobiol Dis.*, 19:183-193.

Weiss, S., Dunne, C., Hewson, J., Wohl, C., Wheatley, M., Peterson, A.C., Reynolds, B.A. (1996) Multipotent CNS stem cells are present in the adult mammalian spinal cord and ventricular neuroaxis. *J Neurosci.*, 16:7599–7609.

Whitman, M.C., Greer, C.A. (2007) Adult-generated neurons exhibit diverse developmental fates. *Dev. Neurobiol.*, 67:1079–1093.

Wilkinson, D.G. (2001) Multiple roles of EPH receptors and ephrins in neural development. Multiple roles of EPH receptors and ephrins in neural development. *Nat Rev Neurosci.*, 2:155-64.

Winkler, C., Fricker, R.A., Gates, M.A., Olsson, M., Hammang, J.P., Carpenter, M.K., Bjorklund, A. (1998) Incorporation and glial differentiation of mouse EGF-responsive neural progenitor cells after transplantation into the embryonic rat brain. *Mol Cell Neurosci.*, 11:99 –116.

World Health Organization (2007) World Health Report ; www.who.int.

Wu, P., Tarasenko, Y.I., Gu, Y., Huang, L.Y., Coggeshall, R.E., Yu, Y. (2002) Region-specific generation of cholinergic neurons from fetal human neural stem cells grafted in adult rat. *Nat Neurosci.*, 5:1271–1278.

Wu, W., Wong, K., Chen, J., Jiang, Z., Dupuis, S., Wu, J.Y., Rao, Y. (1999) Directional guidance of neuronal migration in the olfactory system by the protein Slit. *Nature*, 400:331-336.

Wurmser, A.E., Nakashima, K., Summers, R.G., Toni, N., D'Amour, K.A., Lie, D.C., Gage, F.H. (2004) Cell fusion-independent differentiation of neural stem cells to the endothelial lineage. *Nature*, 430:350 –356.

Yan, J., Xu, L., Welsh, A.M., Hatfield, G., Hazel, T., Johe, K., Koliatsos, V.E. (2007) Extensive neuronal differentiation of human neural stem cell grafts in adult rat spinal cord. *PLoS Med.*, 4:e39.

Yandava, B.D., Billinghurst, L.L., Snyder, E.Y. (1999) "Global" cell replacement is feasible via neural stem cell transplantation: evidence from the dysmyelinated shiverer mouse brain. *Proc Natl Acad Sci U S A*, 96:7029–7034.

Yang, P., Baker, K.A., Hagg, T. (2005) A disintegrin and metalloprotease 21 (ADAM21) is associated with neurogenesis and axonal growth in developing and adult rodent CNS. *J Comp Neurol.,* 490:163–179.

Yang, P., K., Baker, A., Hagg, T. (2006) The ADAMs family: Coordinators of nervous system development, plasticity and repair. *Prog Neurobiol.,* 79:73–94.

Yarden, Y., Sliwkowski, M.X. (2001) Untangling the ErbB signaling network, *Nat Rev Mol Cell Biol.,* 2:127–137.

Young, K.M., Merson, T.D., Sotthibundhu, A., Coulson, E.J., Bartlett, P.F. (2007) p75 neurotrophin receptor expression defines a population of BDNF- responsive neurogenic precursor cells. *J Neurosci.,* 27:5146–5155.

Zhang, H., Vutskits, L., Pepper, M.S., Kiss, J.Z. (2003) VEGF is a chemoattractant for FGF-2-stimulated neural progenitors *J Cell Biol.,* 163:1375–1384.

Zhang, P., Li, J., Liu, Y., Chen, X., Kang, Q. (2009a) Transplanted human embryonic neural stem cells survive, migrate, differentiate and increase endogenous nestin expression in adult rat cortical peri-infarction zone. *Neuropathology,* 29:410–421.

Zhang, P., Li, J., Liu, Y., Chen, X., Kang, Q., Zhao, J., Li, W. (2009b) Human neural stem cell transplantation attenuates apoptosis and improves neurological functions after cerebral ischemia in rats. *Acta Anaesthesiol Scand,* 53:1184-1191.

Zhang, P., Li, J., Liu, Y., Chen, X., Lu, H., Kang, Q., Li, W., Gao, M. (2010) Human embryonic neural stem cell transplantation increases subventricular zone cell proliferation and promotes peri-infarct angiogenesis after focal cerebral ischemia. *Neuropathology,* 39:1440-1789.

Zhang, R.L., Zhang, Z.G., Zhang, L., Chopp, M. (2001) Proliferation and differentiation of progenitor cells in the cortex and the subventricular zone in the adult rat after focal cerebral ischemia. *Neuroscience,* 105:33-41.

Zhao, C., Deng, W., Gage, F.H. (2008) Mechanisms and functional implications of adult neurogenesis. *Cell,* 132:645-60.

Zhao, L.R., Duan, W.M., Reyes, M., Keene, C.D., Verfaillie, C.M., Low, W.C. (2002) Human bone marrow stem cells exhibit neural phenotypes and ameliorate neurological deficits after grafting into the ischemic brain of rats *Exp. Neurol.,* 174:11–20.

Zigova, T., Pencea, V., Wiegand, S.J., Luskin, M.B. (1998) Intraventricular administration of BDNF increases the number of newly generated neurons in the adult olfactory bulb. *Mol Cell Neurosci.,* 11:234–245.

4

Endogenous Neural Stem/Progenitor Cells and Regenerative Responses to Brain Injury

Maria Dizon
Northwestern University/Children's Memorial Hospital
USA

1. Introduction

Neural stem and/or progenitor cells (NSPCs) have generated much excitement because of their envisioned potential to treat a variety of central nervous system diseases that span the human lifetime. This chapter is meant as a general introduction to the topic of NSPCs and how they might be thought of in the context of disease, with a particular focus on endogenous NSPCs. My bias is to focus on endogenous NSPCs as an introduction because the transplantation of NSPCs entails its own complex set of problems including, but not limited to, the effects of in vitro culture conditions, problems of delivery to desired anatomical sites and rejection of foreign cells. Endogenous NSPC populations, on the other hand, change with regard to their distribution, rates of proliferation and fate restriction at different points in brain development. Thus, the cells available to respond to disease necessarily differ depending on whether fetal, neonatal, pediatric or adult brain is affected.

Stem cells are defined by their ability to self-renew indefinitely and by their ability to give rise to cells of many phenotypes. True neural stem cells are tripotential and give rise to neurons, oligodendrocytes and astrocytes. Although stem cells, they are restricted in their fate potential as compared, for example, to pluripotent embryonic stem cells that can give rise to an even wider range of cell phenotypes from endoderm, mesoderm and ectoderm. In turn, embryonic stem cells are restricted in their fate potential in comparison to the totipotent cells from a blastocyst. These cells are able to give rise to any cell of an entire organism; indeed they can give rise to the entire organism itself. In contrast, progenitor cells can self-renew, but only for a limited number of generations, and they give rise to cells of limited phenotypes. For example, glial restricted progenitors can give rise only to astrocytes or oligodendrocytes, neuroblasts can give rise only to neurons, and oligodendrocyte progenitor cells can give rise only to oligodendrocytes.

2. Postnatal neurogenesis and neural stem cells discovered

Prior to the second half of the twentieth century, the dogma was that neurogenesis did not occur postnatally, much less in adult animals. This idea was based largely on the lack of observed neurons with mitotic figures in adult birds and adult mammals. This stance, firmly taken by the father of neuroscience Dr. Ramon y Cajal, likely led to its endurance for almost a century (Ming and Song, 2005). Starting in the 1940s, evidence began to emerge in a number of different species that neurogenesis did indeed occur after development.

2.1 Earliest evidence is human

Some of the earliest evidence for the birth of new neurons after development was actually from human studies. It had been known that a mitotically active region from which the cerebral cortex developed, called the subependymal layer, existed embryonically. In studying ependymomas from autopsies, Drs. Globus and Kuhlenheck noted histologic connections and similarities of features between these neoplasms and the subependymal layer of children and adults, and proposed that the tumors had arisen from undifferentiated cells in the subependymal region. This suggested the persistence of what they termed a bipotential mother cell throughout postnatal life. (Globus and Kuhlenheck, 1944).

2.2 Lower vertebrate evidence

Starting in the 1950s, it was shown that lower vertebrates, including fish, amphibians and lizards (Zupanc, 2008) could regenerate spinal cord (Anderson and Waxman, 1983), optic nerve (Meyer et al., 1985) and even brain (Zupanc, 1999), (Zupanc and Zupanc, 1992).

2.3 Rodent evidence

A breakthrough was made in 1961 when Dr. Smart applied the new technique of labeling dividing cells with tritiated thymidine to 3 day old and adult mice and showed that the subependymal layer of the brain retains its ability to form new cells indefinitely. Standard histologic techniques suggested that these mitotic cells gave rise to neuroblasts and spongioblasts (glial precursors) (Smart, 1961). Shortly thereafter, Dr. Altman began to assemble an impressive body of evidence showing that a large number of interneurons were made postnatally in rat. Like Smart, he used tritiated thymidine, but in contrast he labeled mitotic granule cells within the hippocampus. He showed that these hippocampal granule cells declined from birth with a transient increase at 15 days. Importantly, the decline corresponded with an increase in differentiated granule cells. Later, he extended observations to the olfactory bulb. In both the hippocampus and the olfactory bulb, new interneurons were found continuously at a low rate and were likely born near the ventricles. In contrast, in the cerebellum newly born interneurons were limited to the first three weeks of life. Interneurons were identified both histologically and electrophysiologically. (Altman, 1963; Altman and Das, 1965a; Altman and Das, 1965b; Altman and Das, 1966).

2.4 Avian evidence

By the 1980s, Dr. Nottebohm and colleagues had also clearly demonstrated neurogenesis within the brain of adult birds. Again using tritiated thymidine, they showed that a forebrain nucleus of songbirds (the hyperstriatum ventralis pars caudalis (HVc)), varied greatly in size depending on sex and stage of song development, and that this change in size was related to the birth of new neurons. Cells were identified as neurons ultrastructurally and electrophysiologically. Because labeling was heaviest in the ventricular zone, neurons were presumed to have been born in this zone and to have migrated into the overlying HVc (Goldman and Nottebohm, 1983; Nottebohm, 1985) Interestingly it was Dr. Alvarez-Buylla, who had previously worked on songbirds with Dr. Nottebohm, who revisited the subependymal origin of new neurons in rodent olfactory bulb in the 1990s, and more precisely characterized this region (Lois and Alvarez-Buylla, 1993; Lois and Alvarez-Buylla, 1994).

2.5 Primate evidence

Unfortunately, despite the accumulating evidence, widely held beliefs predominated. As adult neurogenesis was conceded to vertebrates, and even mammals, scientists continued to hold the view that primates were different. Perhaps related to the sensitivity of tritiated thymidine studies, as late as 1985 Dr. Rakic asserted that neurogenesis was limited to development and early postnatal life in primates (Rakic, 1985). It was not until the late 1990s that this view was debunked by Dr. Gould using the thymidine analogue BrdU in adult macaques to show neurogenesis in the hippocampus (Gould et al., 1999a) and even in the neocortex (association cortex) (Gould et al., 1999b). Existence of adult neurogenesis in humans was finally widely embraced by the scientific community in the late twentieth century when Dr. Gage's group demonstrated neurogenesis in adult human dentate gyrus using tissue from cancer victims who had been treated with BrdU (Eriksson et al., 1998). They also formally studied human neocortex using similarly BrdU-treated cancer victims combined with carbon 14 exposure from Cold War above ground nuclear bomb tests and ruled out neocortical neurogenesis after development (Bhardwaj et al., 2006). Recently, a human rostral migratory stream of neuroblasts from subventricular zone to the olfactory bulb was demonstrated by Dr. Curtis (Curtis et al., 2007).

2.6 Neurogenesis indicates neural stem cells

Implicit in the concept of neurogenesis is the existence of a precursor cell capable of giving rise to a neuron. This precursor cell's fate might be limited to neurons, e.g. a restricted neuronal progenitor. Alternatively, the precursor cell might be capable of giving rise to neurons and another cell type such as an oligodendrocyte, e.g. a less restricted bipotential progenitor. Or it might even be capable of giving rise to neurons, oligodendrocytes or astrocytes, e.g. a multipotential neural stem cell. Thus, the firm establishment of postnatal neurogenesis indicates the existence of postnatal neural stem/progenitor cells (NSPCs).

3. Regional distribution of NSPCs

We will discuss the distribution of neural stem cells and more restricted progenitors and how their distribution changes over time. Rodent development is discussed as the bulk of experimental evidence to date derives from rodent studies. Rat brain development has been shown to correlate with mouse brain development. Furthermore, P7 rodent brain development has been shown to correlate with preterm human brain development (Craig et al., 2003). Much insight has been gained from in vitro culture experiments. However, data from in vivo studies including fate mapping experiments using Cre-lox transgenic mouse technology overcomes the uncertainty introduced by culture effects, so the focus here will be on data gleaned from in vivo work. The overarching theme is that earlier in development, precursors tend to be multipotential but become more restricted with time.

3.1 Embryonic period

3.1.1 Early embryonic period

During embryogenesis, the open neural plate folds to form the neural tube. As a result, the primary germinal matrix or neuroepithelium comes to line the lumen that will become the ventricles. Initially, the primary neuroepithelium is a simple columnar epithelium composed of so-called radial glial cells that span from the ventricle to the pial surface. Radial glial cells are more than just glia but are, in fact, "mother cells." They divide after interkinetic nuclear migration from basal surface to the pial surface and back again. Internuclear kinetic migration gives the appearance of a pseudo-stratified epithelium (Altman and Bayer, 1991; Altman and Bayer, 2011). Radial glia divide either symmetrically to form two identical cells, or asymmetrically to give rise to one stem cell and one neuroblast. The neuroblast, using the radial glia's process as a guide, migrates radially toward the pial surface and differentiates into a projection neuron after reaching its destination (Rakic, 1971; Malatesta et al., 2000; Noctor et al., 2001). At E13 the primary neuroepithelium can be subdivided into a more compact zone adjacent to the ventricle called the ventricular zone (VZ), a less cell-dense area more distant from the ventricle called the mantle, and a cell poor area most distant from the ventricle called the marginal zone (Globus and Kuhlenheck, 1944; Altman, 2011). Generally, later migrating neuroblasts move past previously migrated neuroblasts, thus forming the six cortical layers in an inside-out fashion (although Layer I lies closest to the pial surface) (Altman and Bayer, 1991; Altman and Bayer, 2011). During the early embryonic period, the VZ is the most important source of NSPCs and gives rise to projection neurons. The VZ also is the source of cells that create the subsequent germinal matrices.

3.1.2 Mid-late embryonic period

The secondary germinal matrix, termed the subventricular zone (SVZ), begins to evolve as the lateral ganglionic eminence and medial ganglionic eminence enlarge between E12 and E14 as a result of mitotic cells contributed by the VZ, adjacent to it but more distant from the ventricle. NSPCs continue to expand within the SVZ creating a truly stratified epithelium that differs from the VZ. Here the NSPCs do not undergo interkinetic nuclear migration. Nor are the cleavage planes of the mitotic cells oriented in any particular way with regard to the ventricle, so the SVZ does not fit neatly within the symmetrical v. asymmetrical explanation for expansion of NSPCs (Altman and Bayer, 1991; Altman and Bayer, 2011). SVZ NSPCs are tripotential.

During mid-gestation, the SVZ gives rise to neuroblasts that migrate radially to the cortex where they differentiate into interneurons (Altman and Bayer, 2011). The SVZ also gives rise to some OPCs that migrate to the striatum, subcortical white matter and neocortex (Levison and Goldman, 1997; Suzuki and Goldman, 2003) where they persist as oligodendroglial progenitors (OPCs) or differentiate into mature oligodendrocytes (Dawson et al., 2003). Simultaneously the VZ is also a source of OPCs. Distinct populations of VZ NSPCs contribute OPCs at different timepoints in development. Between E11.5 and E14.5, Nkx2.1-expressing NSPCs in the ventral VZ overlying the medial ganglionic eminence and the anterior entopeduncular area give rise to OPCs that migrate radially to the cortex. Later by E16.5, Gsh-2-expressing NSPCs from VZ overlying the lateral ganglionic eminence and caudal ganglionic eminence give rise to OPCs that migrate radially to the cortex (Kessaris et al., 2006).

Starting at approximately E14, radial glial cells start to gradually transform into astrocytes. Nonetheless, the VZ peaks in size at E17 and decreases in size between E18 to E21. Thus the VZ transiently coexists with the SVZ (Temple, 2001).

A tertiary germinal matrix can be found in the hippocampus at E16. Starting at E14.5, NSPCs proliferate at the dentate notch, then differentiate into neuroblasts that migrate along radial glia before differentiating further into granule cell neurons to form the blades of the dentate gyrus. Subsequently, more neuroblasts migrate along the same path but accumulate as mitotic progenitors to form the hilus of the dentate gyrus. Thus, the dentate gyrus is essentially a specialized subventricular zone. The true tertiary germinal matrix is the border between the granule cell layer and the hilus, also known as the subgranular zone (SGZ) (Li and Pleasure, 2005). NSPCs residing at the SGZ give rise to granule cell neurons (Ray et al., 1993).

The SVZ is fully formed by E15-16, and becomes larger than the VZ by E18. The peak of neurogenesis takes place between E14-E17 with the VZ and the SVZ both contributing neurons at this time. Thus, during mid gestation, both the VZ and SVZ are important sources of NSPCs that generate projection neurons and interneurons respectively. By late embryonic life NSPCs are restricted to the SVZ and the SGZ and their fate is further restricted to either a glial or a neuronal fate in the SVZ and a neuronal fate in the SGZ. By late gestation, the SVZ becomes the most important source of NSPCs capable of generating interneurons and oligodendrocytes.

3.2 Postnatal period

At the time of birth, cortical neurogenesis has ended. The VZ no longer exists and has been replaced by the ependyma. The SVZ and SGZ persists postnatally throughout childhood into adulthood. Evidence shows an SVZ containing NSPCs exists in adult humans as well.

3.2.1 Early postnatal period

Postnatally, neurogenesis is confined to the olfactory system and the hippocampus. SVZ neuroblasts no longer migrate radially, but have changed direction and now migrate tangentially through the rostral migratory stream to the olfactory bulb where they differentiate into interneurons (Marshall et al., 2003). By P10, the SGZ is well established and NSPCs here continue to give rise to hippocampal granule cell neurons (Li and Pleasure, 2005).

Oligodendrogenesis, on the other hand, continues to be widespread during the first postnatal week and their source is diverse. At birth, Nkx2.1-derived OPCs are abundant in the cortex. Postnatally, Emx1-expressing NSPCs located dorsally in the cortex give rise to OPCs that populate the corpus callosum and cortex. By P10, the majority of OPCs and oligodendrocytes derive from Emx-1- and Gsh-2-expressing NSPCs, but very few OPCs derive from Nkx2.1-expressing NSPCs remain (Kessaris et al., 2006). As well, OPCs migrate from the SVZ to the striatum, white matter and medial, dorsal and lateral regions of the cortex where they reside as progenitors or differentiate into mature oligodendrocytes. A small proportion the OPCs in the corpus callosum comes from the SVZ (Rivers, 2008). This wave of migration ends by P14.

Also around the time of birth a distinct population of cells migrates from the SVZ to striatum, white matter and medial, dorsal and lateral regions of the cortex to form astrocytes.

In summary, the bulk of neurogenesis occurs prenatally while the bulk of oligodendrogenesis occurs postnatally with a peak in mouse between P7-P14 (Wright et al., 2010). As in late gestation, in the postnatal period the SVZ remains the most important source of NSPCs for the generation of olfactory interneurons and oligodendrocytes throughout the brain. The SGZ remains an important source of NSPCs for the generation of granule cell neurons within the hippocampus.

3.2.2 Adult period

Neurogenesis during adulthood is confined to the olfactory system and the hippocampus. As mentioned above, some of the OPCs that migrated in the late embryonic period and early postnatal period persist within the striatum, white matter and cortex as progenitors (Dawson et al., 2003). Thus, OPCs are found throughout the adult brain. OPCs are characterized by expression of markers including Olig2, PDGFRA and NG2. It is controversial whether NG2+/PDGFRA+ cells scattered throughout the neocortex are truly restricted oligodendrocyte progenitors. Recently, NG2 cells were shown to have characteristics of NSPCs, giving rise to both gray and white matter. In fact, there is some evidence that they are tripotential. This issue has been explored in vivo using Cre conditional mutants and Cre conditional inducible mutants. Using the NG2CreBAC:Z/EG mouse, Zhu et al., showed that EGFP+ cells residing in white matter give rise to OL, whereas those residing in gray matter give rise to OL and some astrocytes (Zhu et al., 2008). As NG2+ cells in adult mice co-express PDGFRA and vice versa, Rivers et al., showed using the PDGFRACreERT2;Rosa26-YFP mouse, that cells that had expressed PDGFRA and their progeny give rise to myelinating oligodendrocytes in the corpus callosum and to projection neurons in the piriform cortex but never astrocytes (Rivers et al., 2008). As NG2+ cells also express Olig2 and vice versa, Dimou et al, showed using the Olig2CreER mouse, that cells that had expressed Olig2 and their progeny give rise to myelinating oligodendrocytes in white matter but not gray matter and became post-mitotic in gray matter, suggesting a non-progenitor function in these regions (Dimou et al., 2008). Interestingly, both ventrally derived (Gsh2-derived) and dorsally derived (Emx1-derived) precursors contribute equally to dividing and non-dividing subpopulations of NG2 cells (Psachoulia, 2009). The conclusion is that the overwhelming progeny of NG2 cells are oligodendrocytes but much less often are astrocytes and neurons. NG2 cells may be a class of cells with a unique function in their own right.

Developmental Period	Location	Differentiated Progeny Phenotype
Early Embryonic	VZ	Projection Neurons, OPCs
Mid-Late Embryonic	VZ, SVZ, SGZ	Projection Neurons, OPCs/NG2 cells, Cortical Interneurons, Hippocampal Granule Cell Neurons, Oligodendrocytes
Postnatal	SVZ, SGZ, striatum, corpus callosum, cortex	Olfactory Cortical Interneurons, Hippocampal Granule Cell Neurons, OPCs/NG2 cells, Oligodendrocytes
Adulthood	SVZ, SGZ, striatum, corpus callosum, cortex	Olfactory Cortical Interneurons, Hippocampal Granule Cell Neurons, OPCs/NG2 cells, Oligodendrocytes

Table 1. Distribution and progeny of NSPCs during development.

In adulthood, the SVZ remains an important source of NSPCs for the generation of olfactory interneurons and the SGZ remains an important source of NSPCs for the generation of granule cell neurons. In addition, widely spread throughout the brain are NG2 cells that are accepted as OPCs but may also be source NSPCs for projection neurons in the piriform cortex and for gray matter astrocytes.

Precursor Cell Phenotype	Markers
Neural stem cells	Nestin, GFAP, Sox2
Neuroblasts	Dcx
Oligodendrocyte Progenitor Cells	Olig2, NG2, PDGFRA, Sox10

Table 2. Markers of neural stem cells and restricted progenitors.

4. NSPCs in perinatal hypoxia-ischemia

Despite the restricted fate for progenitors in development, it seems that injury can provoke a relaxation of this fate restriction. We will review how SVZ cells respond to perinatal hypoxia-ischemia in terms of proliferation, fate commitment and migration. The response of NSPCs to stroke is covered elsewhere in this book.

In vitro data suggest that the SVZ responds to perinatal hypoxia-ischemia by attempting to regenerate lost cells through increased proliferation and also a shift in fate potential. Neurospheres generated from the SVZ of neonatal rats subjected to hypoxia-ischemia yield oligodendrocytes more often than neurospheres generated from non-lesioned rats (Felling et al., 2006; Yang and Levison, 2006). In vivo data also support a regenerative response by the SVZ that includes increased emigration as well. Plane et al. showed an increase in neuroblasts (BrdU+/Doublecortin+ cells) in SVZ and striatum 2 weeks after perinatal hypoxia-ischemia in the mouse, however no mature neurons (BrdU+/NeuN+ cells) 3 weeks after injury (Plane et al., 2004). Similarly in rat, Ong et al. showed an increase in SVZ neuroblasts (BrdU+/Doublecortin+ cells) 2-3 weeks after perinatal hypoxia-ischemia but no increase in mature neurons (BrdU+/NeuN+ cells) in striatum 4 weeks after injury (Ong et al., 2005). By contrast, Yang and Levison did show an increase in neuroblasts (BrdU+/Doublecortin+ cells) and mature neurons (BrdU+/NeuN+ cells) up to 5 months after perinatal hypoxia-ischemia in the rat. They also marked SVZ cells with Retroviral-AP and showed that these newly born neuroblasts and mature neurons originated from the SVZ (Yang and Levison, 2007). Several groups have shown that, 4 weeks after perinatal hypoxic-ischemic injury, newly born oligodendrocytes (BrdU+/MBP+ cells, BrdU+/carbonic anhydrase+ cells, and BrdU+/RIP+ cells) are found in the striatum, corpus callosum and infarcted cortex (Back et al., 2002; Zaidi et al., 2004; Ong et al, 2005).

By contrast our work, focusing on the oligodendroglial lineage, did not show an increase in emigration of OPCs from SVZ after perinatal hypoxia-ischemia. Like others, we showed an increase in neural progenitors in SVZ in response to perinatal HI; specifically, we showed an increase in OPCs in vivo (Figure 1) (Dizon et al., 2010).

Given that OPCs are actively migrating during the timing of perinatal hypoxic-ischemic injury, we expected to see an increase in OPC migration. Rather, using multi-photon microscopy to image OPCs in slice cultures derived from lesioned Olig1-EGFP mice, we showed a paucity of OPC emigration from SVZ. Nonetheless, we showed an increase of Olig1-EGFP+ cells within cortex and striatum in response to perinatal HI (Figure 2) (Dizon et al., 2010).

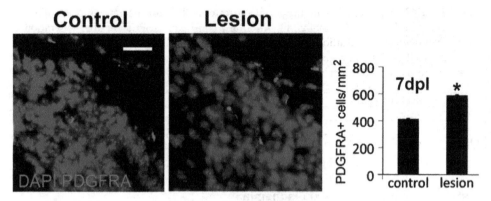

Fig. 1. Perinatal hypoxia-ischemia causes an increase in OPCs marked by PDGFRA within the SVZ by 7 days post lesion (dpl). Scale bar = 50 microns. *p=0.013.

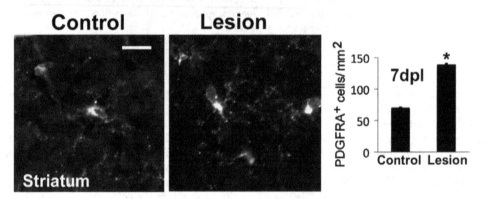

Fig. 2. Perinatal hypoxia-ischemia causes an increase in OPCs marked by PDGFRA within the striatum by 7 days post lesion (dpl). Scale bar = 50 microns. *p=0.003.

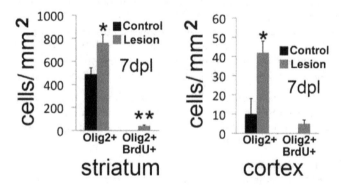

Fig. 3. Increases in OPCs marked by Olig2 result from increased proliferation of OPCs in the striatum but not in the cortex as evidenced by doublemarking with BrdU. Striatum: *p=0.044, **p=0.031. Cortex: *p=0.037.

We also found an increase in OPCs within the cortex. Interestingly, by marking newly born cells with BrdU, we showed that increased OPCs in the striatum arise through proliferation but this is not true for the cortex (Figure 3).

Therefore, we speculated that increased OPCs may arise via increased fate commitment of uncommitted neural progenitors. Thus, we have turned our attention to local neural progenitors and strategies to augment endogenous regenerative responses to white matter injury, specifically toward manipulation of regulators of NSPC fate, namely bone morphogenetic proteins (BMPs). BMPs negatively regulate an oligodendroglial fate choice by NSPCs. Recently, using a transgenic mouse that overexpresses the BMP antagonist noggin during the period of oligodendrogliogenesis, we were able to obtain increased OPCs and myelinating oligodendrocytes as well as improved motor function in lesioned noggin overexpressing mice compared to lesioned wildtype mice (Dizon et al., 2011). Subsequently, another group has independently shown improved outcomes in a rabbit model of perinatal hypoxia-ischemia when pups were treated with recombinant noggin protein after injury (Dummula et al., 2011). We are currently targeting BMP receptor subunits to more precisely downregulate signaling in in vivo experiments utilizing conditional inducible ablation of BMP receptor subunits BMPR1a, BMPR1b and BMPR2 following injury. We would anticipate that our strategies, if successful, could be applied to other diseases of white matter at other developmental timepoints including congenital dysmyelination and multiple sclerosis.

In conclusion, the abundance and fate restriction of available neural precursors to address disease states varies depending on the time during development. Nonetheless, manipulation of endogenous progenitors may be a more promising therapy than transplanted progenitors as there is no need to overcome problems with rejection.

5. Conclusions

In conclusion, the endogenous NSPC cell populations capable of replacing cells lost to disease are specific to the period of development during which injury is sustained as well as to the location of injury. Unlike NSPCs from SVZ or SGZ, NSPCs of the NG2 type are not restricted to these regions but reside in the many brain regions that may be injured throughout the lifetime. Thus, NG2 cells likely reside more proximal to injured regions and might more readily respond, so they may be the more appropriate target for research efforts rather than SVZ cells. In addition, more specific groups of NG2 cells might be targeted. For example, Emx1-derived NSPCs might give rise to OPCs that are capable of compensating for lost white matter in an adult animal, while Nkx2.1-derived NSPCs would more appropriately be targeted to regenerate white matter in newborns; these cells would not be present so could not be exploited in adult onset diseases. Rational therapy would target restricted population of NSPCs, thereby confining therapies to the cells best able to effect regeneration while also minimizing unwanted side effects.

6. References

Altman, J. (1963). Autoradiographic investigation of cell proliferation in the brains of rats and cats. *Anatomical Record.* 145, 573-91.

Altman, J., Das, G. D. (1965a). Autoradiographic and histological evidence of postnatal hippocampal neurogenesis in rats. *Journal of Comparative Neurolology.* 124, 319-35.

Altman, J., Das, G. D. (1965b). Post-natal origin of microneurones in the rat brain. *Nature*. 207, 953-6.

Altman, J., Das, G. D. (1966). Autoradiographic and histological studies of postnatal neurogenesis. I. A longitudinal investigation of the kinetics, migration and transformation of cells incorporating tritiated thymidine in neonate rats, with special reference to postnatal neurogenesis in some brain regions. *Journal of Comparative Neurology*. 126, 337-89.

Anderson, M. J., Waxman, S. G. (1983). Caudal spinal cord of the teleost Sternarchus albifrons resembles regenerating cord. *Anatomical Record*. 205, 85-92.

Bayer, S.A., and Altman, J. (1991). *Neocortical Development*, Raven Press, Retrieved from: <http://neurondevelopment.org>

Bayer, S.A., and Altman, J. (2011a) Laboratory Memoir, In: *Neuron Development*, Available from: <http://neurondevelopment.org>

Back, S.A., Han B.H., Luo, N.L., Chricton, C.A. Zanthoudakis, S., Tam, J. , Arvin, K.L., Holtzman, D.M. (2002). Selective vulnerabiliry of late oligodendrocyte progenitors to hypoxia-ischemia. *Journal of Neuroscience*. 22: 455-463.

Bhardwaj, R. D., Curtis, M.A., Spalding, K.L., Buchholz, B.A,, Fink, D., Bjork-Erikkson, T., Nordborg, C., Gage, F.H., Druid, H., Erikkson, P.S., Frisen, J.. (2006). Neocortical neurogenesis in humans is restricted to development. *Proceedings of the National Academy of Science U S A*. 103, 12564-8.

Craig, A., Ling, L.N., Beardsley, D.J., Wingate-Pearse, N., Walker, D.W., Hohimer, A.R., Back, S.A. (2003). Quantitative analysis of perinatal rodent oligodendrocyte lineage progression and its correlation with human. *Experimental Neurology*. 181, 231-40.

Curtis, M. A., Kam, M., Nannmark, U., Anderson, M.F., Axell, M.Z., Wikkelso, C., Holtas, S., van Roon-Mom, W.M., Bjork-Eriksson, T., Nordberg, C., Fresn, J., Dragunow, M., Faull, R.L., Eriksson, P.S. (2007). Human neuroblasts migrate to the olfactory bulb via a lateral ventricular extension. *Science*. 315, 1243-9.

Dawson., M.R., Polito, A., Levine, J.M., Reynolds, R. (2003). NG2-expressing glial progenitors cells: an abundant and widespread population of cycling cells in the adult rat CNS. *Molecular and Cellular Neuroscience*. 24:476-488.

Dimou, L., Simon, C., Kirchoff, F., Takebayashi, H., Gotz, M. (2008). Progeny of Olig2-expressing progenitors in gray and white matter of the adult mouse cerebral cortex. *Journal of Neuroscience*. 28, 10434-42.

Dizon, M., Szele, F., Kessler, J.A. (2010). Hypoxia-ischemia induces an endogenous reparative response by local neural progenitors in the postnatal mouse telencephalon. *Developmental Neuroscience*. 32, 173-83.

Dizon, M.L., Maa, T., Kessler, J.A. (2011).The bone morphogenetic protein antagonist noggin protects white matter after perinatal hypoxia-ischemia. *Neurobiology of Disease*. 42, 318.26.

Dummula, K., Vinukonda, G., Chu, P., Xing, Y., Hu, F., Mailk, S., Csiszar, A., Chua, C., Mouton, P., Kayton, R.J., Brumberg, J.C., Bansal, R., Ballabh, P. (2011). Bone morphogenetic protein inhibition promotes neurological recovery after intraventricular hemorrhage. *Journal of Neuroscience*. 31:12068-12082.

Eriksson, P. S., Perfilieva, E., Bjork-Eriksson, T., Alborn, A.M., Nordborg, C., Peterson, D.A., Gage, F.H. (1998). Neurogenesis in the adult human hippocampus. *Nature Medicine*. 4, 1313-7.

Felling, R.J., Snyder, M.J., Romanko, M.J., Rothstein R.P., Zeigler, A.N., Yang, Z. Givogri, M.I., Bongarzone, E.R., Levison, S.W. (2006). Neural stem/progenitor cells participate in the regenerative response to perinatal hypoxia/ischemia. *Journal of Neuroscience*. 26, 4359-4369.

Globus, J.H., Kuhlenbeck, H. (1944). The subependymal cell plate (matrix) and its relationship to brain tumors of the ependymal type. *Journal of Neuropathology and Experimental Neurology*. 3:1-35.

Goldman, S. A., Nottebohm, F. (1983). Neuronal production, migration, and differentiation in a vocal control nucleus of the adult female canary brain. *Proceedings of the National Academy of Sciences U S A*. 80, 2390-4.

Gould, E., Reeves, A.J., Fallah, M., Tanapat, P., Gross, C.G., Fuchs, E. (1999a). Hippocampal neurogenesis in adult Old World primates. *Proceedings of the National Academy of Sciences U S A*. 96, 5263-7.

Gould, E., Reeves, A.J., Graziano, M.S., Gross, C.G. (1999b). Neurogenesis in the neocortex of adult primates. *Science*. 286, 548-52.

Kessaris, N., Fogarty, M., Iannarelli, P., Grist, M., Wegner, M., Richardson, W.D. (2006). Competing waves of oligodendrocytes in the forebrain and postnatal elimination of an embryonic lineage. *Nature Neuroscience*. 9, 173-179.

Levison, S.W. and Goldman, J.E. (1997). Multipotential and lineage restricted precursors coexist in the mammalian perinatal subventricular zone. *Journal of Neuroscience Research*. 48, 83-94.

Li, G., and Pleasure, S.J. (2005). Morphogenesis of the dentate gyrus: what we are learning from mouse mutants. *Developmental Neuroscience*. 27:93-99.

Lois, C., Alvarez-Buylla, A. (1993). Proliferating subventricular zone cells in the adult mammalian forebrain can differentiate into neurons and glia. *Proceedings of the National Academy of Sciences U S A*. 90, 2074-7.

Lois, C., Alvarez-Buylla, A. (1994). Long-distance neuronal migration in the adult mammalian brain. *Science*. 264, 1145-8.

Malatesta, P., Hartfuss, E., Gotz, M. (2000) Isolation of radial glial cells by fluorescent-activated cell sorting reveals a neuronal lineage. *Development*. 127:5253-63.

Marshall, C. A., et al., (2003). Gliogenic and neurogenic progenitors of the subventricular zone: who are they, where did they come from, and where are they going? *Glia*. 43, 52-61.

Menn, B., Garcia-Verdugo, J.M., Yaschine, C., Gonzalez-Perez, O., Rowtich, D., Alvarez-Buylla, A. (2006). Origin of oligodendrocytes in the subventricular zone of the adult brain. *Journal of Neuroscience*. 26, 7907-7918.

Meyer, R. L., et al., (1985). Topography of regenerating optic fibers in goldfish traced with local wheat germ injections into retina: evidence for discontinuous microtopography in the retinotectal projection. *Journal of Comparative Neurology*. 239, 27-43.

Ming, G. L.and Song, H. (2005). Adult neurogenesis in the mammalian central nervous system. *Annual Reviews of Neuroscience*. 28, 223-50.

Noctor, S.C., Flint, A.C., Weissman, T.A., Dammerman, R.S., Kriegstein, A.R. (2001). Neurons derived from radial glial cells establish radial units in neocortex. *Nature*. 409, 714-720.

Nottebohm, F. (1985). Neuronal replacement in adulthood. Annals of the New York Academy of Sciences. 457, 143-61.

Ong, J., Plane, J.M., Parent, J.M., Silverstein, F.S. (2005). Hypoxic-ischemic injury stimulates subventricular zone proliferation and neurogenesis in the neonatal rat. *Pediatric Research*. 58:600-606.

Plane, J.M., Liu, R., Wang, T.W., Silverstein, F.S., Parent, J.M. (2004). Neonatal hypoxic-ischemic injury increases forebrain subventricular zone neurogenesis in the mouse. Neurobiology of Disease 16:585-595.

Psachoulia, K., Jamen, F., Young, K.M., Richardson, W.D. (2009). Cell cycle dynamics of NG2 cells in the postnatal and ageing brain. *Neuron Glia Biology*. 5, 57-67.

Ray, J., Peterson, D.A., Schinstine M., Gage, F.H.(1993). Proliferation, differentiation, and long term culture of primary hippocampal neurons. *Proceedings of the National Academy of Sciences*. 90:3602-6.

Rakic, P. (1971). Guidance of neurons migrating to the fetal monkey neocortex. *Brain Research*. 33, 471-476.

Rakic, P. (1985). Limits of neurogenesis in primates. *Science*. 227, 1054-6.

Rivers, L.E., Young, K.M., Rizzi, M., Jamen, F., Psachoulia, K., Wade, A., Kessaris, N., Richardson, W.D. (2008). PDGFRA/NG2 glia generate myelinating oligodendrocytes and piriform projection neurons in adult mice. Nature Neuroscience. 11: 1392-401.

Smart, I., (1961). The subependymal layer of the mouse brain and its cell production as shown by autography after [H^3]-thymidine injection. *Journal of Comparative Neurology*. 116:325-27.

Suzuki, S.O., and Goldman, J.E. (2003). Multiple cell populations in the early postnatal subventricular zone take distinct migratory pathways: a dynamic study of glial and neuronal progenitor migration. *Journal of Neuroscience*. 23. 4240-4250.

Wright, J. Zhang, G., Yu, T.S., Kernie, S.G. (2010). Age related changes in the oligodendrocyte progenitor pool influence brain remodeling after injury. *Developmental Neuroscience*. 32:499-509.

Yang, Z., and Levison, S.W. (2006). Hypoxia/ischemia expands the regenerative capacity of progenitors in the perinatal subventricular zone. Neuroscience. 139:555-64.

Yang, Z., and Levison, S.W. (2007). Perinatal hyposic-ischemic brain injury induces persistent production of striatal neurons from subventricular zone progenitors. *Developmental Neuroscience*. 29:331-340.

Zaidi, A.U., Bessert, D.A., Ong, J.E., Xu, H., Barks, J.D., Silverstein, F.S., Skoff, R.P. (2004). New oligodendrocytes are generated after neonatal hypoxic-ischemic brain injury in rodents. *Glia*. 46:380-390.

Zhu, X., Bergles, D.E., Nishiyama, A. (2008). Ng2 cells generate oligodendrocytes and gray matter astrocytes. *Development*. 135:145-157.

Zupanc, G. K. (1999). Neurogenesis, cell death and regeneration in the adult gymnotiform brain. *Journal of Experimental Biology*. 202, 1435-46.

Zupanc, G. K. (2008). Adult neurogenesis and neuronal regeneration in the brain of teleost fish. *Journal of Physiology Paris*. 102, 357-73.

5

Ischemia-Induced Neural Stem/Progenitor Cells Within the Post-Stroke Cortex in Adult Brains

Takayuki Nakagomi and Tomohiro Matsuyama
Institute for Advanced Medical Sciences,
Hyogo College of Medicine
Hyogo,
Japan

1. Introduction

Stroke is one of the major causes of death and disability in developed countries. The central nervous system (CNS) is known for its limited reparative capacity, but several studies demonstrated that the CNS has some reparative potential and cerebral ischemia is followed by activation of endogenous neurogenesis (Nakatomi et al., 2002; Taguchi et al., 2004). It is well-known that new neurons are continuously generated in specific brain regions such as the subventricular zones (SVZ) (Alvarez-Buylla et al., 2002) and the subgranular zone within the dentate gyrus of the hippocampus (SGZ) (Kuhn et al., 1996). Although adult cerebral cortical neurogenesis remains controversial, accumulating evidence has shown that under pathological conditions, new neurons are generated in the adult mammalian cerebral cortex (Magavi et al., 2000; Jiang et al., 2001; Jin et al., 2006; Yang et al., 2007). This suggests that neural stem/progenitor cells (NSPCs) can be activated in the cortex by brain injury such as ischemic stroke. In support of this notion, we demonstrated that NSPCs develop in the post-stroke area of the cortex in the adult murine (Nakagomi et al., 2009a; Nakagomi et al., 2009b; Nakano-Doi et al., 2010; Saino et al., 2010) and human brain (Nakayama et al., 2010), and we referred to these as ischemia/injury-induced NSPCs (iNSPCs). These cells express markers of NSPCs, such as nestin and Sox2. They also form neurospheres that have the capacity for self-renewal, and differentiate into electrophysiologically functional neurons, astrocytes, and myelin-producing oligodendrocytes (Nakagomi et al., 2009a; Nakagomi et al., 2009b; Nakano-Doi et al., 2010; Clausen et al., 2011). In addition, we demonstrated that iNSPCs originate, at least in part, from within the cerebral cortex, but not from SVZ cells (Nakagomi et al., 2009b). However, the detailed origin and identity of the iNSPCs remains unclear. In this chapter, we introduce the characterization and possible origin of iNSPCs based on our reports and recent viewpoint, and compare them to other previously reported types of CNS stem/progenitor cells, including SVZ astrocytes (Doetsch et al., 1999), ependymal cells (Moreno-Manzano et al., 2009), reactive astrocytes (Shimada et al., 2010), resident glia (Zawadzka et al., 2010), and oligodendrocyte precursor cells (OPCs) (Kondo et al., 2000). We also refer to the possible cortical neurogenesis by iNSPCs and to the therapeutic potential of iNSPC transplantation in stroke patients.

2. NSPCs in the adult cortex

In the CNS of adult mammals, it is well-known that NSPCs are present in the SVZ and SVG, and that ongoing neurogenesis is retained in these two zones. However, accumulating evidence suggests that NSPCs reside in many parts of the adult brain including the cortex (Arsenijevic et al., 2001; Joh et al., 2005; Kallur et al., 2006; Jiao et al., 2008; Willaime-Morawek et al., 2008), striatum (Kallur et al., 2006; Willaime-Morawek et al., 2008), subcortical white matter (Nunes et al., 2003), and spinal cord (Weiss et al., 1996; Parr et al., 2008). These observations suggest that NSPCs are widely distributed throughout the adult CNS. In this chapter, we introduce iNSPCs, which are induced within the post-stroke cortex after brain injury/ischemia in adult brains.

2.1 Cortical development in the embryonic stage: comparison to iNSPCs in the cortex

In the embryonic stage, neurogenesis was observed throughout the CNS including the cortex. Mignone and colleagues traced nestin-expressing NSPCs, and showed that green fluorescent protein (GFP) expression in developing transgenic nestin-GFP mice was evident on as early as day 7 of embryonic development (e7). At e8, a GFP signal was observed predominantly in the neural plate, and by e10 intense GFP fluorescence was observed throughout the neuroepithelium. At e10 to e12, GFP signals marked the entire thickness of the cerebral wall, but GFP expression became weaker near the pial surface and stronger in the ventricular zones starting from e12. Finally, in the adult brain, GFP was selectively expressed in the SVZ and SGZ in areas related to continuous neurogenesis (Mignone et al., 2004). Thus, in the postnatal CNS, constitutive neurogenesis is known to be retained in only two regions the SVZ (Alvarez-Buylla et al., 2002) and SGZ (Kuhn et al., 1996). However, under pathological conditions, neurogenesis may occur again in the adult cerebral cortex (Magavi et al., 2000; Jiang et al., 2001; Jin et al., 2006; Yang et al., 2007). Supporting their observations, nestin-positive NSPCs were observed after brain injury/ischemia in nonconventional neurogenic zones, such as the cortex (Nakagomi et al., 2009b; Nakayama et al., 2010). Because they were rarely observed in the absence of brain injury (Nakagomi et al., 2009b), cortical neurogenesis may reoccur only in the case of brain injury. These findings suggest that in adult mammalian brains, NSPC activation and neuronal homeostasis are maintained under physiological conditions, at least in part, in specific brain regions, such as the SVZ and SGZ. However, after brain injury, it appears that regional NSPCs are mobilized to accelerate tissue repair by a mechanism similar to embryonic neurogenesis. Taken together, these observations suggest that ischemia/hypoxia is essential for the induction of NSPCs in the adult cortex, although we remain unaware of the required signaling and/or factors.

2.1.1 Characteristics of iNSPCs from the post-stroke cortex

To confirm the possible adult neurogenesis induced by brain injury, we have sought to isolate NSPCs from the injured area of the post-stroke cortex. Previously, we established a highly reproducible murine model of cortical infarction using CB-17/Icr-+/+Jcl and CB-17/Icr-Scid/scid Jcl mice. The infarct area in mice of this background has been limited to the ipsilateral cerebral cortex of the territory occupied by the middle cerebral artery (MCA) (Taguchi et al., 2004; Taguchi et al., 2007; Nakagomi et al., 2009a; Nakagomi et al., 2009b;

Nakano-Doi *et al.*, 2010; Saino *et al.*, 2010; Taguchi *et al.*, 2010). Following MCA occlusion, abundant nestin-positive cells emerged within the post-stroke cortex, although they were rarely observed in the non-ischemic cortex (Nakagomi *et al.*, 2009b; Nakano-Doi *et al.*, 2010; Saino *et al.*, 2010). To examine whether these cells showed stem cell-characteristics, we cultured cells isolated from the post-stroke cortex under conditions that promoted the formation of neurospheres (Reynolds *et al.*, 1992). In brief, tissue from the ischemic core of the post-infarct cerebral cortex was obtained on day 7 after MCA occlusion. Cells were dissociated by passage through 23 and 27 gauge needles, and cell suspensions were incubated in tissue culture flasks with DMEM containing epidermal growth factor (EGF), basic fibroblast growth factor (bFGF) and N2 supplement. This procedure allowed us to obtain nestin-positive neurosphere-like cell clusters (iNSPCs) (Nakagomi *et al.*, 2009a; Nakagomi *et al.*, 2009b; Nakano-Doi *et al.*, 2010) (Fig. 1).

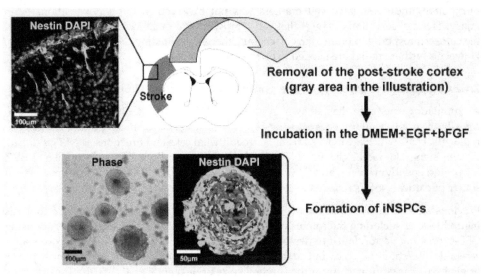

Fig. 1. Isolation of nestin-positive iNSPCs developing within the post-stroke cortex

However, iNSPCs were rarely obtained in the absence of brain injury. Notably, because we could not obtain iNSPCs from the peri-stroke cortex, it is possible that these cells are generated within the degenerating cortical tissue after ischemic stroke.

Uptake of 5-bromo-2'-deoxyuridine (BrdU) by iNSPCs was confirmed *in vivo* (Nakano-Doi *et al.*, 2010; Saino *et al.*, 2010) and *in vitro* (Nakagomi *et al.*, 2009a; Nakagomi *et al.*, 2009b), showing that they have the proliferative activity. They possessed self-renewal capacity, which was confirmed by a clonal assay. However, in contrast to the embryonic stem cells, the cluster formation in the same medium at a clonal density was limited to between three and five cell passages (Nakagomi *et al.*, 2009b; Nakano-Doi *et al.*, 2010), consistent with other adult candidates of stem cells, such as neurospheres derived from hippocampus (Bull *et al.*, 2005) and subcortical white matter (Nunes *et al.*, 2003). These observations suggest that cortex-derived iNSPCs are more likely to be neural progenitors than neural stem cells (NSCs). However, they certainly differentiated into electrophysiologically functional neurons, astrocytes, and myelin-producing oligodendrocytes (Nakagomi *et al.*, 2009a; Nakagomi *et al.*, 2009b; Nakano-Doi *et al.*, 2010), indicating that iNSPCs have a stemness-capacity similar to other adult NSPCs. Interestingly, they predominantly differentiated into neurons (approximately 35%) and oligodendrocytes (approximately 30%) rather than astrocytes (approximately 5%) (Nakagomi *et al.*, 2009a; Nakano-Doi *et al.*, 2010; Nakagomi *et al.*, 2011) with characteristics discriminating from other adult NSPCs such as SVZ astrocytes, most of which are known to differentiate into astrocytes. These findings suggest that iNSPCs have a strong potential of contributing to cortical neurogenesis compared to NSPCs derived from other origins, especially under the conditions of brain injury.

Consistent with the SVZ-derived NSPCs (Kim *et al.*, 2009b), cortical iNSPCs expressed several pluripotent/undifferentiated cell markers, including Sox2, Klf4, c-myc and Nanog (Nakagomi *et al.*, 2009b; Nakagomi *et al.*, 2011). However, expression of various pluripotent/undifferentiated cell markers was not observed in the cortex without brain injury. These observations suggest that cell reprogramming may occur in unknown cells of the cortex in response to brain injury/ischemia, thereby promoting the induction of iNSPCs. However, further studies are needed to clarify this hypothesis.

2.1.2 Comparison to other types of reported CNS stem/progenitor cells

Accumulating evidence has shown several candidates for adult NSPCs, which can contribute to adult neurogenesis in the cerebral cortex. One of these candidates may be radial glia cells, which are derived from neuroepithelial cells and functions as NSPCs during development. The radial glia are able to develop into several types of NSPCs, such as SVZ astrocytes, ependymal cells, and OPCs in adult (Kriegstein *et al.*, 2009). However, precise cell source of cortical NSPCs remains unclear, especially in the injured brain.

Previous studies demonstrated that SVZ astrocytes have the capacity to migrate towards injured lesions, including the cerebral cortex (Goings *et al.*, 2004). However, our study using GFP-expressing vector, failed to demonstrate cell migration from the SVZ to the cortex after cerebral infarction *in vivo*, but demonstrated that iNSPCs in the post-stroke cortex originated, at least in part, from the cerebral cortex (Nakagomi *et al.*, 2009b). Consistently, subsequent studies showed that NSPCs developing within and around the post-stroke cortex are derived from locally activated stem/progenitor cells, but not from SVZ cells (Ohira *et al.*, 2010; Shimada *et al.*, 2010). To answer which cells can be activated by cerebral injury, some studies proposed the reactive astrocytes as a source of injury-induced NSPCs (Oki *et al.*, 2010; Shimada *et al.*, 2010), because NSPCs express the astrocyte marker, GFAP. However, we could not detect GFAP- (Nakagomi *et al.*, 2011) and S100β-positive astrocytes within the post-stroke cortex (Nakagomi *et al.*, 2009b). Eventually, the isolated iNSPCs from the infarct cortex rarely expressed GFAP and developed few astrocytic traits even after differentiation (Nakagomi *et al.*, 2011). In addition, although we found some nestin and GFAP double-positive reactive astrocyte-like cells in the peri-infarct area, we could not obtain neurospheres from these areas. These findings strongly suggest that the source of iNSPCs within the infarct cortex is distinct from reactive astrocytes.

Currently, it is still highly controversial whether periventricular NSPCs can be derived from SVZ astrocytes, ependymal cells, or both (Chojnacki *et al.*, 2009). Ependymal cells were originally considered to be the resident stem cell population in the wall of the lateral ventricle, in which they locate nearby perivascular cells (Pfenninger *et al.*, 2007; Coskun *et al.*, 2008). Although it is controversial whether ependymal cells have NSPC activity or not, recent studies confirmed that ependymal cells do not play a role in adult neurogenesis under normal conditions, but do possess NSPC activity and can differentiate into neurons, astrocytes, and oligodendrocytes in response to the CNS injuries including ischemic stroke (Carlen *et al.*, 2009; Moreno-Manzano *et al.*, 2009). Furthermore, ependymal cells express PDGFRα (Danilov *et al.*, 2009) and NG2 (Moreno-Manzano *et al.*, 2009), and have the structure of lipid droplets, microvilli, and cilia (Coskun *et al.*, 2008; Danilov *et al.*, 2009). Consistent with the traits of ependymal cells, iNSPCs express PDGFRα and NG2, but do not possess microvilli-like structures (Nakagomi *et al.*, 2011). These findings indicate that iNSPCs do not have completely identical characteristics to those of ependymal cells.

Adult OPCs comprise approximately 5%–8% of the glial cell population in the CNS. Their function in the CNS remains unknown, although accumulating evidence has shown that they have NSPC activity (Kondo *et al.*, 2000; Gaughwin *et al.*, 2006), in addition to myelin-producing abilities (Sundberg *et al.*, 2010). OPCs are known to express NG2 (Ulrich *et al.*, 2008) and PDGFRα (Hall *et al.*, 1996), and OPCs expressing A2B5 have NSPC activity (Kondo *et al.*, 2000; Gaughwin *et al.*, 2006). To investigate whether iNSPCs are derived from OPCs, we analyzed OPC markers expressed by iNSPCs *in vivo* and *in vitro*. Although iNSPCs express some OPC markers such as NG2 and PDGFRα, they do not possess A2B5 or even Olig2 (another OPC marker) (Billon *et al.*, 2002). These observations indicate that iNSPCs are different from reported multipotent OPCs (Kondo *et al.*, 2000; Gaughwin *et al.*, 2006). However, when iNSPCs were incubated in OPC-promoting medium (Chen *et al.*, 2007), they began to express Olig2. In addition, almost all cells developed from iNSPCs in this medium differentiated into O4- and/or myelin-associated glycoprotein (MAG)-positive oligodendrocytes (Nakagomi *et al.*, 2011). These findings suggest that iNSPCs express some OPC markers during their development/differentiation.

It is well-known that NG2 is not only the marker of OPC, but is also the marker of resident glial cells/glial progenitors (Stallcup *et al.*, 1987). More recently, NG2-positive resident glia was reported to develop NSPC activity after brain injury (Yokoyama *et al.*, 2006; Zawadzka *et al.*, 2010). We demonstrated that cortical iNSPCs express NG2 and PDGFRα in a similar manner to resident glial/progenitor cells. However, neuronal differentiation from NG2- and/or PDGFRα-positive glial cells is rarely observed (Zawadzka *et al.*, 2010; Richardson *et al.*, 2011), suggesting that iNSPCs may be different from these glial cells or belonging to unknown cell type, which expresses some glial markers.

2.1.3 What is the origin of iNSPCs in the cortex?

So far, it seems possible that iNSPCs are different from previously proposed CNS stem/progenitor cells such as SVZ astrocytes, reactive astrocytes, ependymal cells, or OPCs. The essential difference of these cells may be their induction pattern and localization, because iNSPCs were found only after ischemic insult, and in close association with the blood vessels in the cortex. This unique localization allowed us to examine the characteristics of cells nearby blood vessels as a candidate of iNSPCs.

Our studies showed that the nestin-positive iNSPCs developed in the perivascular regions of the post-stroke cortex (Nakano-Doi *et al.*, 2010; Nakayama *et al.*, 2010), where nestin-positive cells express NG2 and PDGFRβ (both of which are the pericyte marker), suggesting that the iNSPCs are derived from pericytes. Pericytes with multipotent progenitor activity have been indentified in various organs (Crisan *et al.*, 2009) as well as in the CNS (Dore-Duffy *et al.*, 2006). In addition, Dore-Duffy and colleagues (Dore-Duffy *et al.*, 2006) showed that pericyte-derived NSPCs can be isolated from the CNS of non-injured animals. However, we hardly obtained iNSPCs from the nonischemic cortex (Nakagomi *et al.*, 2009b), suggesting that pericytes in the cortical tissues increase their stemness activity during the progression of cerebral injury.

Increasing evidence has shown that ischemic insult promotes stem cell activity, and NSPCs (Sirko *et al.*, 2009; Xue *et al.*, 2009) and neuronal progenitors (Ohira *et al.*, 2010) are also induced in response to cortical ischemic injury. These cortical NSPCs are frequently observed at the subpial/cortical layer 1 regions, suggesting that NSPCs can be activated preferentially in the cortical surface. Independent of these studies, we found nestin/Sox2-positive iNSPCs proliferating in the pia mater, which covers the surface of the post-ischemic cortex (Nakagomi *et al.*, 2011). Pia mater is widely distributed throughout the CNS, and is closely associated with the blood vessels. It has been reported that leptomeninges (including pia mater and arachnoid membrane) regulate NSPCs (Sockanathan *et al.*, 2009) and cortical neuron generation (Siegenthaler *et al.*, 2009) in embryonic cortical formation, and function as a niche for stem/progenitor cells with neuronal differentiation potential (Bifari *et al.*, 2009). These findings suggest that pia mater contains NSPCs at embryonic stage. The pial iNSPCs, which we found in the adult brain, partially spread into the cortical parenchyma as perivascular cells/pericytes with expression of pericyte markers such as NG2 and PDGFRβ. In addition, cells isolated from the infarcted area including pia mater and cortex and sorted by magnetic cell sorting (MACS) with a pericyte marker (PDGFRβ) had NSPC activity and differentiated into neurons (Nakagomi *et al.*, 2011). These findings indicate that the microvascular pericytes that distribute from the pia mater to the cortex are a potential source of the iNSPCs (Fig. 2).

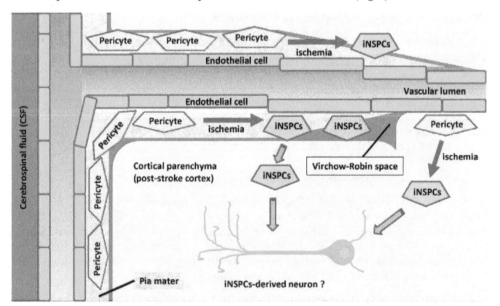

Fig. 2. Schematic representation for the fate of iNSPCs following cortical infarction

Thus, our recent study suggests that pia mater may have the potential to generate NSPCs even in the adult brain. Until now, it has been demonstrated that pia mater, as well as some CNS pericytes, originate from the neural crest (Morse et al., 1984; Etchevers et al., 2001). We recently demonstrated that pial iNSPCs express various neural crest markers, such as Sox9, Sox10, Snail, Slug, and Twist (Aihara et al., 2010; Nakagomi et al., 2011), suggesting that pial iNSPCs are neural crest derivatives. This may provide a novel concept that neural crest-derived cells play a crucial role in the CNS repair following cortical infarction by a similar mechanism to the CNS formation in development. Considering that the neural crest has stem cell potential (neural crest-derived stem cells) (Teng et al., 2006) with differentiation into a variety of cell types including neurons and glia (Nagoshi et al., 2009), this hypothesis would not be surprising. In addition, this might explain why Schwann cells, which have neural crest origin, are induced in the injured CNS (Zawadzka et al., 2010). However, the precise source, lineage, and traits of iNSPCs warrants further investigation. This may be clarified through experiment of lineage labeling by genetic means.

2.2 Potential contribution of endogenous iNSPCs to cortical neurogenesis

Although iNSPCs are generated within the post-stroke area following cortical infarction, almost all of them can undergo apoptotic cell death (Saino et al., 2010). Subsequently, appropriate support for survival of iNSPCs is essential in maintaining post-stroke neurogenesis. Because iNSPCs developed in close association with the blood vessels from the pia mater to the cortex, they must be influenced by the vascular microenvironment, consisting of endothelial cells (ECs) (Palmer et al., 2000; Louissaint et al., 2002) and inflammatory cells infiltrated after cerebral injury (Saino et al., 2010).

ECs are a component of the blood brain barrier (BBB) and also function as a vascular niche (Shen et al., 2008). It has been reported that although inflammation exacerbates post-stroke neuronal damage, inflammation is a strong stimulus for activation of neurogenesis. Such inflammatory reactions may happen in perivascular (Virchow-Robin) spaces (Hutchings et al., 1986), in which inflammatory cells such as macrophage and lymphocytes infiltrate and may affect angiogenesis and neurogenesis after brain injury. These factors should be considered when observing cortical neurogenesis through iNSPCs after ischemic stroke.

NSPCs reside in a vascular niche and the vasculature is regarded as a key element, especially in the adult SVZ (Tavazoie et al., 2008). ECs are believed to make valuable contribution to this vascular microenvironment (Palmer et al., 2000; Louissaint et al., 2002). In support of this viewpoint, co-culture experiments showed that ECs increase proliferation of NSPCs derived from the adult SVZ (Shen et al., 2004; Teng et al., 2008). Furthermore, we demonstrated both in vitro and in vivo, that the presence of ECs enhances survival, proliferation, migration, and differentiation of iNSPCs (Nakagomi et al., 2009a), indicating that augmentation of ECs (e.g., proliferation of ECs [angiogenesis]) can promote neurogenesis by enhancing the proliferation of endogenous iNSPCs.

Thus, therapeutic angiogenesis may enhance endogenous neurogenesis even after cerebral injury (Hamano et al., 2000; Chen et al., 2003). It has been reported that bone marrow cells (BMCs) such as bone marrow mononuclear cells (BMMCs) (Li et al., 2006; Kim et al., 2009a; Ribeiro-Resende et al., 2009) and mesenchymal stem cells (MSCs) (Labouyrie et al., 1999; Mahmood et al., 2004; Kurozumi et al., 2005) induce angiogenic effects by secreting multiple growth factors including vascular endothelial growth factor (VEGF), glia-derived neurotrophic factor (GDNF), brain-derived neurotrophic factor (BDNF), nerve growth factor (NGF), and hepatocyte growth factor (HGF). We showed that BMMCs can contribute to the proliferation of endogenous iNSPCs through vascular niche regulation, which includes EC proliferation following cortical infarction (Nakano-Doi et al., 2010).

In addition to ECs, astrocytes are also reported to be important niche cells for NSPCs in the SVZ (Song et al., 2002), SGZ (Lim et al., 1999) and cortex (Jiao et al., 2008). Our study already showed that astrocytes, as well as ECs, promote the proliferation of iNSPCs (Nakagomi et al., 2009a), suggesting that astrocytes function as a niche for cortex-derived iNSPCs. Although astrocytes were not observed within the post-stroke cortex after permanent ischemia (Nakagomi et al., 2011), astrocytes are resistant to hypoxia/ischemia and they can still survive after transient ischemia (Li et al., 1995). These findings might explain the reason why new-born neurons are frequently found in the post-stroke cortex after mild transient ischemia (Ohira et al., 2010), but are not seen after severe permanent ischemia (Nakagomi et al., 2009b).

Regulation of the immune system has also been proposed as one of the key factors in enhancing neurogenesis and functional recovery after stroke. Our studies showed that T lymphocytes, mainly CD4- but not CD8-positive T cells, induce apoptosis in iNSPCs (Saino et al., 2010; Takata et al., 2011). The details of the mechanism are still under investigation, but these findings suggest that the immune response and/or enhanced inflammation triggered by CD4-positive T cells, are major deteriorating modulators of post-stroke neurogenesis. These findings, at least in part, are consistent with previous results demonstrating that transplantation of mesenchymal cells accelerates endogenous neurogenesis after stroke (Li et al., 2008; Yoo et al., 2008), because such treatment is known to suppress the immune response in graft-versus-host disease.

2.3 Exogenous iNSPC transplantation after cerebral infarction

Compared to the strategy focusing on enhanced endogenous neurogenesis, exogenous NSPC transplantation may have some advantages in treating stroke patients; this therapy allows a longer therapeutic time window to administer larger numbers of stem cells, and to repeat the treatment. The therapeutic time window to enhance the endogenous neurogenesis may be limited, because we observed that neurogenesis peaks for several days and ends within a few weeks after stroke onset in patients (Nakayama et al., 2010).

Until now, various cell sources for exogenous NSPC transplantation have been proposed; e.g., fetal brain (Ishibashi et al., 2004; Kelly et al., 2004; Cayre et al., 2006; Darsalia et al., 2007), adult brain tissue obtained from the SVZ (Cayre et al., 2006; Hicks et al., 2007; Kameda et al., 2007), gene transfected bone marrow cells (Dezawa et al., 2004), immortalized tumor cell lines (Staines et al., 1994), embryonic stem (ES) cells/induced pluripotent stem cell (iPS) cells (Bjorklund et al., 2002; Wei et al., 2005; Buhnemann et al., 2006) and ex vivo expanded cortex-derived iNSPCs (Nakagomi et al., 2009a; Nakagomi et al., 2009b; Nakano-Doi et al., 2010). Transplantation of exogenous NSPCs can be performed even at the chronic stage of post-stroke. In experimental models of stroke using fetal NSPCs, transplanted cells were reported to survive within the host brain, migrate into the injured area, and maintain their multipotency (Ishibashi et al., 2004; Kelly et al., 2004; Darsalia et al., 2007). However, there are some issues to be solved for clinical application of exogenous NSPC transplantation in stroke patients; e.g., survival, safety and suitability of transplanted cells, and their capacity to repair injured adult brain. Indeed, the other lines of experiment using NSPCs derived from adult mammalian brains showed that only a small population of grafted cells can survive in the injured brain (Toda *et al.*, 2001; Hicks *et al.*, 2007; Kameda *et al.*, 2007; Takahashi *et al.*, 2008). Consistent with these reports, we showed that the majority of transplanted iNSPCs, which are derived from the adult cortex, cannot survive in the injured cortex (Nakagomi *et al.*, 2009a).

A higher survival rate of transplanted NSPCs carrying the property of neoplasm (such as ES/iPS-derived NSPCs) can be expected, because survival is often attributed to a lack of apoptotic signaling. However, this property may be directly linked to a high risk of tumorigenesis. Whether the transplanted fetal NSPCs will be able to contribute to reconstitution of the adult brain is also an issue to be addressed, because they are the cells destined to form the infant brain. Therefore, we must achieve significant recovery of impaired neurological functions of the adult brain to determine the suitability of transplanted cells.

Our study showed that iNSPCs from the injured cortex differentiate into functional neurons with less tumorigenesis, suggesting that these cells are one of the most suitable NSPCs for transplantation. Therefore, we may choose alternative ways to continue the survival of transplanted iNSPCs. Recently, we reported that co-transplantation of iNSPCs with ECs as a vascular niche, enhances functional recovery after cortical infarction with longer survival of transplanted cells (Nakagomi *et al.*, 2009a). This suggests that the microenvironment around the transplants has to be considered for cell therapy. From another point of view, as differentiated cells are more resistant to apoptotic cell death, enhancing differentiation of NSPCs into mature neurons may be a choice in maintaining the transplant. Recent studies showed that transplantation of NSPCs with valproic acid, which inhibits proliferation but enhances differentiation of transplanted stem cells to functional neurons, significantly improves motor function in a spinal cord injury model (Abematsu *et al.*, 2010). These results may indicate a future direction for the clinical application of exogenous NSPC transplantation for patients after cerebral infarction.

Another problem regarding cell transplantation is the difficulty in regulating the differentiation of transplanted NSPCs *in vivo*. It is well-known that a variety of chemical mediators/cytokines are produced/activated at the site of brain injury, and among these, IL-6, CNTF, and BMPs promote differentiation of NSPCs into the astrocytic phenotype (Nakashima *et al.*, 1999; Okada *et al.*, 2004). Our previous studies showed that transplanted iNSPCs largely differentiated into glial cells *in vivo*, although they predominantly differentiated into neuronal cells *in vitro* (Nakagomi *et al.*, 2009a). These results suggest that the neurogenesis-oriented regulation of transplanted iNSPCs might accomplish a real functional restoration of stroke patients in the future.

3. Conclusion

In conclusion, we demonstrated that iNSPCs, which are the potential cell sources for neocortical neurogenesis, develop in the murine post-stroke cortex (Nakagomi *et al.*, 2009a; Nakagomi *et al.*, 2009b; Nakano-Doi *et al.*, 2010; Saino *et al.*, 2010). Furthermore, we demonstrat that iNSPCs develop within the post-stroke pia mater, suggesting that pia mater is an important target for cortical neurogenesis. In the field of cardiology, accumulating evidence has shown that cardiac stem/progenitor cells reside in epicardium, termed as "epicardial progenitor cells" (Zhou *et al.*, 2008; Smart *et al.*, 2011). These findings may raise a possibility that stem/progenitor cells are present in the surface of multiple organs as well as those observed in the brain and heart. In addition, deposition of several materials including cell sheets onto infarcted heart could improve cardiac repair and functions after myocardial infarction (Zakharova *et al.*; Miyahara *et al.*, 2006; Derval *et al.*, 2008). Thus, patches of cell sheets carrying bioactive substances on post-stroke pia mater may promote cortical repair/neurogenesis without parenchymal damage, due to the intracerebral approach of cell transplantation.

In the past, cerebral infarction was believed to be a region occupied only by necrotic tissue and inflammatory cells. However, we detected viable cells with the capacity for proliferation, differentiation, and multipotency within the post-stroke cortex and pia mater in an experimental murine model of ischemic stroke. Because similar iNSPCs were detected in the post-stroke human cortex (Nakayama *et al.*, 2010), further investigation will establish novel therapeutic neurogenesis for stroke patients by iNSPCs.

4. Acknowledgement

Our series of studies were partially supported by a Grant-in-Aid for Scientific Research from the Ministry of Education, Culture, Sports, Science and Technology [(18800071 and 21700363; to T. Nakagomi) and (21500359; to T. Matsuyama)], Hyogo Science and Technology Association (2009), Takeda Science Foundation (2009) and Grant-in-Aid for Researchers, Hyogo College of Medicine (2006 and 2011). We would like to thank Dr. A. Nakano-Doi, Y. Okinaka, Y. Tanaka, Y. Tatsumi, Dr. O. Saino, Dr. Y. Momota, Dr. M. Takata, Dr. N. Nakagomi, Y. Kasahara, Dr. A. Taguchi and Prof. Z. Molnár for helpful assistances.

5. References

Abematsu, M., Tsujimura, K., Yamano, M., et al (2010) Neurons derived from transplanted neural stem cells restore disrupted neuronal circuitry in a mouse model of spinal cord injury. *J Clin Invest*, 120, 3255-3266.

Aihara, Y., Hayashi, Y., Hirata, M., et al (2010) Induction of neural crest cells from mouse embryonic stem cells in a serum-free monolayer culture. *Int J Dev Biol*, 54, 1287-1294.

Alvarez-Buylla, A. & Garcia-Verdugo, J.M. (2002) Neurogenesis in adult subventricular zone. *J Neurosci*, 22, 629-634.

Arsenijevic, Y., Villemure, J.G., Brunet, J.F., et al (2001) Isolation of multipotent neural precursors residing in the cortex of the adult human brain. *Exp Neurol*, 170, 48-62.

Bifari, F., Decimo, I., Chiamulera, C., et al (2009) Novel stem/progenitor cells with neuronal differentiation potential reside in the leptomeningeal niche. *J Cell Mol Med*, 13, 3195-3208.

Billon, N., Jolicoeur, C., Ying, Q.L., et al (2002) Normal timing of oligodendrocyte development from genetically engineered, lineage-selectable mouse ES cells. *J Cell Sci*, 115, 3657-3665.

Bjorklund, L.M., Sanchez-Pernaute, R., Chung, S., et al (2002) Embryonic stem cells develop into functional dopaminergic neurons after transplantation in a Parkinson rat model. *Proc Natl Acad Sci U S A*, 99, 2344-2349.

Buhnemann, C., Scholz, A., Bernreuther, C., et al (2006) Neuronal differentiation of transplanted embryonic stem cell-derived precursors in stroke lesions of adult rats. *Brain*, 129, 3238-3248.

Bull, N.D. & Bartlett, P.F. (2005) The adult mouse hippocampal progenitor is neurogenic but not a stem cell. *J Neurosci*, 25, 10815-10821.

Carlen, M., Meletis, K., Goritz, C., et al (2009) Forebrain ependymal cells are Notch-dependent and generate neuroblasts and astrocytes after stroke. *Nat Neurosci*, 12, 259-267.

Cayre, M., Bancila, M., Virard, I., et al (2006) Migrating and myelinating potential of subventricular zone neural progenitor cells in white matter tracts of the adult rodent brain. *Mol Cell Neurosci*, 31, 748-758.

Chen, J., Li, Y., Katakowski, M., et al (2003) Intravenous bone marrow stromal cell therapy reduces apoptosis and promotes endogenous cell proliferation after stroke in female rat. *J Neurosci Res*, 73, 778-786.

Chen, Y., Balasubramaniyan, V., Peng, J., et al (2007) Isolation and culture of rat and mouse oligodendrocyte precursor cells. *Nat Protoc*, 2, 1044-1051.

Chojnacki, A.K., Mak, G.K. & Weiss, S. (2009) Identity crisis for adult periventricular neural stem cells: subventricular zone astrocytes, ependymal cells or both? *Nat Rev Neurosci*, 10, 153-163.

Clausen, M., Nakagomi, T., Nakano-Doi, A., et al. (2011) Ischemia-induced neural stem/progenitor cells express pyramidal cells markers. Neuroreport, 22, 789-794.

Coskun, V., Wu, H., Blanchi, B., et al (2008) CD133+ neural stem cells in the ependyma of mammalian postnatal forebrain. *Proc Natl Acad Sci U S A*, 105, 1026-1031.

Crisan, M., Chen, C.W., Corselli, M., et al (2009) Perivascular multipotent progenitor cells in human organs. *Ann N Y Acad Sci*, 1176, 118-123.

Danilov, A.I., Gomes-Leal, W., Ahlenius, H., et al (2009) Ultrastructural and antigenic properties of neural stem cells and their progeny in adult rat subventricular zone. *Glia*, 57, 136-152.

Darsalia, V., Kallur, T. & Kokaia, Z. (2007) Survival, migration and neuronal differentiation of human fetal striatal and cortical neural stem cells grafted in stroke-damaged rat striatum. *Eur J Neurosci*, 26, 605-614.

Derval, N., Barandon, L., Dufourcq, P., et al (2008) Epicardial deposition of endothelial progenitor and mesenchymal stem cells in a coated muscle patch after myocardial infarction in a murine model. *Eur J Cardiothorac Surg*, 34, 248-254.

Dezawa, M., Kanno, H., Hoshino, M., et al (2004) Specific induction of neuronal cells from bone marrow stromal cells and application for autologous transplantation. *J Clin Invest*, 113, 1701-1710.

Doetsch, F., Caille, I., Lim, D.A., et al (1999) Subventricular zone astrocytes are neural stem cells in the adult mammalian brain. *Cell*, 97, 703-716.

Dore-Duffy, P., Katychev, A., Wang, X., et al (2006) CNS microvascular pericytes exhibit multipotential stem cell activity. *J Cereb Blood Flow Metab*, 26, 613-624.

Etchevers, H.C., Vincent, C., Le Douarin, N.M., et al (2001) The cephalic neural crest provides pericytes and smooth muscle cells to all blood vessels of the face and forebrain. *Development*, 128, 1059-1068.

Gaughwin, P.M., Caldwell, M.A., Anderson, J.M., et al (2006) Astrocytes promote neurogenesis from oligodendrocyte precursor cells. *Eur J Neurosci*, 23, 945-956.

Goings, G.E., Sahni, V. & Szele, F.G. (2004) Migration patterns of subventricular zone cells in adult mice change after cerebral cortex injury. *Brain Res*, 996, 213-226.

Hall, A., Giese, N.A. & Richardson, W.D. (1996) Spinal cord oligodendrocytes develop from ventrally derived progenitor cells that express PDGF alpha-receptors. *Development*, 122, 4085-4094.

Hamano, K., Li, T.S., Kobayashi, T., et al (2000) Angiogenesis induced by the implantation of self-bone marrow cells: a new material for therapeutic angiogenesis. *Cell Transplant*, 9, 439-443.

Hicks, A.U., Hewlett, K., Windle, V., et al (2007) Enriched environment enhances transplanted subventricular zone stem cell migration and functional recovery after stroke. *Neuroscience*, 146, 31-40.

Hutchings, M. & Weller, R.O. (1986) Anatomical relationships of the pia mater to cerebral blood vessels in man. *J Neurosurg*, 65, 316-325.

Ishibashi, S., Sakaguchi, M., Kuroiwa, T., et al (2004) Human neural stem/progenitor cells, expanded in long-term neurosphere culture, promote functional recovery after focal ischemia in Mongolian gerbils. *J Neurosci Res*, 78, 215-223.

Jiang, W., Gu, W., Brannstrom, T., et al (2001) Cortical neurogenesis in adult rats after transient middle cerebral artery occlusion. *Stroke*, 32, 1201-1207.

Jiao, J. & Chen, D.F. (2008) Induction of neurogenesis in nonconventional neurogenic regions of the adult central nervous system by niche astrocyte-produced signals. *Stem Cells*, 26, 1221-1230.

Jin, K., Wang, X., Xie, L., et al (2006) Evidence for stroke-induced neurogenesis in the human brain. *Proc Natl Acad Sci U S A*, 103, 13198-13202.

Joh, T., Sasaki, M., Kataoka, H., et al (2005) Helicobacter pylori eradication decreases the expression of glycosylphosphatidylinositol-anchored complement regulators, decay-accelerating factor and homologous restriction factor 20, in human gastric epithelium. *J Gastroenterol Hepatol*, 20, 1344-1351.

Kallur, T., Darsalia, V., Lindvall, O., et al (2006) Human fetal cortical and striatal neural stem cells generate region-specific neurons in vitro and differentiate extensively to neurons after intrastriatal transplantation in neonatal rats. *Journal of neuroscience research*, 84, 1630-1644.

Kameda, M., Shingo, T., Takahashi, K., et al (2007) Adult neural stem and progenitor cells modified to secrete GDNF can protect, migrate and integrate after intracerebral transplantation in rats with transient forebrain ischemia. *Eur J Neurosci*, 26, 1462-1478.

Kelly, S., Bliss, T.M., Shah, A.K., et al (2004) Transplanted human fetal neural stem cells survive, migrate, and differentiate in ischemic rat cerebral cortex. *Proc Natl Acad Sci U S A*, 101, 11839-11844.

Kim, H., Park, J.S., Choi, Y.J., et al (2009a) Bone Marrow Mononuclear Cells Have Neurovascular Tropism and Improve Diabetic Neuropathy. *Stem Cells*, 27, 1686-1696.

Kim, J.B., Sebastiano, V., Wu, G., et al (2009b) Oct4-induced pluripotency in adult neural stem cells. *Cell*, 136, 411-419.

Kondo, T. & Raff, M. (2000) Oligodendrocyte precursor cells reprogrammed to become multipotential CNS stem cells. *Science*, 289, 1754-1757.

Kriegstein, A. & Alvarez-Buylla, A. (2009) The glial nature of embryonic and adult neural stem cells. *Annu Rev Neurosci*, 32, 149-184.

Kuhn, H.G., Dickinson-Anson, H. & Gage, F.H. (1996) Neurogenesis in the dentate gyrus of the adult rat: age-related decrease of neuronal progenitor proliferation. *J Neurosci*, 16, 2027-2033.

Kurozumi, K., Nakamura, K., Tamiya, T., et al (2005) Mesenchymal stem cells that produce neurotrophic factors reduce ischemic damage in the rat middle cerebral artery occlusion model. *Mol Ther*, 11, 96-104.

Labouyrie, E., Dubus, P., Groppi, A., et al (1999) Expression of neurotrophins and their receptors in human bone marrow. *Am J Pathol*, 154, 405-415.

Li, T.S., Furutani, A., Takahashi, M., et al (2006) Impaired potency of bone marrow mononuclear cells for inducing therapeutic angiogenesis in obese diabetic rats. *Am J Physiol Heart Circ Physiol*, 290, H1362-1369.

Li, W.Y., Choi, Y.J., Lee, P.H., et al (2008) Mesenchymal stem cells for ischemic stroke: changes in effects after ex vivo culturing. *Cell Transplant*, 17, 1045-1059.

Li, Y., Chopp, M., Zhang, Z.G., et al (1995) Expression of glial fibrillary acidic protein in areas of focal cerebral ischemia accompanies neuronal expression of 72-kDa heat shock protein. *J Neurol Sci*, 128, 134-142.

Lim, D.A. & Alvarez-Buylla, A. (1999) Interaction between astrocytes and adult subventricular zone precursors stimulates neurogenesis. *Proc Natl Acad Sci U S A*, 96, 7526-7531.

Louissaint, A., Jr., Rao, S., Leventhal, C., et al (2002) Coordinated interaction of neurogenesis and angiogenesis in the adult songbird brain. *Neuron*, 34, 945-960.

Magavi, S.S., Leavitt, B.R. & Macklis, J.D. (2000) Induction of neurogenesis in the neocortex of adult mice. *Nature*, 405, 951-955.

Mahmood, A., Lu, D. & Chopp, M. (2004) Intravenous administration of marrow stromal cells (MSCs) increases the expression of growth factors in rat brain after traumatic brain injury. *J Neurotrauma*, 21, 33-39.

Mignone, J.L., Kukekov, V., Chiang, A.S., et al (2004) Neural stem and progenitor cells in nestin-GFP transgenic mice. *J Comp Neurol*, 469, 311-324.

Miyahara, Y., Nagaya, N., Kataoka, M., et al (2006) Monolayered mesenchymal stem cells repair scarred myocardium after myocardial infarction. *Nat Med*, 12, 459-465.

Moreno-Manzano, V., Rodriguez-Jimenez, F.J., Garcia-Rosello, M., et al (2009) Activated spinal cord ependymal stem cells rescue neurological function. *Stem Cells*, 27, 733-743.

Morse, D.E. & Cova, J.L. (1984) Pigmented cells in the leptomeninges of the cat. *Anat Rec*, 210, 125-132.

Nagoshi, N., Shibata, S., Nakamura, M., et al (2009) Neural crest-derived stem cells display a wide variety of characteristics. *J Cell Biochem*, 107, 1046-1052.

Nakagomi, N., Nakagomi, T., Kubo, S., et al (2009a) Endothelial cells support survival, proliferation, and neuronal differentiation of transplanted adult ischemia-induced neural stem/progenitor cells after cerebral infarction. *Stem Cells*, 27, 2185-2195.

Nakagomi, T., Molnár, Z., Nakano-Doi, A., et al (2011) Ischemia-induced neural stem/progenitor cells in the pia mater following cortical infarction. *Stem Cells and Development*, 20, 2037-2051.

Nakagomi, T., Taguchi, A., Fujimori, Y., et al (2009b) Isolation and characterization of neural stem/progenitor cells from post-stroke cerebral cortex in mice. *Eur J Neurosci*, 29, 1842-1852.

Nakano-Doi, A., Nakagomi, T., Fujikawa, M., et al (2010) Bone Marrow Mononuclear Cells Promote Proliferation of Endogenous Neural Stem Cells Through Vascular Niches After Cerebral Infarction. *Stem Cells*, 28, 1292-1302.

Nakashima, K., Yanagisawa, M., Arakawa, H., et al (1999) Synergistic signaling in fetal brain by STAT3-Smad1 complex bridged by p300. *Science*, 284, 479-482.

Nakayama, D., Matsuyama, T., Ishibashi-Ueda, H., et al (2010) Injury-induced neural stem/progenitor cells in post-stroke human cerebral cortex. *Eur J Neurosci*, 31, 90-98.

Nunes, M.C., Roy, N.S., Keyoung, H.M., et al (2003) Identification and isolation of multipotential neural progenitor cells from the subcortical white matter of the adult human brain. *Nat Med*, 9, 439-447.

Ohira, K., Furuta, T., Hioki, H., et al (2010) Ischemia-induced neurogenesis of neocortical layer 1 progenitor cells. *Nat Neurosci*, 13, 173-179.

Okada, S., Nakamura, M., Mikami, Y., et al (2004) Blockade of interleukin-6 receptor suppresses reactive astrogliosis and ameliorates functional recovery in experimental spinal cord injury. *J Neurosci Res*, 76, 265-276.

Oki, K., Kaneko, N., Kanki, H., et al (2010) Musashi1 as a marker of reactive astrocytes after transient focal brain ischemia. *Neurosci Res*, 66, 390-395.

Palmer, T.D., Willhoite, A.R. & Gage, F.H. (2000) Vascular niche for adult hippocampal neurogenesis. *J Comp Neurol*, 425, 479-494.

Parr, A.M., Kulbatski, I., Zahir, T., et al (2008) Transplanted adult spinal cord-derived neural stem/progenitor cells promote early functional recovery after rat spinal cord injury. *Neuroscience*, 155, 760-770.

Pfenninger, C.V., Roschupkina, T., Hertwig, F., et al (2007) CD133 is not present on neurogenic astrocytes in the adult subventricular zone, but on embryonic neural stem cells, ependymal cells, and glioblastoma cells. *Cancer Res*, 67, 5727-5736.

Reynolds, B.A. & Weiss, S. (1992) Generation of neurons and astrocytes from isolated cells of the adult mammalian central nervous system. *Science*, 255, 1707-1710.

Ribeiro-Resende, V.T., Pimentel-Coelho, P.M., Mesentier-Louro, L.A., et al (2009) Trophic activity derived from bone marrow mononuclear cells increases peripheral nerve regeneration by acting on both neuronal and glial cell populations. *Neuroscience*, 159, 540-549.

Richardson, W.D., Young, K.M., Tripathi, R.B., et al (2011) NG2-glia as Multipotent Neural Stem Cells: Fact or Fantasy? *Neuron*, 70, 661-673.

Saino, O., Taguchi, A., Nakagomi, T., et al (2010) Immunodeficiency reduces neural stem/progenitor cell apoptosis and enhances neurogenesis in the cerebral cortex after stroke. *J Neurosci Res*, 88, 2385-2397.

Shen, Q., Goderie, S.K., Jin, L., et al (2004) Endothelial cells stimulate self-renewal and expand neurogenesis of neural stem cells. *Science*, 304, 1338-1340.

Shen, Q., Wang, Y., Kokovay, E., et al (2008) Adult SVZ stem cells lie in a vascular niche: a quantitative analysis of niche cell-cell interactions. *Cell Stem Cell*, 3, 289-300.

Shimada, I.S., Peterson, B.M. & Spees, J.L. (2010) Isolation of locally derived stem/progenitor cells from the peri-infarct area that do not migrate from the lateral ventricle after cortical stroke. *Stroke*, 41, e552-560.

Siegenthaler, J.A., Ashique, A.M., Zarbalis, K., et al (2009) Retinoic acid from the meninges regulates cortical neuron generation. *Cell*, 139, 597-609.

Sirko, S., Neitz, A., Mittmann, T., et al (2009) Focal laser-lesions activate an endogenous population of neural stem/progenitor cells in the adult visual cortex. *Brain*, 132, 2252-2264.

Smart, N., Bollini, S., Dube, K.N., et al (2011) De novo cardiomyocytes from within the activated adult heart after injury. *Nature*, 474, 640-644.

Sockanathan, S. & Gaiano, N. (2009) Preview. Meninges Play a RAdical Role in Embryonic Neural Stem Cell Regulation. *Cell Stem Cell*, 5, 455-456.

Song, H., Stevens, C.F. & Gage, F.H. (2002) Astroglia induce neurogenesis from adult neural stem cells. *Nature*, 417, 39-44.

Staines, W.A., Morassutti, D.J., Reuhl, K.R., et al (1994) Neurons derived from P19 embryonal carcinoma cells have varied morphologies and neurotransmitters. *Neuroscience*, 58, 735-751.

Stallcup, W.B. & Beasley, L. (1987) Bipotential glial precursor cells of the optic nerve express the NG2 proteoglycan. *J Neurosci*, 7, 2737-2744.

Sundberg, M., Skottman, H., Suuronen, R., et al (2010) Production and isolation of NG2+ oligodendrocyte precursors from human embryonic stem cells in defined serum-free medium. *Stem Cell Res*, 5, 91-103.

Taguchi, A., Kasahara, Y., Nakagomi, T., et al (2010) A Reproducible and Simple Model of Permanent Cerebral Ischemia in CB-17 and SCID Mice. *J Exp Stroke Transl Med*, 3, 28-33.

Taguchi, A., Soma, T., Tanaka, H., et al (2004) Administration of CD34+ cells after stroke enhances neurogenesis via angiogenesis in a mouse model. *J Clin Invest*, 114, 330-338.

Taguchi, A., Wen, Z., Myojin, K., et al (2007) Granulocyte colony-stimulating factor has a negative effect on stroke outcome in a murine model. *Eur J Neurosci*, 26, 126-133.

Takahashi, K., Yasuhara, T., Shingo, T., et al (2008) Embryonic neural stem cells transplanted in middle cerebral artery occlusion model of rats demonstrated potent therapeutic effects, compared to adult neural stem cells. *Brain Res*, 1234, 172-182.

Takata, M., Nakagomi, T., Kashiwamura, S., et al. (2011) Glucocorticoid-induced TNF receptor-triggered T cells are key modulators for survival/death of neural stem/progenitor cells induced by ischemic stroke. Cell death and Differentiation, in press.

Tavazoie, M., Van der Veken, L., Silva-Vargas, V., et al (2008) A specialized vascular niche for adult neural stem cells. *Cell stem cell*, 3, 279-288.

Teng, H., Zhang, Z.G., Wang, L., et al (2008) Coupling of angiogenesis and neurogenesis in cultured endothelial cells and neural progenitor cells after stroke. *J Cereb Blood Flow Metab*, 28, 764-771.

Teng, L. & Labosky, P.A. (2006) Neural crest stem cells. *Adv Exp Med Biol*, 589, 206-212.

Toda, H., Takahashi, J., Iwakami, N., et al (2001) Grafting neural stem cells improved the impaired spatial recognition in ischemic rats. *Neurosci Lett*, 316, 9-12.

Ulrich, R., Seeliger, F., Kreutzer, M., et al (2008) Limited remyelination in Theiler's murine encephalomyelitis due to insufficient oligodendroglial differentiation of nerve/glial antigen 2 (NG2)-positive putative oligodendroglial progenitor cells. *Neuropathol Appl Neurobiol*, 34, 603-620.

Wei, L., Cui, L., Snider, B.J., et al (2005) Transplantation of embryonic stem cells overexpressing Bcl-2 promotes functional recovery after transient cerebral ischemia. *Neurobiol Dis*, 19, 183-193.

Weiss, S., Dunne, C., Hewson, J., et al (1996) Multipotent CNS stem cells are present in the adult mammalian spinal cord and ventricular neuroaxis. *J Neurosci*, 16, 7599-7609.

Willaime-Morawek, S. & van der Kooy, D. (2008) Cortex- and striatum- derived neural stem cells produce distinct progeny in the olfactory bulb and striatum. *The European journal of neuroscience*, 27, 2354-2362.

Xue, J.H., Yanamoto, H., Nakajo, Y., et al (2009) Induced spreading depression evokes cell division of astrocytes in the subpial zone, generating neural precursor-like cells and new immature neurons in the adult cerebral cortex. *Stroke*, 40, e606-613.

Yang, Z., Covey, M.V., Bitel, C.L., et al (2007) Sustained neocortical neurogenesis after neonatal hypoxic/ischemic injury. *Ann Neurol*, 61, 199-208.

Yokoyama, A., Sakamoto, A., Kameda, K., et al (2006) NG2 proteoglycan-expressing microglia as multipotent neural progenitors in normal and pathologic brains. *Glia*, 53, 754-768.

Yoo, S.W., Kim, S.S., Lee, S.Y., et al (2008) Mesenchymal stem cells promote proliferation of endogenous neural stem cells and survival of newborn cells in a rat stroke model. *Exp Mol Med*, 40, 387-397.

Zakharova, L., Mastroeni, D., Mutlu, N., et al Transplantation of cardiac progenitor cell sheet onto infarcted heart promotes cardiogenesis and improves function. *Cardiovasc Res.*

Zawadzka, M., Rivers, L.E., Fancy, S.P., et al (2010) CNS-resident glial progenitor/stem cells produce Schwann cells as well as oligodendrocytes during repair of CNS demyelination. *Cell Stem Cell*, 6, 578-590.

Zhou, B., Ma, Q., Rajagopal, S., et al (2008) Epicardial progenitors contribute to the cardiomyocyte lineage in the developing heart. *Nature*, 454, 109-113.

6

Assessing the Influence of Neuroinflammation on Neurogenesis: *In Vitro* Models Using Neural Stem Cells and Microglia as Valuable Research Tools

Bruno P. Carreira[1], Maria Inês Morte[1],
Caetana M. Carvalho[1] and Inês M. Araújo[1,2]
[1]*Center for Neuroscience and Cell Biology, Neuroendocrinology and Neurogenesis Group,
University of Coimbra, Coimbra,*
[2]*Regenerative Medicine Program, Department of Biomedical Sciences and Medicine
University of Algarve, Faro,
Portugal*

1. Introduction

1.1 Neural stem cells

Neural stem cells are localized in two limited regions of the adult mammalian brain: the subgranular zone of the dentate gyrus (DG) of the hippocampus, a cell layer located between the granule cell layer and the hilus (Eriksson *et al.*, 1998; Limke and Rao, 2002), and the subventricular zone (SVZ), located next to the ependyma of the lateral walls of the lateral ventricles (Doetsch and Scharff, 2001; Curtis *et al.*, 2007). These regions are thought to provide a specific microenvironment, the stem cell niche, characterized by the presence of several agents involved in the maintenance of self-renewal and/or multipotency of neural stem cells (Alvarez-Buylla and Lim, 2004).

Although neurogenesis has been intensively studied over the past decades, only recently it has been established that newly formed neurons in the adult mammalian brain are functional and integrate into the existing neuronal network (Carlen *et al.*, 2002). The several stages of adult neurogenesis include proliferation of adult neural stem cells, fate determination, migration, integration and maturation of the newborn neurons. Using specific cell markers it is possible to independently investigate the different phases of development. Hippocampal neurogenesis plays an important role in normal hippocampal function, learning and memory (Gould *et al.*, 1999a; Shors *et al.*, 2001; Drapeau *et al.*, 2007). Newborn cells emerging from the SVZ migrate through the rostral migratory stream and integrate into the neuronal network of the olfactory bulb, establish functional synaptic connections and develop electrophysiological properties of mature neurons (Carlen *et al.*, 2002; Petreanu and Alvarez-Buylla, 2002; Belluzzi *et al.*, 2003). Furthermore, neurogenesis in the olfactory bulb is involved in important functions such as odor memory and discrimination (Gheusi *et al.*, 2000; Rochefort *et al.*, 2002; Shingo *et al.*, 2003). Under physiological conditions, neural stem cells are tightly controlled contributing for the maintenance of brain homeostasis (Morshead et al., 1994; Morshead et al., 1998), however they seem to be also involved in neuronal replacement in response to pathophysiological conditions, particularly in conditions associated with neuroinflammation. Although little is known about the molecular mechanisms involved in the regulation of neural stem cells, several factors, both intrinsic and extrinsic, have been described to modulate the neurogenic process, such as hormones, trophic factors, neurotransmitters, neuromodulators and glial cells (for review see Ming and Song, 2005).

The existence of neurogenesis in areas beyond the SVZ and the DG of the adult mammalian brain have also been reported, namely in the neocortex (Gould et al., 1999b; Dayer et al., 2005), striatum, amygdala (Bernier et al., 2002), hypothalamus (Gould et al., 2001; Xu et al., 2005), mesencephalon (Zhao et al., 2003) and spinal cord (Yamamoto et al., 2001). However, these findings need further experimental support, thus more studies need to be conducted.

1.2 Neuroinflammation

The central nervous system (CNS) was considered an immunologically privileged site, not susceptible to immune activation, due to its protection by the blood-brain barrier, which selectively allows certain inflammatory agents to enter and/or exit (Lucas et al., 2006). Nowadays it is well established that immune surveillance takes place in the CNS due to the selective permeability of the blood-brain barrier to immune cells such as T cells, macrophages and dendritic cells (Hickey, 1999). Following injury or exposure to pathogens, an inflammatory response is driven by the activation of two types of immune cells: CNS resident cells, such as microglial cells and astrocytes, and CNS infiltrating cells, such as lymphocytes, monocytes and macrophages from the hematopoietic system (Stoll and Jander, 1999; Streit et al., 1999). The activation of immune cells leads to the production and release of a plethora of regulatory substances, like cytokines, chemokines, neurotransmitters, reactive oxygen species and reactive nitrogen species (reviewed by Whitney et al., 2009). These inflammatory mediators are essential for the recruitment of immune cells, particularly microglial cells, but also for changing the permeability of the blood-brain barrier and recruitment of monocytes and lymphocytes from the hematopoietic system to the compromised area (Hickey, 1999; Lossinsky and Shivers, 2004; Taupin, 2008), which creates a positive feedback loop to the inflammatory response.

Microglia, frequently referred to as the resident macrophages of the brain parenchyma, play a central role in the inflammatory response. Unlike astrocytes, oligodendrocytes and ependymal cells, microglial cells derive from the mesodermal germ layer. During adult life, the microglial cell pool is renewed by division of CNS resident cells. Moreover, microglia are distributed throughout the CNS with distinct densities (Lawson et al., 1990). In the healthy brain, microglia are present in a resting state assuming a typical and dynamic morphology, whose function has been clarified by different studies (Davalos et al., 2005; Nimmerjahn et al., 2005; Davalos et al., 2008). This resting state consists of a constant surveillance activity of the brain parenchyma, which enables microglial cells to screen different brain regions without disturbing the neuronal network (Hanisch and Kettenmann, 2007). Therefore, microglial cells can rapidly react to subtle homeostatic variations by changing morphology and acquiring an array of functions that allow the targeted migration into a site of injury and release of inflammatory mediators (Gehrmann, 1996; Kreutzberg, 1996; Haynes et al., 2006). Reactive microglia have the ability to rapidly upregulate a large number of receptor types, like cytokine receptors, toll-like receptors or cell adhesion molecules, but also to release a plethora of inflammatory agents (for review see Block and Hong, 2005). In fact, chemokines released by reactive microglial cells attract more microglia that, following activation, contribute to further propagate the neuroinflammatory event (Whitney et al., 2009).

Astrocytes constitute the majority of glial cells in the CNS, and play an important structural function, providing support for neurons, playing also regulatory functions, including maintenance of extracellular ion balance, signaling to neurons, repair and scarring process of the CNS (Svendsen, 2002). During inflammation, astrocytes also become activated and release inflammatory factors, growth factors and excitatory amino acids, such as glutamate, which are involved in the regulation of the inflammatory response (Song et al., 2002).

1.3 Neuroinflammation and neurogenesis

Neuroinflammation is a complex event with different outcomes in the neurogenic process, which can therefore enhance or suppress neurogenesis. The secreted products during inflammation have been shown to act as pro- or anti-neurogenic agents, contributing to beneficial or detrimental outcomes of neuroinflammation on the different steps of neurogenesis. Moreover, these effects seem to be particularly dependent on how and for how long microglial cells are activated. Inflammation and microglia activation were initially thought to inhibit adult neurogenesis (Ekdahl et al., 2003; Monje et al., 2003), while recent evidence indicates that microglia under certain circumstances can support neurogenic events (reviewed by Hanisch and Kettenmann, 2007). It has been suggested that mediators released by reactive microglia, such as cytokines and nitric oxide (NO), can inhibit adult neurogenesis in inflammatory conditions (Vallieres et al., 2002; Monje et al., 2003; Liu et al., 2006). On the other hand, neurogenesis seems to be induced by microglial cells activated by IL-4 or low level of IFN-gamma, which has been associated with increased neuroprotection (Wong et al., 2004; Song et al., 2005; Baron et al., 2008). Moreover, some inflammatory mediators like NO seem to have opposite roles in regulating neurogenesis in inflammatory conditions (Carreira et al., 2010). Apparently, microglial cells and the factors they release play a dual role in neurogenesis acting as antiproliferative or proliferative agents. Indeed, self-renewal, proliferation, migration, differentiation, integration and, more importantly, survival of newborn neurons is modulated by the local microenvironment characterizing the neuroinflammatory response. Neural stem cells become "activated" following brain injury and migrate into the lesioned areas, which suggests that mediators present in the inflammatory microenvironment can guide the migration of newborn cells (Arvidsson et al., 2002; Nakatomi et al., 2002).

The role of neuroinflammation in regulating neurogenesis and neuroprotection is not clear yet, and is the subject of numerous studies (for comprehensive review see Whitney et al., 2009; and Gonzalez-Perez et al., 2010). There is, however, evidence for some of the most important mediators of the inflammatory response in their role in the regulation of neurogenesis and neuroprotection (Table 1).

Inflammatory factor	Neurogenesis	Neuroprotection	References
IFN-gamma	Pro-neurogenic	Decreased	(Ben-Hur et al., 2003; Wong et al., 2004; Butovsky et al., 2006; Johansson et al., 2008)
Interleukin-6	Anti-neurogenic	Decreased	(Ekdahl et al., 2003; Liu et al., 2005; Nakanishi et al., 2007; Koo and Duman, 2008; Bauer, 2009; Islam et al., 2009)
Interleukin-18			
Nitric oxide	Anti-neurogenic (nNOS) Pro-astrogliogenic (iNOS)	Decreased	(Contestabile et al., 2003; Moreno-Lopez et al., 2004; Matarredona et al., 2005; Ciani et al., 2006; Covacu et al., 2006; Fritzen et al., 2007; Luo et al., 2007; Carreira et al., 2010)
TNF-alpha	Anti-neurogenic (TNF-R1) Pro-neurogenic (TNF-R2)	Decreased or Increased	(Ben-Hur et al., 2003; Wong et al., 2004; Cacci et al., 2005; Heldmann et al., 2005; Liu et al., 2005; Iosif et al., 2006; Bernardino et al., 2008)

Table 1. Effect of some inflammatory factors on neurogenesis and their neuroprotective role.

We are only beginning to understand how inflammatory factors and microglial cells influence neurogenesis in an inflammatory scenario, and the mechanisms, function and modulation of neurogenesis during inflammation require further investigation. This field of work is of particular interest for a better understanding of the mechanisms underlying the effects of neuroinflammation on neurogenesis, and further studies need to be conducted to increase the potential therapeutic value of regulating neuroinflammation in cellular regeneration in the diseased brain.

1.4 Brain repair and stem cell based therapies

Repair of damaged tissues is essential for the survival of living organisms. Each tissue or organ has an intrinsic, albeit limited ability for the replacement of dead cells, and correct integration of the newborn cells that, ideally, should restore the original structure. Cell replacement and correct integration of the newborn cells in the CNS is not so efficient as in other tissues such as skin or bone, which present a higher cell turnover. The CNS, on the other hand, has weak capabilities for both endogenous cell replacement and pattern repair. Some approaches have been used to attempt to develop therapeutic strategies for brain repair, namely transplantation of neural stem cells, stimulation of endogenous neurogenesis, neuroprotective strategies and anti-inflammatory approaches.

Transplantation of neural stem cells is one of the promising methods in study to be used in the reconstruction of neuronal circuits. However, the cells to be transplanted should be phenotypically plastic and able to proliferate *ex vivo* in response to external stimulus (Wang et al., 1998; Sheen et al., 1999). Intracerebral transplantation of SVZ-derived neural stem cells has been successfully used in experimental models of Parkinson's disease (Zigova et al., 1998; Richardson et al., 2005), Huntington's disease (Vazey et al., 2006), and in Multiple Sclerosis (Cayre et al., 2006). Cell replacement could also be achieved by inducing endogenous neural stem cells to differentiate into neurons in the adult CNS, which consists in a less invasive strategy when compared to cell transplantation.

Indeed, in situ stimulation of endogenous adult neural stem cells and modulation of injury-induced neurogenesis is a therapeutic strategy, developed to upregulate endogenous neurogenesis, for instance through the control of the inflammatory response in a safe and efficient way. This approach seems to be a more advantageous strategy for multifocal diseases such as Alzheimer's disease, when compared to grafting strategies. Therefore, increased neurogenesis has been achieved by different strategies, such as administration of mitotic agents or trophic factors (Craig et al., 1996; Kuhn et al., 1997; Zigova et al., 1998), treatment with neuroleptics like olanzepine (Green et al., 2006), administration of NO donors or 5-phosphodiesterase inhibitors (Zhang et al., 2003; Imitola et al., 2004; Sun et al., 2004; Sun et al., 2006).

Other strategies designed to improve brain repair are being investigated, such as neuroprotective approaches consisting in the administration of radical scavengers, apoptosis inhibitors, neurotrophic agents, metal ions chelators and gene therapy, which seem to be useful to limit injury-induced lesion, but also for the enhancement of the survival of newborn cells (Polazzi and Monti, 2010). The use of anti-inflammatory drugs as a strategy to promote neurogenesis has also been explored and, although the chronic use of nonsteroidal anti-inflammatory drugs is detrimental for the gastrointestinal tract, it has also been associated with a decreased risk for neurodegenerative diseases (McGeer and McGeer, 1995; Lim et al., 2000; Chen et al., 2003). In fact, control of the inflammatory response seems to be an important strategy to increase proliferation of neural stem cells and/or differentiation of newborn neurons.

Strategies to promote regeneration of lesioned areas or cell replacement therapies will have to take into account the effects of inflammation on the formation and survival of newly generated neurons, either from the brain's own pool of neural stem cells, or from transplanted neural stem cells. Thus, the understanding of the mechanisms underlying the effect of neuroinflammation in proliferation, fate determination, migration and differentiation of neural stem cells is the first step in the development of specific strategies that could target the deleterious effect of inflammation in neurogenesis. Since the neuroinflammatory event is mostly characterized by the activation of resident microglial cells, the use of in vitro models that allow the study of the effects of microglia activation in the modulation of neural stem cells proliferation, fate determination, migration and differentiation into neurons is of high importance for the development of therapeutic strategies.

2. In vitro models to assess the crosstalk of neurogenesis and neuroinflammation

In vitro culture systems are critical tools for the study of various aspects related to the mechanisms that regulate biological functions. The removal of cells from their native microenvironment allows the study in a more focused way without the restrictions or control of other cell types. When using *in vitro* systems it is essential to recognize that some of the isolated cells must be studied within a short period of time following isolation, or instead, the experimental model must reproduce the microenvironment of the CNS from where cells were isolated. These limitations can, however, be useful to investigate the factors that regulate the phenotype of isolated cells. Different *in vitro* models using neural stem cells and microglial cells may be used, to better understand how inflammation affects the formation of new neurons from neural stem cells.

2.1 Neural stem cell cultures

Reynolds and collaborators performed the first adult neural stem cell culture in the 90's (Reynolds *et al.*, 1992; Reynolds and Weiss, 1992), as free floating cell clusters, commonly referred to as neurospheres. These adult neural stem cells found *in vivo* were dissociated *in vitro* and kept their main properties: self-renewal capacity and multipotency, when in presence of mitogens such as basic fibroblast growth factor (bFGF) and epidermal growth factor (EGF). This cell culture system is extensively used by researchers in neural stem cell biology, and models based on adherent adult neural stem cells cultured in a monolayer on matrix are also widely used (Pollard *et al.*, 2006).

The neural stem cell cultures can be obtained from different regions from the neuroaxis of the adult mammalian CNS, from the olfactory bulb to the spinal cord, and kept in uncoated dishes under serum-free conditions plus mitogens and other essential supplements (Golmohammadi *et al.*, 2008). These adult neural stem cells can be identified based on the expression of specific protein markers such as the transcription factor Sox2, nestin, musashi-1 and the EGF receptor, among others (Kaneko *et al.*, 2000; Ming and Song, 2005). After removal of mitogens these cells can give rise to three different cell types, namely neurons, astrocytes and oligodendrocytes (Levison and Goldman, 1997; Luskin *et al.*, 1997; Palmer *et al.*, 2001; Sanai *et al.*, 2004). Thus, in cultures we can find cells expressing the referred markers but also cells expressing other specific markers, such as glial fibrillary acidic protein (GFAP), polysialylated-neural cell adhesion molecule (PSA-NCAM) and beta-IIII tubulin (Suslov *et al.*, 2002; Ming and Song, 2011).

It is believed that the neurosphere culture may closer resemble the *in vivo* architecture than adherent cultures since it is believed that the stem cell niche is created by clustered cells. On the other hand, the sphere size can be a limitation of this culture in comparison to adherent neural stem cell cultures since the cells that are in the sphere core can have lower access to the nutrients and oxygen, thus undergoing cell death (Ostenfeld *et al.*, 2002; Bez *et al.*, 2003).

Adult neural stem cell culturing systems have been a relevant tool in the study of biological processes within the mammalian nervous system such as neurogenesis and their distinct phases. Cultures are good platforms for expansion of adult neural stem cells, being easily manipulated without loss of function. Additionally, they can be used as experimental models for the study of differentiation and intrinsic specification, and also for screening of drugs with the potential to enhance neurogenesis. However, further investigation should be performed for characterization of stem cells in these models, since a specific marker for neural stem cells is still lacking.

On the other hand, adult stem cell cultures have some limitations, as described next. Cells are sensitive to the culturing protocols, namely the overall number of passages, mitogen

concentration and also to the methodology adopted to dissociate spheres – mechanically or
by enzymatic digestion (Caldwell, 2001; Caldwell et al., 2001; Morshead et al., 2002; Irvin et
al., 2003). The overall size of spheres has been linked to the heterogeneity of sphere
composition, since it increases with sphere size, the artificiality of the cell cultures, since
cells propagate without instructions of their niche, and the fact that all dividing cells
propagate resulting in a mixture of different cell types, are all limitations of the neurosphere
culture (Reynolds and Weiss, 1996; Suslov et al., 2002; Parmar et al., 2003). Moreover, the
non-limited expansion of cultures could be a disadvantage once the proliferative capacity
could be lost by fast dividing cells over multipotent cells or by loss of stem cell capacity over
the number of passages. This situation may occur at the expense of differentiation.
Moreover, long-term culturing emphasizes the tendency for neural stem cells to adopt an
astrocytic phenotype, with reduced capacity to generate oligodendrocytes and neurons
(Chang et al., 2004; Vukicevic et al., 2010). Despite these limitations, free floating neural stem
cell culturing systems have several advantages and are by far the most used tool concerning
the study of neural stem cell biology. The use of neural stem cell cultures allows the easy
access to different stages of adult neurogenesis, including proliferation of neural stem cells
or progenitors, differentiation and fate determination of progenitor cells, migration of
newborn cells and cell survival. By choosing the right tools and correct techniques, these
different stages can be independently studied in vitro.

Adult neurogenesis was initially reported in vivo using autoradiography to track tritiated
([3H])-thymidine. [3H]-thymidine is incorporated in the DNA of dividing cells, thus proving
evidence for the existence of newborn cells in the hippocampus (Altman and Das, 1965) and
later, in the olfactory bulb (Altman, 1969). Proliferation of neural stem cells, the first stage of
neurogenesis, can be also detected in vitro. Different methods have been developed since, such
as the evaluation of 5-bromo-2'deoxyuridine (BrdU) incorporation, a thymidine analogue that
can be incorporated by S-phase cells during DNA synthesis, to detect cell proliferation instead
of [3H]-thymidine (Gratzner, 1982; Nowakowski et al., 1989). BrdU has been the golden
standard in the detection of cell proliferation for the last 20 years both in vivo and in vitro.
Detection of BrdU can be easily performed with antibodies, either by immunocytochemistry,
microplate assay or by flow cytometry. However, BrdU detection requires aggressive
treatment for DNA denaturation, in order to allow exposure of the incorporated BrdU to
antibodies. Such harsh treatment can be a major drawback in the technique, as head or acid
treatment can destroy several epitopes, thus precluding multiplex labeling with other
antibodies, and DNA denaturation causes the loss of binding sites for cell cycle dyes.

The use of 5-ethynyl-2'-deoxyuridine (EdU) has recently been proposed as an alternative to
BrdU, since EdU detection does not require DNA denaturation, thus improving DNA
structural preservation (Salic and Mitchison, 2008). EdU is also a thymidine analog that is
incorporated into DNA by dividing cells during active DNA synthesis, and can be used in vitro
as well as in vivo (Rostovtsev et al., 2002). EdU detection is based on click chemistry, via the
copper-mediated covalent coupling of the ethynyl group of EdU to a fluorescent dye-
conjugated azide (Rostovtsev et al., 2002). Detection can be performed by microscopy, high-
throughput analysis equipment or flow cytometry. Particularly, flow cytometry is extremely
useful for fast cell cycle analysis together with detection of EdU incorporation, while at same
time it is possible to co-label the proliferative cells with other cell-type specific markers. The
use of cell cycle markers (described next) complement detection of proliferation by 3H-
thymidine, BrdU or EdU, allowing for a more accurate timing of the birth of newborn cells

(Eisch and Mandyam, 2007). Other thymidine analogues that can be detected with antibodies are also available, such as iododeoxyuridine (IdU) and chlorodeoxyuridine (CldU).

Proteins related to the cell cycle have different expression patterns in the neurogenic regions accordingly to the phases of the cell cycle: retinoblastoma protein (Rb), a nuclear protein involved in the control of cell cycle progression, has a functional domain that binds to transcription factors and is expressed mostly in late G1 phase (Yoshikawa, 2000). Proliferating cell nuclear antigen (PCNA), a catalytic nuclear protein associated with DNA polymerase δ, is detected throughout all four phases of the cell cycle, however it is most abundant at late G1 and early S and scarce during G2 and M (Kawabe et al., 2002). Ki-67, a nonhistone nuclear protein, is present during G1, S, G2 and M phase (Gerdes et al., 1984). Cyclin-dependent kinase 1 (CDK1) or Cdc2 (the p34cdc2) is one of the mitosis-promoting factors and has an important role in the initiation of mitosis (Draetta et al., 1988; Okano et al., 1993).

Multi-labeling cells with specific cell markers and proliferation makers could easily identify newly generated neurons and glial cells, such as astrocytes and oligodendrocytes, which allows the distinction between these cell types. Proteins such as RNA-binding protein Hu and musashi-1 are exclusively expressed in mitotic active neural precursor cells, and they are absent in fully differentiated neuronal cells (Sakakibara et al., 1996; Akamatsu et al., 1999). The expression pattern of these markers can be detected by immunolabeling or quantitative real-time PCR (qRT-PCR). Mature neurons can be identified by assessing the presence of markers such as beta-III-tubulin, which contributes to microtubule stability in neuronal cell bodies and axons (Lee et al., 1990; Memberg and Hall, 1995), or by evaluating the presence of neuronal nuclear antigen (NeuN) (Mullen et al., 1992). Also the transcription factor NeuroD can be used since it is expressed throughout maturation until new neurons develop dendrites (Seki, 2002). Other markers that are commonly used can also be found in non-neuronal cells, namely PSA-NCAM (Seki and Arai, 1993; Kiss and Rougon, 1997); nestin, which is expressed in newly generated cells that still have the capacity to divide and differentiate into neurons or astrocytes (Reynolds and Weiss, 1992; Daniel et al., 2008); Sox2, a transcription factor essential to maintain self-renewal of stem cells (Pevny and Placzek, 2005); and doublecortin (DCX) which has a transient expression in proliferating progenitor cells and newly generated neuroblasts or glial cells (Brown et al., 2003; Kempermann et al., 2003; Rao and Shetty, 2004). Oligodendrocytes are easily identified by imunolabeling against 2', 3'-cyclic nucleotide 3'-phosphodiesterase (CNPase), APC or O4 (Vernadakis et al., 1984; Wu et al., 2008; Girolamo et al., 2010), while astrocytes can be identified by immunolabeling against GFAP, a specific protein for astrocytes (Bock et al., 1977).

Concerning the migration of newly formed cells, it has been extensively studied in vivo (Kempermann et al., 2003; Rao and Shetty, 2004), but also in vitro, by measuring DCX immunoreactivity (Francis et al., 1999; Cohen et al., 2008). DCX is a microtubule-associated protein having an important role in neuronal migration, by stabilizing microtubules and causing bundling (Sapir et al., 2000). While immunolabeling is currently used, other assays have been developed in order to evaluate migration and simultaneously the mechanisms controlling cell migration, cell protrusion and cell polarization, such as the scratch-wound migration assay (Etienne-Manneville, 2006). Additionally, Durbec and collaborators compared three different assays to evaluate migration of neural stem cells in vitro: matrigel, a three-dimensional substrate mimicking the in vivo extracellular matrix, detection of soluble factors influencing radial migration and the chemotaxis chamber assay, where the researcher can evaluate whether the cells prefer or not a chemical factor (Durbec et al., 2008).

Assessing the Influence of Neuroinflammation on Neurogenesis: In Vitro Models Using Neural Stem Cells and
Microglia as Valuable Research Tools

129

When mature, not all neurons in culture are functional or survive. It is important to check their viability, namely identify functional synapses by morphological, electrophysiological and immunological characterization (Hartley *et al.*, 1999). Several methods have been used, including immunocytochemical assays, Western blotting and qRT-PCR which allow identification and quantification of proteins, neurotransmitters, neurotrophic factors, among others, involved in neuronal or glial neurotransmitter systems (Hartley *et al.*, 1999; Elmariah *et al.*, 2005; Goodfellow *et al.*, 2011). Using patch-clamp techniques *in vitro* the electrophysiological characterization of neural stem cell cultures can be performed by evaluating the formation of action potentials and activity patterns (Li *et al.*, 2008; Cheyne *et al.*, 2011). Also single-cell calcium currents may be evaluated to discriminate neuronal profile and viability in response to different stimuli, as reported by Bernardino and collaborators (Bernardino *et al.*, 2008).

2.2 Microglial cell cultures

Microglial cells may be obtained for culturing by several methods. One of the most used models for the study of microglial cell function consists in the isolation and expansion of microglia from the neonatal brain. However, there are several limitations and criticisms to this approach since it consists in the isolation of microglial cells from the neonatal brain, not the adult brain. One of the main problems associated with the use of microglial cells *in vitro* is related to the characterization of microglia phenotype. Since there are no truly, unique and specific microglial cell markers, microglia phenotype is defined through a combined analysis of morphology and presence or absence of certain antigens. Several works lack a proper evaluation of microglia phenotype that would allow to distinguish microglia from macrophages. In most studies, the presence of microglial cell markers is excluded from cells that are positive for astrocytic or neuronal markers, but do not distinguish between microglia or macrophages. One of the most used immunocytochemical marker of microglial cells that is the ionized calcium binding adapter molecule 1 (Iba1) (Ito *et al.*, 1998). Other markers that have been identified include the beta-integrin marker CD11b (Ling and Wong, 1993; Gonzalez-Scarano and Baltuch, 1999), the glucose transporter 5 (GLUT5) (Sasaki *et al.*, 2004), CD163 (Roberts *et al.*, 2004; Borda *et al.*, 2008), CCR2 (Albright *et al.*, 1999; Zhang *et al.*, 2007), CD34 (Asheuer *et al.*, 2004; Ladeby *et al.*, 2005) and C-type lectin CD209b (Park *et al.*, 2009). Toll-like receptor 2 (TLR2) and Toll-like receptor 4 (TLR4) have been also used as markers of microglial cells as they appear to be involved in determining the phenotype and function of microglia (Li *et al.*, 2009). A combination of several of these markers would allow for a better characterization of microglia phenotype, rather than the use of a single marker, which is the current standard. The use of multiplex detection systems would be the best approach for a full molecular characterization of microglia (Albright and Gonzalez-Scarano, 2004; Duke *et al.*, 2004; Gebicke-Haerter, 2005; Glanzer *et al.*, 2007; Moran *et al.*, 2007).

The most popular protocol to isolate microglial cells is the shaking method described by Guilian and Baker (Giulian and Baker, 1986) and Frei and colleagues (Frei *et al.*, 1986). In this method, microglial cells are separated from confluent primary mixed glial cultures, isolated from the rodent neonatal cortex, by agitation in an orbital shaker. Although this method allows the preparation of highly pure microglial cultures, the yield of this protocol is low. Saura and colleagues described a method to isolate microglial cells from primary mixed glial cultures of rodent brain by a mild trypsinization protocol, which allows the preparation of high purity microglial cultures, with a higher yield when compared to the shaking method (Saura *et al.*, 2003). Similarly to the shaking method, several works describe the isolation of microglia from adult rodents, and the large majority of these studies take advantage from the astrocyte-microglia interaction for the success of cell cultures (Rosenstiel *et al.*, 2001; Ponomarev *et al.*, 2005). These studies showed that microglial cells, when grown on a monolayer of astrocytes, develop a highly branched morphology which seems to be associated with the downregulation of the nuclear factor kappa B (NF-kappaB) (Rosenstiel *et al.*, 2001). It has been shown that microglial cells isolated from the neonatal or adult brain are sensitive to the treatment with granulocyte macrophage colony-stimulating factor (GM-CSF), which induced a differentiation into a phenotype more similar to those of dendritic cells (Suzumura *et al.*, 1990; Aloisi, 2001). On the other hand, the isolation of adult microglial cells and subsequent culture with low concentrations of macrophage colony-stimulating factor (M-CSF) leads to increased proliferation and survival of cells that persists for several weeks (Suzumura *et al.*, 1990; Ponomarev *et al.*, 2005). M-CSF seems to be a key factor for the maintenance and survival of microglial cells *in vitro*, and has been used in several works (Wegiel *et al.*, 1998; Ponomarev *et al.*, 2005; Carreira *et al.*, 2010). Other methods are also described for the isolation of microglial cells, which include isolation from CNS tissue by Percoll gradient (Dick *et al.*, 1995; Ford *et al.*, 1995), isolation from primary cultures by nutritional deprivation (Hao *et al.*, 1991) or by collecting floating cells in mixed glial cultures (Ganter *et al.*, 1992), but the yield is generally very low.

The use of *in vitro* models allows for the understanding of many aspects of the dynamics associated with the biological functions of microglial cells in a quick and simple manner. However, one cannot overlook that the relevance of the observations obtained can only be extrapolated following *in vivo* studies. Several groups work with microglial cell lines, such as BV-2, HAPI or N9, however the use of microglial cell lines should be carefully considered since immortalization could significantly affect cell biology when compared to the use of primary microglial cultures (Corradin *et al.*, 1993; Lockhart *et al.*, 1998; Horvath *et al.*, 2008).

Concerning primary cultures of microglial cells it is always important to assess the purity of the cultures, this parameter being intrinsically linked to the method of isolation adopted. The isolation method described by Saura and collaborators is, therefore, one of the methods that seems to offer the best value yield/purity (Saura *et al.*, 2003). We favor the isolation of microglial cells by shaking from mixed glial cultures treated with low levels of M-CSF as an alternative to the method of Saura (Saura *et al.*, 2003), with a high purity of the microglia obtained (>90%) and, unlike previous methods, with a high yield (Carreira *et al.*, 2010).

When microglial cells become activated in response to immunologic stimuli or brain injury, activation is characterized by changes in microglia morphology (Streit *et al.*, 1988; Kreutzberg, 1996; Streit *et al.*, 1999; Liu and Hong, 2003), from resting ramified into activated amoeboid microglia (Kreutzberg, 1996). There is also a complex cellular response after activation of microglial cells, which is characterized by upregulation of surface molecules, such as complement receptors and major histocompatibility complex molecules (Oehmichen and Gencic, 1975; Graeber *et al.*, 1988). In addition, activated microglia release a large variety of soluble factors, with a pro- or anti- inflammatory nature and potentially cytotoxic (for review see Block and Hong, 2005). It is therefore important, when establishing primary cultures of microglia, to assess whether microglial cells *in vitro* are also responsive to inflammatory stimuli similarly to what occurs *in vivo*. Microglial cells can be challenged with different stimuli *in vitro*, and by far the most widely used stimulus in primary cultures of microglia isolated from rodents is the bacterial endotoxin lipopolysaccharide (LPS) (Qin *et al.*, 2005a; Qin *et al.*, 2005b; Pei *et al.*, 2007). LPS mimics the infection by Gram-negative bacteria, which induces an increase in the synthesis of inflammatory mediators, namely cytokines, such as IL-1, IL-6 and tumor necrosis factor-alpha (TNF-alpha), chemokines, such as stromal derived factor-1 alpha (SDF-1alpha), free radicals and nitric oxide (Block and Hong, 2005). Other stimuli may consist in the use of ATP, interleukins, IFN-gamma or LPS plus IFN-gamma (Wollmer *et al.*, 2001; Saura *et al.*, 2003).

To characterize the activation of microglial cells after an inflammatory stimulus, we suggest to define at least three parameters to evaluate the activation of microglial cells following exposure to an inflammatory stimulus, including: change to an amoeboid morphology (Suzumura *et al.*, 1991; Wollmer *et al.*, 2001), the expression of NF-kappaB (Heyen *et al.*, 2000; Wollmer *et al.*, 2001), expression of the inducible nitric oxide synthase (iNOS) and subsequent evaluation of the production of NO (Boje and Arora, 1992; Chao *et al.*, 1992b), or the release of TNF-alpha (Sawada *et al.*, 1989; Chao *et al.*, 1992a). The various mechanisms by which microglial cells are activated and the identity of the inflammatory factors released by microglia have been studied and characterized, but there still is a great controversy whether these factors are neuroprotective or neurotoxic when released. The hypothesis that seems to be more acceptable is that, depending on the aggressiveness of the inflammatory response, the activation of microglial cells may shift from a beneficial to a harmful outcome for neurogenesis.

2.3 Combination of neural stem cells and microglial cell cultures

The study of the link between brain inflammation and neurogenesis, in particular the role of microglia in the modulation of the various steps of the neurogenic process, is of particular relevance. In order to operate at a therapeutic level there is an urgent need to understand the crosstalk between microglia and neural stem cells and the implications of the inflammatory response for the neurogenic outcome. Several studies *in vivo* have been developed in recent years, but the potential of *in vitro* studies becomes indisputable when the aim is to study the effect of a particular inflammatory factor or a very specific parameter related to the inflammatory response and its effect on neurogenesis. Whether the function of microglial cells is pro- or anti-neurogenic and whether it is possible to control microglial activation in order to reach a beneficial effect are important questions that need to be answered. Thus, the development of basic models for the *in vitro* study of these issues is an asset to the studies in this area. The use of combined primary neuronal and microglial cell cultures has been a very useful tool in studying the effect of the inflammatory response on neurons from different brain regions. In fact, there are numerous published studies where different approaches have been adopted for the study of the crosstalk between microglial cells and neurons *in vitro* (Boje and Arora, 1992; Lambertsen *et al.*, 2009). Here we describe the use of three different *in vitro* models, which address different aspects of the effects of inflammatory factors released by microglial cells in the neurogenic process.

2.3.1 Co-cultures of neural stem cells with microglia

The inflammatory response has been identified as responsible for the down-regulation of neurogenesis. This hypothesis has been supported by several studies *in vivo* (Ekdahl *et al.*, 2003; Monje *et al.*, 2003), but also by *in vitro* studies where the survival of new neurons is compromised when these are co-cultured with microglial cells activated by LPS (Monje *et al.*, 2003; Cacci *et al.*, 2005; Liu *et al.*, 2005; Cacci *et al.*, 2008). Co-cultures of neural stem cells with microglia, without physical contact between the two cell types, is an experimental model that allows the researcher to assess the role of soluble neuroinflammatory factors using co-cultures of microglial cells seeded in membrane inserts placed on top of multiwell plates containing neural stem cells. The use of techniques of immunodepletion, but also the use of genetically modified animals, allowed to correlate this anti-neurogenic inflammatory response to different interleukins produced during the activation of microglial cells, including IL-6 and IL-1beta (Vallieres *et al.*, 2002; Monje *et al.*, 2003; Nakanishi *et al.*, 2007; Goshen *et al.*, 2008; Koo and Duman, 2008; Spulber *et al.*, 2008). Other factors involved in the inflammatory response appear to contribute to the inhibition of neurogenesis. For example, the increased production of TNF-alpha by microglial cells appears to reduce the survival and differentiation of neural stem cells (Vezzani *et al.*, 2002; Monje *et al.*, 2003; Liu *et al.*, 2005; Iosif *et al.*, 2006).

Although some studies have described IFN-gamma as having a deleterious effect on neurogenesis, it has been demonstrated that microglia stimulated with low levels of IFN-gamma can support the neurogenic process, promoting neuronal differentiation *in vitro* (Butovsky *et al.*, 2006). In other studies it was observed that IFN-gamma is involved in the modulation of proliferation and differentiation of neural stem cells into neurons (Wong *et al.*, 2004; Song *et al.*, 2005; Baron *et al.*, 2008). Recent *in vitro* studies based on the establishment of co-cultures of microglia and neural stem cells, without physical contact between cells, reported that microglia might have a more complex role in neurogenesis contrarily to initial thoughts. Microglia seems to play a dual role in adult neurogenesis, being detrimental or beneficial and support the different steps in neurogenesis, such as stem cell proliferation, differentiation, migration and survival (reviewed in Ekdahl *et al.*, 2009). This dual effect becomes associated to different soluble factors produced by activated microglial cells, such as TNF-alpha or nitric oxide.

The establishment of experimental models such as co-cultures of microglia and neural stem cells allows to mimic the chemical microenvironment that surrounds the SVZ and/or the DG during inflammatory conditions when microglial cells are recruited and activated. On the other hand, the fact that both cell types share the same culture environment is important to determine the effect of factors produced by microglial cells on neural stem cells. The fact that this is a system without physical contact between the two cell types also allows determining more quickly, and using more economic approaches, the modulation of the multistep neurogenic process mediated by the inflammatory response. Thus, experimental approaches to determine cell proliferation and cell cycle, such as flow cytometry, cell migration, could be performed without the need for prior characterization to distinguish neural stem cells from microglial cells as in mixed cultures. Moreover, signaling pathways present in both cell types can be studied this way, as is the case of TLR4 that directly modulates self-renewal and the decision-cell-fate in neural stem cells (Rolls *et al.*, 2007) and in microglial cells is involved in its activation, particularly in the regulation of gene expression of iNOS (Graeber and Streit, 2010).

However, there are also some disadvantages associated with the use of this experimental methodology. Firstly, the fact that it does not allow an easy processing of microglia cells, which are placed in membrane inserts, after experimental treatment. In fact, simple experimental procedures such as protein, RNA or DNA extraction from microglial cells becomes difficult to perform. On the other hand, it is not possible to perform immunostaining techniques for subsequent microscopic analysis of microglial cells plated in inserts. In addition, this model does not answer a question that seems to be increasingly important which is the influence of cell-to-cell contact in the modulation of neurogenesis by the inflammatory response (Song et al., 2002; Aarum et al., 2003; Alvarez-Buylla and Lim, 2004). Despite these disadvantages, the use of co-cultures of neural stem cells with microglia, without physical contact between the two cell types, is a good approach for some studies.

2.3.2 Neural stem cell cultures exposed to microglia-conditioned medium

The production of cytokines and other molecules by activated microglial cells with implications in cellular processes has been demonstrated in many studies based on *in vitro* models (Banati et al., 1993; Minghetti and Levi, 1998; Gebicke-Haerter et al., 2001; Hanisch, 2002; Hausler et al., 2002). However, there is still much to be learned about how cellular pathways in neural stem cells are regulated by these soluble factors from microglial origin. It is therefore important to assess how these diffusible factors influence phenomena as diverse as proliferation, differentiation, migration or cell survival.

Culturing neural stem cells with microglia conditioned medium, obtained from a separate microglia culture, allows the isolation of the unidirectional communication between activated microglia and neural stem cells, with further investigation of soluble inflammatory factors. According to studies using this experimental model, the conditioned medium of microglial cells acutely challenged with LPS reduced the survival of neural stem cells, preventing their differentiation into neurons (Monje et al., 2003; Cacci et al., 2008). One of the inflammatory agents reported to be responsible for this antineurogenic effect is the cytokine IL-6, as evidenced by the works of Monje and collaborators or Nakanishi and colleagues that by using a specific antibody against IL-6 rescued neurogenesis (Monje et al., 2003; Nakanishi et al., 2007). On the other hand, several *in vitro* studies described a pro-neurogenic effect of microglial cells and their conditioned medium, in which neural stem cells grow (Aarum et al., 2003; Morgan et al., 2004; Walton et al., 2006; Nakanishi et al., 2007).

Despite the advantages of this experimental model, namely the fact that it allows a study of the unidirectional effect of microglia on neural stem cells, there are also some disadvantages. This model does not allow inferring any conclusion about the influence of cell-to-cell contact between microglia and neural stem cells, an event that has been described to occur between glial cells and neural stem cells (Song et al., 2002; Aarum et al., 2003; Alvarez-Buylla and Lim, 2004). On the other hand, this model completely neglects the fact that some of the factors released by microglial cells have physical characteristics that do not allow their study in a conditioned medium transferred from a cell culture to another. Particularly nitric oxide, a gaseous molecule with a short half-life, cannot be studied because it is highly reactive in aqueous solution at 37 °C and physiological pH (pH = 7.4). Thus, although stable end products of NO can be detected in conditioned medium from activated microglial cell cultures, the effect of NO in the neural stem cells cannot be analyzed. These are negative aspects that must be taken into account when a researcher decides to select this experimental model. Despite these aspects, the use of conditioned medium of microglia in cultures of neural stem cells is a good model to further study the influence of inflammation on neurogenesis. This model is useful to complement other *in vitro* approaches, including co-cultures of microglia and neural stem cells, with or without physical contact.

2.3.3 Mixed cultures of neural stem cells with microglia

The progression of the neurogenic process until the differentiation of neural stem cells into neurons appears to be regulated by the inflammatory microenvironment but also by cell-to-cell interactions involved (Arvidsson *et al.*, 2002; Nakatomi *et al.*, 2002; Ben-Hur *et al.*, 2003; Thored *et al.*, 2006; Thored *et al.*, 2009). Therefore, the optimization of an *in vitro* system that allows the study of physical interactions between microglia and neural stem cells is of great interest to understand how both cell types crosstalk in inflammatory conditions.

Mixed cultures are co-cultures of neural stem cells with microglia with physical contact between the two cell types. In this culture model, the role of physical contacts between microglia and neural stem cells can be studied. The mixed culture system is, probably, the *in vitro* approach that more closely mimics what happens *in vivo*, where microglial cells physically contact with the neural stem cells from neurogenic areas. Adopting this experimental model, the researcher can study the influence of the inflammatory response on the several steps of the neurogenic process, but also cell-cell interactions, which is an advantage compared to the *in vitro* models already described. An example of a mixed culture of neural stem cells cultured together with forebrain microglia is shown in Fig. 1. Enhanced green fluorescent protein (EGFP)-positive SVZ cells were isolated from the SVZ of postnatal day 1-3 actin-EGFP C57Bl6 mice, thus being readily distinguishable from microglia isolated from wild-type mice (Fig. 1A).

The mixed culture model allows simultaneous evaluation of microglia and neural stem cells. Thus, following stimulation of microglial cells, the researcher can evaluate the activation of these cells as well as several biological processes of neural stem cells, such as proliferation, differentiation and/or survival. Moreover, multi-labeling experiments of proliferation markers, such as BrdU or EdU (Fig. 1B), with microglia-specific (Iba-1 or CD11b), neuron-specific (NeuN or Tuj-1) or glia-specific (GFAP) proteins by confocal microscopy or flow cytometry are a good way to determine the phenotype of proliferating cells (Nixon and Crews, 2004). In addition, it is also possible to evaluate the effect of diffusible factors that are produced following activation of microglial cells. Separation of the two cell populations for posterior analysis (e.g. of protein or nucleic acids) is possible using a cell sorter. The researcher can confirm whether the effects observed in mixed cultures are caused by physical interactions or by diffusible factors released by microglial cells by combining such experiments with a comparative study using co-cultured cells without physical contact.

A

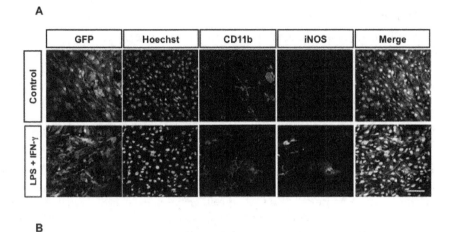

B

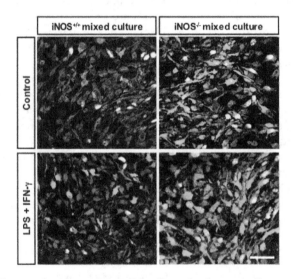

Fig. 1. Mixed cultures of primary microglial cells and subventricular zone (SVZ)-derived
neural stem cells. SVZ cells (isolated from transgenic mice expressing green fluorescence
protein (GFP) under the actin promoter (shown in white) are readily distinguishable from
CD11b-positive microglia (red) (A). Microglia (red) cultured with GFP-positive SVZ cells
(white) show immunoreactivity for inducible nitric oxide synthase (iNOS, green), following
treatment with lipopolysaccharide (LPS; 100 ng/ml) plus interferon-gamma (IFN-gamma;
0.5 ng/ml), for 24 h. Nuclei are labeled with Hoechst 33342 (blue). Scale bar: 20 μm. B)
Stimulation with LPS plus IFN-gamma decreases the proliferation of GFP-positive SVZ-
derived neural stem cells (green), in mixed cultures of SVZ and microglia obtained from
wild type mice (iNOS+/+), which are CD11b-positive (red). Cell proliferation was assessed
by 5-ethynyl-2'-deoxyuridine (EdU) incorporation (white). The antiproliferative effect of
LPS plus IFN-gamma on EdU incorporation is abolished in mixed cultures in which the
microglia was obtained from iNOS-knockout mice (iNOS-/-). Scale bar: 20 μm.

3. Summary and future directions

Microglial cells may cause different effects on the neurogenic process, promoting or inhibiting it. Experimental evidence has been presented indicating that microglia, depending on their activation status and phenotype, could favor or hinder adult neurogenesis, in physiological or pathophysiological conditions. In fact, microglia can have a dual role in different steps of the neurogenic process, namely in the formation, maturation and integration of newly formed neurons. Therefore the need to explore in more detail how microglia regulate adult neurogenesis in physiological and pathophysiological conditions is of particular importance (Graeber and Streit, 2010).

Genetic mouse models in which the researcher can selectively ablate genes have already been described as useful strategies to study the involvement of particular effectors of the neuroinflammatory response on neural stem cells. Experimental models may have as an objective the determination of how modulation of microglial cell activation can be used as a therapeutic target to regulate neurogenesis in the adult brain (Ekdahl et al., 2009; Whitney et al., 2009; Polazzi and Monti, 2010). These models are suitable to evaluate the neurogenic potential of anti-inflammatory drugs or identify pro-neurogenic targets. Thus, these experimental approaches will allow the design of therapeutic strategies to enhance the formation, proper migration, differentiation, integration and survival of new neuronal cells in the injured nervous system. Moreover, all culture models are suitable for pharmacological or genetic manipulation, including obtaining the cells used in the cultures from wild-type or genetically modified animals, and can be adapted for high-throughput analysis and drug screening. The use of anti-inflammatory drugs with a selective mechanism of action at the level of microglial cells, or the use of anti-inflammatory drugs which may release molecules that may enhance the neurogenesis are strategies under investigation (Keeble and Moore, 2002; Napoli and Ignarro, 2003; Ajmone-Cat et al., 2008; Koc and Kucukguzel, 2009). In order to develop more specific therapeutic interventions in the future, it is necessary to identify the mechanisms and factors that regulate the switch between the enhancing or detrimental effect of the inflammatory response on neurogenic events. The in vitro strategies discussed here are important as a first step in identifying and characterizing these events (Table 2).

Experimental model	Parameters evaluated			
	Diffusible/soluble factors	Cell-to-cell interaction	Cellular characterization	Protein, RNA and DNA content
Co-culture	Very Good	-	Very Good	Very Good
Conditioned medium	Good	-	Very Good	Very Good
Mixed culture	Very Good	Very Good	Good (requires multiplex analysis)	Good (requires cell sorting)

Table 2. Evaluation of experimental in vitro models using neural stem cells and microglial cells as research tools to evaluate the effect of neuroinflammation in the neurogenesis.

4. References

Aarum J, Sandberg K, Haeberlein SL and Persson MA (2003). "Migration and differentiation of neural precursor cells can be directed by microglia." *Proc Natl Acad Sci U S A* 100(26): 15983-8.

Ajmone-Cat MA, Cacci E and Minghetti L (2008). "Non steroidal anti-inflammatory drugs and neurogenesis in the adult mammalian brain." *Curr Pharm Des* 14(14): 1435-42.

Akamatsu W, Okano HJ, Osumi N, Inoue T, Nakamura S, Sakakibara S, Miura M, Matsuo N, Darnell RB and Okano H (1999). "Mammalian ELAV-like neuronal RNA-binding proteins HuB and HuC promote neuronal development in both the central and the peripheral nervous systems." *Proc Natl Acad Sci U S A* 96(17): 9885-90.

Albright AV and Gonzalez-Scarano F (2004). "Microarray analysis of activated mixed glial (microglia) and monocyte-derived macrophage gene expression." *J Neuroimmunol* 157(1-2): 27-38.

Albright AV, Shieh JT, Itoh T, Lee B, Pleasure D, O'Connor MJ, Doms RW and Gonzalez-Scarano F (1999). "Microglia express CCR5, CXCR4, and CCR3, but of these, CCR5 is the principal coreceptor for human immunodeficiency virus type 1 dementia isolates." *J Virol* 73(1): 205-13.

Aloisi F (2001). "Immune function of microglia." *Glia* 36(2): 165-79.

Altman J (1969). "Autoradiographic and histological studies of postnatal neurogenesis. IV. Cell proliferation and migration in the anterior forebrain, with special reference to persisting neurogenesis in the olfactory bulb." *J Comp Neurol* 137(4): 433-57.

Altman J and Das GD (1965). "Autoradiographic and histological evidence of postnatal hippocampal neurogenesis in rats." *J Comp Neurol* 124(3): 319-35.

Alvarez-Buylla A and Lim DA (2004). "For the long run: maintaining germinal niches in the adult brain." *Neuron* 41(5): 683-6.

Arvidsson A, Collin T, Kirik D, Kokaia Z and Lindvall O (2002). "Neuronal replacement from endogenous precursors in the adult brain after stroke." *Nat Med* 8(9): 963-70.

Asheuer M, Pflumio F, Benhamida S, Dubart-Kupperschmitt A, Fouquet F, Imai Y, Aubourg P and Cartier N (2004). "Human CD34+ cells differentiate into microglia and express recombinant therapeutic protein." *Proc Natl Acad Sci U S A* 101(10): 3557-62.

Banati RB, Gehrmann J, Schubert P and Kreutzberg GW (1993). "Cytotoxicity of microglia." *Glia* 7(1): 111-8.

Baron R, Nemirovsky A, Harpaz I, Cohen H, Owens T and Monsonego A (2008). "IFN-gamma enhances neurogenesis in wild-type mice and in a mouse model of Alzheimer's disease." *Faseb J* 22(8): 2843-52.

Bauer S (2009). "Cytokine control of adult neural stem cells." *Ann N Y Acad Sci* 1153: 48-56.

Belluzzi O, Benedusi M, Ackman J and LoTurco JJ (2003). "Electrophysiological differentiation of new neurons in the olfactory bulb." *J Neurosci* 23(32): 10411-8.

Ben-Hur T, Ben-Menachem O, Furer V, Einstein O, Mizrachi-Kol R and Grigoriadis N (2003). "Effects of proinflammatory cytokines on the growth, fate, and motility of multipotential neural precursor cells." *Mol Cell Neurosci* 24(3): 623-31.

Bernardino L, Agasse F, Silva B, Ferreira R, Grade S and Malva JO (2008). "Tumor necrosis factor-alpha modulates survival, proliferation, and neuronal differentiation in neonatal subventricular zone cell cultures." *Stem Cells* 26(9): 2361-71.

Bernier PJ, Bedard A, Vinet J, Levesque M and Parent A (2002). "Newly generated neurons in the amygdala and adjoining cortex of adult primates." *Proc Natl Acad Sci U S A* 99(17): 11464-9.

Bez A, Corsini E, Curti D, Biggiogera M, Colombo A, Nicosia RF, Pagano SF and Parati EA (2003). "Neurosphere and neurosphere-forming cells: morphological and ultrastructural characterization." *Brain Res* 993(1-2): 18-29.

Block ML and Hong JS (2005). "Microglia and inflammation-mediated neurodegeneration: multiple triggers with a common mechanism." *Prog Neurobiol* 76(2): 77-98.

Bock E, Moller M, Nissen C and Sensenbrenner M (1977). "Glial fibrillary acidic protein in primary astroglial cell cultures derived from newborn rat brain." *FEBS Lett* 83(2): 207-11.

Boje KM and Arora PK (1992). "Microglial-produced nitric oxide and reactive nitrogen oxides mediate neuronal cell death." *Brain Res* 587(2): 250-6.

Borda JT, Alvarez X, Mohan M, Hasegawa A, Bernardino A, Jean S, Aye P and Lackner AA (2008). "CD163, a marker of perivascular macrophages, is up-regulated by microglia in simian immunodeficiency virus encephalitis after haptoglobin-hemoglobin complex stimulation and is suggestive of breakdown of the blood-brain barrier." *Am J Pathol* 172(3): 725-37.

Brown JP, Couillard-Despres S, Cooper-Kuhn CM, Winkler J, Aigner L and Kuhn HG (2003). "Transient expression of doublecortin during adult neurogenesis." *J Comp Neurol* 467(1): 1-10.

Butovsky O, Ziv Y, Schwartz A, Landa G, Talpalar AE, Pluchino S, Martino G and Schwartz M (2006). "Microglia activated by IL-4 or IFN-gamma differentially induce neurogenesis and oligodendrogenesis from adult stem/progenitor cells." *Mol Cell Neurosci* 31(1): 149-60.

Cacci E, Ajmone-Cat MA, Anelli T, Biagioni S and Minghetti L (2008). "In vitro neuronal and glial differentiation from embryonic or adult neural precursor cells are differently affected by chronic or acute activation of microglia." *Glia* 56(4): 412-25.

Cacci E, Claasen JH and Kokaia Z (2005). "Microglia-derived tumor necrosis factor-alpha exaggerates death of newborn hippocampal progenitor cells in vitro." *J Neurosci Res* 80(6): 789-97.

Caldwell MA (2001). "Recent advances in neuralstem cell technologies." *Trends Neurosci* 24(2): 72-4.

Caldwell MA, He X, Wilkie N, Pollack S, Marshall G, Wafford KA and Svendsen CN (2001). "Growth factors regulate the survival and fate of cells derived from human neurospheres." *Nat Biotechnol* 19(5): 475-9.

Carlen M, Cassidy RM, Brismar H, Smith GA, Enquist LW and Frisen J (2002). "Functional integration of adult-born neurons." *Curr Biol* 12(7): 606-8.

Carreira BP, Morte MI, Inacio A, Costa G, Rosmaninho-Salgado J, Agasse F, Carmo A, Couceiro P, Brundin P, Ambrosio AF, Carvalho CM and Araujo IM (2010). "Nitric oxide stimulates the proliferation of neural stem cells bypassing the epidermal growth factor receptor." *Stem Cells* 28(7): 1219-30.

Cayre M, Bancila M, Virard I, Borges A and Durbec P (2006). "Migrating and myelinating potential of subventricular zone neural progenitor cells in white matter tracts of the adult rodent brain." *Mol Cell Neurosci* 31(4): 748-58.

Chang MY, Park CH, Lee SY and Lee SH (2004). "Properties of cortical precursor cells
    cultured long term are similar to those of precursors at later developmental stages."
    Brain Res Dev Brain Res 153(1): 89-96.
Chao CC, Hu S, Close K, Choi CS, Molitor TW, Novick WJ and Peterson PK (1992a).
    "Cytokine release from microglia: differential inhibition by pentoxifylline and
    dexamethasone." J Infect Dis 166(4): 847-53.
Chao CC, Hu S, Molitor TW, Shaskan EG and Peterson PK (1992b). "Activated microglia
    mediate neuronal cell injury via a nitric oxide mechanism." J Immunol 149(8): 2736-
    41.
Chen H, Zhang SM, Hernan MA, Schwarzschild MA, Willett WC, Colditz GA, Speizer FE
    and Ascherio A (2003). "Nonsteroidal anti-inflammatory drugs and the risk of
    Parkinson disease." Arch Neurol 60(8): 1059-64.
Cheyne JE, Grant L, Butler-Munro C, Foote JW, Connor B and Montgomery JM (2011).
    "Synaptic integration of newly generated neurons in rat dissociated hippocampal
    cultures." Mol Cell Neurosci 47(3): 203-14.
Ciani E, Calvanese V, Crochemore C, Bartesaghi R and Contestabile A (2006). "Proliferation
    of cerebellar precursor cells is negatively regulated by nitric oxide in newborn rat."
    J Cell Sci 119(Pt 15): 3161-70.
Cohen D, Segal M and Reiner O (2008). "Doublecortin supports the development of
    dendritic arbors in primary hippocampal neurons." Dev Neurosci 30(1-3): 187-99.
Contestabile A, Monti B and Ciani E (2003). "Brain nitric oxide and its dual role in
    neurodegeneration/neuroprotection: understanding molecular mechanisms to
    devise drug approaches." Curr Med Chem 10(20): 2147-74.
Corradin SB, Mauel J, Donini SD, Quattrocchi E and Ricciardi-Castagnoli P (1993).
    "Inducible nitric oxide synthase activity of cloned murine microglial cells." Glia 7(3):
    255-62.
Covacu R, Danilov AI, Rasmussen BS, Hallen K, Moe MC, Lobell A, Johansson CB, Svensson
    MA, Olsson T and Brundin L (2006). "Nitric oxide exposure diverts neural stem cell
    fate from neurogenesis towards astrogliogenesis." Stem Cells 24(12): 2792-800.
Craig CG, Tropepe V, Morshead CM, Reynolds BA, Weiss S and van der Kooy D (1996). "In
    vivo growth factor expansion of endogenous subependymal neural precursor cell
    populations in the adult mouse brain." J Neurosci 16(8): 2649-58.
Curtis MA, Eriksson PS and Faull RL (2007). "Progenitor cells and adult neurogenesis in
    neurodegenerative diseases and injuries of the basal ganglia." Clin Exp Pharmacol
    Physiol 34(5-6): 528-32.
Daniel C, Albrecht H, Ludke A and Hugo C (2008). "Nestin expression in repopulating
    mesangial cells promotes their proliferation." Lab Invest 88(4): 387-97.
Davalos D, Grutzendler J, Yang G, Kim JV, Zuo Y, Jung S, Littman DR, Dustin ML and Gan
    WB (2005). "ATP mediates rapid microglial response to local brain injury in vivo."
    Nat Neurosci 8(6): 752-8.
Davalos D, Lee JK, Smith WB, Brinkman B, Ellisman MH, Zheng B and Akassoglou K (2008).
    "Stable in vivo imaging of densely populated glia, axons and blood vessels in the
    mouse spinal cord using two-photon microscopy." J Neurosci Methods 169(1): 1-7.
Dayer AG, Cleaver KM, Abouantoun T and Cameron HA (2005). "New GABAergic
    interneurons in the adult neocortex and striatum are generated from different
    precursors." J Cell Biol 168(3): 415-27.

Dick AD, Ford AL, Forrester JV and Sedgwick JD (1995). "Flow cytometric identification of a minority population of MHC class II positive cells in the normal rat retina distinct from CD45lowCD11b/c+CD4low parenchymal microglia." *Br J Ophthalmol* 79(9): 834-40.

Doetsch F and Scharff C (2001). "Challenges for brain repair: insights from adult neurogenesis in birds and mammals." *Brain Behav Evol* 58(5): 306-22.

Draetta G, Brizuela L, Moran B and Beach D (1988). "Regulation of the vertebrate cell cycle by the cdc2 protein kinase." *Cold Spring Harb Symp Quant Biol* 53 Pt 1: 195-201.

Drapeau E, Montaron MF, Aguerre S and Abrous DN (2007). "Learning-induced survival of new neurons depends on the cognitive status of aged rats." *J Neurosci* 27(22): 6037-44.

Duke DC, Moran LB, Turkheimer FE, Banati R and Graeber MB (2004). "Microglia in culture: what genes do they express?" *Dev Neurosci* 26(1): 30-7.

Durbec P, Franceschini I, Lazarini F and Dubois-Dalcq M (2008). "In vitro migration assays of neural stem cells." *Methods Mol Biol* 438: 213-25.

Eisch AJ and Mandyam CD (2007). "Adult neurogenesis: can analysis of cell cycle proteins move us "Beyond BrdU"?" *Curr Pharm Biotechnol* 8(3): 147-65.

Ekdahl CT, Claasen JH, Bonde S, Kokaia Z and Lindvall O (2003). "Inflammation is detrimental for neurogenesis in adult brain." *Proc Natl Acad Sci U S A* 100(23): 13632-7.

Ekdahl CT, Kokaia Z and Lindvall O (2009). "Brain inflammation and adult neurogenesis: the dual role of microglia." *Neuroscience* 158(3): 1021-9.

Elmariah SB, Oh EJ, Hughes EG and Balice-Gordon RJ (2005). "Astrocytes regulate inhibitory synapse formation via Trk-mediated modulation of postsynaptic GABAA receptors." *J Neurosci* 25(14): 3638-50.

Eriksson PS, Perfilieva E, Bjork-Eriksson T, Alborn AM, Nordborg C, Peterson DA and Gage FH (1998). "Neurogenesis in the adult human hippocampus." *Nat Med* 4(11): 1313-7.

Etienne-Manneville S (2006). "In vitro assay of primary astrocyte migration as a tool to study Rho GTPase function in cell polarization." *Methods Enzymol* 406: 565-78.

Ford AL, Goodsall AL, Hickey WF and Sedgwick JD (1995). "Normal adult ramified microglia separated from other central nervous system macrophages by flow cytometric sorting. Phenotypic differences defined and direct ex vivo antigen presentation to myelin basic protein-reactive CD4+ T cells compared." *J Immunol* 154(9): 4309-21.

Francis F, Koulakoff A, Boucher D, Chafey P, Schaar B, Vinet MC, Friocourt G, McDonnell N, Reiner O, Kahn A, McConnell SK, Berwald-Netter Y, Denoulet P and Chelly J (1999). "Doublecortin is a developmentally regulated, microtubule-associated protein expressed in migrating and differentiating neurons." *Neuron* 23(2): 247-56.

Frei K, Bodmer S, Schwerdel C and Fontana A (1986). "Astrocyte-derived interleukin 3 as a growth factor for microglia cells and peritoneal macrophages." *J Immunol* 137(11): 3521-7.

Fritzen S, Schmitt A, Koth K, Sommer C, Lesch KP and Reif A (2007). "Neuronal nitric oxide synthase (NOS-I) knockout increases the survival rate of neural cells in the hippocampus independently of BDNF." *Mol Cell Neurosci* 35(2): 261-71.

Ganter S, Northoff H, Mannel D and Gebicke-Harter PJ (1992). "Growth control of cultured microglia." *J Neurosci Res* 33(2): 218-30.

Gebicke-Haerter PJ (2005). "Microarrays and expression profiling in microglia research and in inflammatory brain disorders." *J Neurosci Res* 81(3): 327-41.

Gebicke-Haerter PJ, Spleiss O, Ren LQ, Li H, Dichmann S, Norgauer J and Boddeke HW (2001). "Microglial chemokines and chemokine receptors." *Prog Brain Res* 132: 525-32.

Gehrmann J (1996). "Microglia: a sensor to threats in the nervous system?" *Res Virol* 147(2-3): 79-88.

Gerdes J, Lemke H, Baisch H, Wacker HH, Schwab U and Stein H (1984). "Cell cycle analysis of a cell proliferation-associated human nuclear antigen defined by the monoclonal antibody Ki-67." *J Immunol* 133(4): 1710-5.

Gheusi G, Cremer H, McLean H, Chazal G, Vincent JD and Lledo PM (2000). "Importance of newly generated neurons in the adult olfactory bulb for odor discrimination." *Proc Natl Acad Sci U S A* 97(4): 1823-8.

Girolamo F, Strippoli M, Errede M, Benagiano V, Roncali L, Ambrosi G and Virgintino D (2010). "Characterization of oligodendrocyte lineage precursor cells in the mouse cerebral cortex: a confocal microscopy approach to demyelinating diseases." *Ital J Anat Embryol* 115(1-2): 95-102.

Giulian D and Baker TJ (1986). "Characterization of ameboid microglia isolated from developing mammalian brain." *J Neurosci* 6(8): 2163-78.

Glanzer JG, Enose Y, Wang T, Kadiu I, Gong N, Rozek W, Liu J, Schlautman JD, Ciborowski PS, Thomas MP and Gendelman HE (2007). "Genomic and proteomic microglial profiling: pathways for neuroprotective inflammatory responses following nerve fragment clearance and activation." *J Neurochem* 102(3): 627-45.

Golmohammadi MG, Blackmore DG, Large B, Azari H, Esfandiary E, Paxinos G, Franklin KB, Reynolds BA and Rietze RL (2008). "Comparative analysis of the frequency and distribution of stem and progenitor cells in the adult mouse brain." *Stem Cells* 26(4): 979-87.

Gonzalez-Perez O, Jauregui-Huerta F and Galvez-Contreras AY (2010). "Immune system modulates the function of adult neural stem cells." *Curr Immunol Rev* 6(3): 167-173.

Gonzalez-Scarano F and Baltuch G (1999). "Microglia as mediators of inflammatory and degenerative diseases." *Annu Rev Neurosci* 22: 219-40.

Goodfellow CE, Graham SE, Dragunow M and Glass M (2011). "Characterization of NTera2/D1 cells as a model system for the investigation of cannabinoid function in human neurons and astrocytes." *J Neurosci Res.*

Goshen I, Kreisel T, Ben-Menachem-Zidon O, Licht T, Weidenfeld J, Ben-Hur T and Yirmiya R (2008). "Brain interleukin-1 mediates chronic stress-induced depression in mice via adrenocortical activation and hippocampal neurogenesis suppression." *Mol Psychiatry* 13(7): 717-28.

Gould E, Beylin A, Tanapat P, Reeves A and Shors TJ (1999a). "Learning enhances adult neurogenesis in the hippocampal formation." *Nat Neurosci* 2(3): 260-5.

Gould E, Reeves AJ, Graziano MS and Gross CG (1999b). "Neurogenesis in the neocortex of adult primates." *Science* 286(5439): 548-52.

Gould E, Vail N, Wagers M and Gross CG (2001). "Adult-generated hippocampal and neocortical neurons in macaques have a transient existence." *Proc Natl Acad Sci U S A* 98(19): 10910-7.

Graeber MB and Streit WJ (2010). "Microglia: biology and pathology." *Acta Neuropathol* 119(1): 89-105.

Graeber MB, Streit WJ and Kreutzberg GW (1988). "The microglial cytoskeleton: vimentin is localized within activated cells in situ." *J Neurocytol* 17(4): 573-80.

Gratzner HG (1982). "Monoclonal antibody to 5-bromo- and 5-iododeoxyuridine: A new reagent for detection of DNA replication." *Science* 218(4571): 474-5.

Green W, Patil P, Marsden CA, Bennett GW and Wigmore PM (2006). "Treatment with olanzapine increases cell proliferation in the subventricular zone and prefrontal cortex." *Brain Res* 1070(1): 242-5.

Hanisch UK (2002). "Microglia as a source and target of cytokines." *Glia* 40(2): 140-55.

Hanisch UK and Kettenmann H (2007). "Microglia: active sensor and versatile effector cells in the normal and pathologic brain." *Nat Neurosci* 10(11): 1387-94.

Hao C, Richardson A and Fedoroff S (1991). "Macrophage-like cells originate from neuroepithelium in culture: characterization and properties of the macrophage-like cells." *Int J Dev Neurosci* 9(1): 1-14.

Hartley RS, Margulis M, Fishman PS, Lee VM and Tang CM (1999). "Functional synapses are formed between human NTera2 (NT2N, hNT) neurons grown on astrocytes." *J Comp Neurol* 407(1): 1-10.

Hausler KG, Prinz M, Nolte C, Weber JR, Schumann RR, Kettenmann H and Hanisch UK (2002). "Interferon-gamma differentially modulates the release of cytokines and chemokines in lipopolysaccharide- and pneumococcal cell wall-stimulated mouse microglia and macrophages." *Eur J Neurosci* 16(11): 2113-22.

Haynes SE, Hollopeter G, Yang G, Kurpius D, Dailey ME, Gan WB and Julius D (2006). "The P2Y12 receptor regulates microglial activation by extracellular nucleotides." *Nat Neurosci* 9(12): 1512-9.

Heldmann U, Thored P, Claasen JH, Arvidsson A, Kokaia Z and Lindvall O (2005). "TNF-alpha antibody infusion impairs survival of stroke-generated neuroblasts in adult rat brain." *Exp Neurol* 196(1): 204-8.

Heyen JR, Ye S, Finck BN and Johnson RW (2000). "Interleukin (IL)-10 inhibits IL-6 production in microglia by preventing activation of NF-kappaB." *Brain Res Mol Brain Res* 77(1): 138-47.

Hickey WF (1999). "Leukocyte traffic in the central nervous system: the participants and their roles." *Semin Immunol* 11(2): 125-37.

Horvath RJ, Nutile-McMenemy N, Alkaitis MS and Deleo JA (2008). "Differential migration, LPS-induced cytokine, chemokine, and NO expression in immortalized BV-2 and HAPI cell lines and primary microglial cultures." *J Neurochem* 107(2): 557-69.

Imitola J, Raddassi K, Park KI, Mueller FJ, Nieto M, Teng YD, Frenkel D, Li J, Sidman RL, Walsh CA, Snyder EY and Khoury SJ (2004). "Directed migration of neural stem cells to sites of CNS injury by the stromal cell-derived factor 1alpha/CXC chemokine receptor 4 pathway." *Proc Natl Acad Sci U S A* 101(52): 18117-22.

Iosif RE, Ekdahl CT, Ahlenius H, Pronk CJ, Bonde S, Kokaia Z, Jacobsen SE and Lindvall O (2006). "Tumor necrosis factor receptor 1 is a negative regulator of progenitor proliferation in adult hippocampal neurogenesis." *J Neurosci* 26(38): 9703-12.

Irvin DK, Dhaka A, Hicks C, Weinmaster G and Kornblum HI (2003). "Extrinsic and intrinsic factors governing cell fate in cortical progenitor cultures." *Dev Neurosci* 25(2-4): 162-72.

Islam O, Gong X, Rose-John S and Heese K (2009). "Interleukin-6 and neural stem cells: more than gliogenesis." *Mol Biol Cell* 20(1): 188-99.

Ito D, Imai Y, Ohsawa K, Nakajima K, Fukuuchi Y and Kohsaka S (1998). "Microglia-specific localisation of a novel calcium binding protein, Iba1." *Brain Res Mol Brain Res* 57(1): 1-9.

Johansson S, Price J and Modo M (2008). "Effect of inflammatory cytokines on major histocompatibility complex expression and differentiation of human neural stem/progenitor cells." *Stem Cells* 26(9): 2444-54.

Kaneko Y, Sakakibara S, Imai T, Suzuki A, Nakamura Y, Sawamoto K, Ogawa Y, Toyama Y, Miyata T and Okano H (2000). "Musashi1: an evolutionally conserved marker for CNS progenitor cells including neural stem cells." *Dev Neurosci* 22(1-2): 139-53.

Kawabe T, Suganuma M, Ando T, Kimura M, Hori H and Okamoto T (2002). "Cdc25C interacts with PCNA at G2/M transition." *Oncogene* 21(11): 1717-26.

Keeble JE and Moore PK (2002). "Pharmacology and potential therapeutic applications of nitric oxide-releasing non-steroidal anti-inflammatory and related nitric oxide-donating drugs." *Br J Pharmacol* 137(3): 295-310.

Kempermann G, Gast D, Kronenberg G, Yamaguchi M and Gage FH (2003). "Early determination and long-term persistence of adult-generated new neurons in the hippocampus of mice." *Development* 130(2): 391-9.

Kiss JZ and Rougon G (1997). "Cell biology of polysialic acid." *Curr Opin Neurobiol* 7(5): 640-6.

Koc and Kucukguzel SG (2009). "Medicinal chemistry and anti-inflammatory activity of nitric oxide-releasing NSAI drugs." *Mini Rev Med Chem* 9(5): 611-9.

Koo JW and Duman RS (2008). "IL-1beta is an essential mediator of the antineurogenic and anhedonic effects of stress." *Proc Natl Acad Sci U S A* 105(2): 751-6.

Kreutzberg GW (1996). "Microglia: a sensor for pathological events in the CNS." *Trends Neurosci* 19(8): 312-8.

Kuhn HG, Winkler J, Kempermann G, Thal LJ and Gage FH (1997). "Epidermal growth factor and fibroblast growth factor-2 have different effects on neural progenitors in the adult rat brain." *J Neurosci* 17(15): 5820-9.

Ladeby R, Wirenfeldt M, Dalmau I, Gregersen R, Garcia-Ovejero D, Babcock A, Owens T and Finsen B (2005). "Proliferating resident microglia express the stem cell antigen CD34 in response to acute neural injury." *Glia* 50(2): 121-31.

Lambertsen KL, Clausen BH, Babcock AA, Gregersen R, Fenger C, Nielsen HH, Haugaard LS, Wirenfeldt M, Nielsen M, Dagnaes-Hansen F, Bluethmann H, Faergeman NJ, Meldgaard M, Deierborg T and Finsen B (2009). "Microglia protect neurons against ischemia by synthesis of tumor necrosis factor." *J Neurosci* 29(5): 1319-30.

Lawson LJ, Perry VH, Dri P and Gordon S (1990). "Heterogeneity in the distribution and morphology of microglia in the normal adult mouse brain." *Neuroscience* 39(1): 151-70.

Lee MK, Rebhun LI and Frankfurter A (1990). "Posttranslational modification of class III beta-tubulin." *Proc Natl Acad Sci U S A* 87(18): 7195-9.

Levison SW and Goldman JE (1997). "Multipotential and lineage restricted precursors coexist in the mammalian perinatal subventricular zone." *J Neurosci Res* 48(2): 83-94.

Li T, Jiang L, Chen H and Zhang X (2008). "Characterization of excitability and voltage-gated ion channels of neural progenitor cells in rat hippocampus." *J Mol Neurosci* 35(3): 289-95.

Li W, Gao G, Guo Q, Jia D, Wang J, Wang X, He S and Liang Q (2009). "Function and phenotype of microglia are determined by toll-like receptor 2/toll-like receptor 4 activation sequence." *DNA Cell Biol* 28(10): 493-9.

Lim GP, Yang F, Chu T, Chen P, Beech W, Teter B, Tran T, Ubeda O, Ashe KH, Frautschy SA and Cole GM (2000). "Ibuprofen suppresses plaque pathology and inflammation in a mouse model for Alzheimer's disease." *J Neurosci* 20(15): 5709-14.

Limke TL and Rao MS (2002). "Neural stem cells in aging and disease." *J Cell Mol Med* 6(4): 475-96.

Ling EA and Wong WC (1993). "The origin and nature of ramified and amoeboid microglia: a historical review and current concepts." *Glia* 7(1): 9-18.

Liu B and Hong JS (2003). "Role of microglia in inflammation-mediated neurodegenerative diseases: mechanisms and strategies for therapeutic intervention." *J Pharmacol Exp Ther* 304(1): 1-7.

Liu BF, Gao EJ, Zeng XZ, Ji M, Cai Q, Lu Q, Yang H and Xu QY (2006). "Proliferation of neural precursors in the subventricular zone after chemical lesions of the nigrostriatal pathway in rat brain." *Brain Res* 1106(1): 30-9.

Liu YP, Lin HI and Tzeng SF (2005). "Tumor necrosis factor-alpha and interleukin-18 modulate neuronal cell fate in embryonic neural progenitor culture." *Brain Res* 1054(2): 152-8.

Lockhart BP, Cressey KC and Lepagnol JM (1998). "Suppression of nitric oxide formation by tyrosine kinase inhibitors in murine N9 microglia." *Br J Pharmacol* 123(5): 879-89.

Lossinsky AS and Shivers RR (2004). "Structural pathways for macromolecular and cellular transport across the blood-brain barrier during inflammatory conditions. Review." *Histol Histopathol* 19(2): 535-64.

Lucas SM, Rothwell NJ and Gibson RM (2006). "The role of inflammation in CNS injury and disease." *Br J Pharmacol* 147 Suppl 1: S232-40.

Luo CX, Zhu XJ, Zhou QG, Wang B, Wang W, Cai HH, Sun YJ, Hu M, Jiang J, Hua Y, Han X and Zhu DY (2007). "Reduced neuronal nitric oxide synthase is involved in ischemia-induced hippocampal neurogenesis by up-regulating inducible nitric oxide synthase expression." *J Neurochem* 103(5): 1872-82.

Luskin MB, Zigova T, Soteres BJ and Stewart RR (1997). "Neuronal progenitor cells derived from the anterior subventricular zone of the neonatal rat forebrain continue to proliferate in vitro and express a neuronal phenotype." *Mol Cell Neurosci* 8(5): 351-66.

Matarredona ER, Murillo-Carretero M, Moreno-Lopez B and Estrada C (2005). "Role of nitric oxide in subventricular zone neurogenesis." *Brain Res Brain Res Rev* 49(2): 355-66.

McGeer PL and McGeer EG (1995). "The inflammatory response system of brain: implications for therapy of Alzheimer and other neurodegenerative diseases." *Brain Res Brain Res Rev* 21(2): 195-218.

Memberg SP and Hall AK (1995). "Dividing neuron precursors express neuron-specific tubulin." *J Neurobiol* 27(1): 26-43.

Ming GL and Song H (2005). "Adult neurogenesis in the mammalian central nervous system." *Annu Rev Neurosci* 28: 223-50.

Ming GL and Song H (2011). "Adult neurogenesis in the mammalian brain: significant answers and significant questions." *Neuron* 70(4): 687-702.

Minghetti L and Levi G (1998). "Microglia as effector cells in brain damage and repair: focus on prostanoids and nitric oxide." *Prog Neurobiol* 54(1): 99-125.

Assessing the Influence of Neuroinflammation on Neurogenesis: In Vitro Models Using Neural Stem Cells and Microglia as Valuable Research Tools

145

Monje ML, Toda H and Palmer TD (2003). "Inflammatory blockade restores adult hippocampal neurogenesis." *Science* 302(5651): 1760-5.

Moran LB, Duke DC and Graeber MB (2007). "The microglial gene regulatory network activated by interferon-gamma." *J Neuroimmunol* 183(1-2): 1-6.

Moreno-Lopez B, Romero-Grimaldi C, Noval JA, Murillo-Carretero M, Matarredona ER and Estrada C (2004). "Nitric oxide is a physiological inhibitor of neurogenesis in the adult mouse subventricular zone and olfactory bulb." *J Neurosci* 24(1): 85-95.

Morgan SC, Taylor DL and Pocock JM (2004). "Microglia release activators of neuronal proliferation mediated by activation of mitogen-activated protein kinase, phosphatidylinositol-3-kinase/Akt and delta-Notch signalling cascades." *J Neurochem* 90(1): 89-101.

Morshead CM, Benveniste P, Iscove NN and van der Kooy D (2002). "Hematopoietic competence is a rare property of neural stem cells that may depend on genetic and epigenetic alterations." *Nat Med* 8(3): 268-73.

Morshead CM, Craig CG and van der Kooy D (1998). "In vivo clonal analyses reveal the properties of endogenous neural stem cell proliferation in the adult mammalian forebrain." *Development* 125(12): 2251-61.

Morshead CM, Reynolds BA, Craig CG, McBurney MW, Staines WA, Morassutti D, Weiss S and van der Kooy D (1994). "Neural stem cells in the adult mammalian forebrain: a relatively quiescent subpopulation of subependymal cells." *Neuron* 13(5): 1071-82.

Mullen RJ, Buck CR and Smith AM (1992). "NeuN, a neuronal specific nuclear protein in vertebrates." *Development* 116(1): 201-11.

Nakanishi M, Niidome T, Matsuda S, Akaike A, Kihara T and Sugimoto H (2007). "Microglia-derived interleukin-6 and leukaemia inhibitory factor promote astrocytic differentiation of neural stem/progenitor cells." *Eur J Neurosci* 25(3): 649-58.

Nakatomi H, Kuriu T, Okabe S, Yamamoto S, Hatano O, Kawahara N, Tamura A, Kirino T and Nakafuku M (2002). "Regeneration of hippocampal pyramidal neurons after ischemic brain injury by recruitment of endogenous neural progenitors." *Cell* 110(4): 429-41.

Napoli C and Ignarro LJ (2003). "Nitric oxide-releasing drugs." *Annu Rev Pharmacol Toxicol* 43: 97-123.

Nimmerjahn A, Kirchhoff F and Helmchen F (2005). "Resting microglial cells are highly dynamic surveillants of brain parenchyma in vivo." *Science* 308(5726): 1314-8.

Nixon K and Crews FT (2004). "Temporally specific burst in cell proliferation increases hippocampal neurogenesis in protracted abstinence from alcohol." *J Neurosci* 24(43): 9714-22.

Nowakowski RS, Lewin SB and Miller MW (1989). "Bromodeoxyuridine immunohistochemical determination of the lengths of the cell cycle and the DNA-synthetic phase for an anatomically defined population." *J Neurocytol* 18(3): 311-8.

Oehmichen W and Gencic M (1975). "Experimental studies on kinetics and functions of monuclear phagozytes of the central nervous system." *Acta Neuropathol Suppl* Suppl 6: 285-90.

Okano HJ, Pfaff DW and Gibbs RB (1993). "RB and Cdc2 expression in brain: correlations with 3H-thymidine incorporation and neurogenesis." *J Neurosci* 13(7): 2930-8.

Ostenfeld T, Joly E, Tai YT, Peters A, Caldwell M, Jauniaux E and Svendsen CN (2002). "Regional specification of rodent and human neurospheres." *Brain Res Dev Brain Res* 134(1-2): 43-55.

Palmer TD, Schwartz PH, Taupin P, Kaspar B, Stein SA and Gage FH (2001). "Cell culture. Progenitor cells from human brain after death." *Nature* 411(6833): 42-3.

Park JY, Choi HJ, Prabagar MG, Choi WS, Kim SJ, Cheong C, Park CG, Chin CY and Kang YS (2009). "The C-type lectin CD209b is expressed on microglia and it mediates the uptake of capsular polysaccharides of Streptococcus pneumoniae." *Neurosci Lett* 450(3): 246-51.

Parmar M, Sjoberg A, Bjorklund A and Kokaia Z (2003). "Phenotypic and molecular identity of cells in the adult subventricular zone. in vivo and after expansion in vitro." *Mol Cell Neurosci* 24(3): 741-52.

Pei Z, Pang H, Qian L, Yang S, Wang T, Zhang W, Wu X, Dallas S, Wilson B, Reece JM, Miller DS, Hong JS and Block ML (2007). "MAC1 mediates LPS-induced production of superoxide by microglia: the role of pattern recognition receptors in dopaminergic neurotoxicity." *Glia* 55(13): 1362-73.

Petreanu L and Alvarez-Buylla A (2002). "Maturation and death of adult-born olfactory bulb granule neurons: role of olfaction." *J Neurosci* 22(14): 6106-13.

Pevny L and Placzek M (2005). "SOX genes and neural progenitor identity." *Curr Opin Neurobiol* 15(1): 7-13.

Polazzi E and Monti B (2010). "Microglia and neuroprotection: from in vitro studies to therapeutic applications." *Prog Neurobiol* 92(3): 293-315.

Pollard SM, Conti L, Sun Y, Goffredo D and Smith A (2006). "Adherent neural stem (NS) cells from fetal and adult forebrain." *Cereb Cortex* 16 Suppl 1: i112-20.

Ponomarev ED, Novikova M, Maresz K, Shriver LP and Dittel BN (2005). "Development of a culture system that supports adult microglial cell proliferation and maintenance in the resting state." *J Immunol Methods* 300(1-2): 32-46.

Qin H, Wilson CA, Lee SJ, Zhao X and Benveniste EN (2005a). "LPS induces CD40 gene expression through the activation of NF-kappaB and STAT-1alpha in macrophages and microglia." *Blood* 106(9): 3114-22.

Qin L, Li G, Qian X, Liu Y, Wu X, Liu B, Hong JS and Block ML (2005b). "Interactive role of the toll-like receptor 4 and reactive oxygen species in LPS-induced microglia activation." *Glia* 52(1): 78-84.

Rao MS and Shetty AK (2004). "Efficacy of doublecortin as a marker to analyse the absolute number and dendritic growth of newly generated neurons in the adult dentate gyrus." *Eur J Neurosci* 19(2): 234-46.

Reynolds BA, Tetzlaff W and Weiss S (1992). "A multipotent EGF-responsive striatal embryonic progenitor cell produces neurons and astrocytes." *J Neurosci* 12(11): 4565-74.

Reynolds BA and Weiss S (1992). "Generation of neurons and astrocytes from isolated cells of the adult mammalian central nervous system." *Science* 255(5052): 1707-10.

Reynolds BA and Weiss S (1996). "Clonal and population analyses demonstrate that an EGF-responsive mammalian embryonic CNS precursor is a stem cell." *Dev Biol* 175(1): 1-13.

Richardson RM, Broaddus WC, Holloway KL and Fillmore HL (2005). "Grafts of adult subependymal zone neuronal progenitor cells rescue hemiparkinsonian behavioral decline." *Brain Res* 1032(1-2): 11-22.

Roberts ES, Masliah E and Fox HS (2004). "CD163 identifies a unique population of ramified microglia in HIV encephalitis (HIVE)." *J Neuropathol Exp Neurol* 63(12): 1255-64.

Rochefort C, Gheusi G, Vincent JD and Lledo PM (2002). "Enriched odor exposure increases the number of newborn neurons in the adult olfactory bulb and improves odor memory." *J Neurosci* 22(7): 2679-89.

Rolls A, Shechter R, London A, Ziv Y, Ronen A, Levy R and Schwartz M (2007). "Toll-like receptors modulate adult hippocampal neurogenesis." *Nat Cell Biol* 9(9): 1081-8.

Rosenstiel P, Lucius R, Deuschl G, Sievers J and Wilms H (2001). "From theory to therapy: implications from an in vitro model of ramified microglia." *Microsc Res Tech* 54(1): 18-25.

Rostovtsev VV, Green LG, Fokin VV and Sharpless KB (2002). "A stepwise huisgen cycloaddition process: copper(I)-catalyzed regioselective "ligation" of azides and terminal alkynes." *Angew Chem Int Ed Engl* 41(14): 2596-9.

Sakakibara S, Imai T, Hamaguchi K, Okabe M, Aruga J, Nakajima K, Yasutomi D, Nagata T, Kurihara Y, Uesugi S, Miyata T, Ogawa M, Mikoshiba K and Okano H (1996). "Mouse-Musashi-1, a neural RNA-binding protein highly enriched in the mammalian CNS stem cell." *Dev Biol* 176(2): 230-42.

Salic A and Mitchison TJ (2008). "A chemical method for fast and sensitive detection of DNA synthesis in vivo." *Proc Natl Acad Sci U S A* 105(7): 2415-20.

Sanai N, Tramontin AD, Quinones-Hinojosa A, Barbaro NM, Gupta N, Kunwar S, Lawton MT, McDermott MW, Parsa AT, Manuel-Garcia Verdugo J, Berger MS and Alvarez-Buylla A (2004). "Unique astrocyte ribbon in adult human brain contains neural stem cells but lacks chain migration." *Nature* 427(6976): 740-4.

Sapir T, Horesh D, Caspi M, Atlas R, Burgess HA, Wolf SG, Francis F, Chelly J, Elbaum M, Pietrokovski S and Reiner O (2000). "Doublecortin mutations cluster in evolutionarily conserved functional domains." *Hum Mol Genet* 9(5): 703-12.

Sasaki A, Yamaguchi H, Horikoshi Y, Tanaka G and Nakazato Y (2004). "Expression of glucose transporter 5 by microglia in human gliomas." *Neuropathol Appl Neurobiol* 30(5): 447-55.

Saura J, Tusell JM and Serratosa J (2003). "High-yield isolation of murine microglia by mild trypsinization." *Glia* 44(3): 183-9.

Sawada M, Kondo N, Suzumura A and Marunouchi T (1989). "Production of tumor necrosis factor-alpha by microglia and astrocytes in culture." *Brain Res* 491(2): 394-7.

Seki T (2002). "Hippocampal adult neurogenesis occurs in a microenvironment provided by PSA-NCAM-expressing immature neurons." *J Neurosci Res* 69(6): 772-83.

Seki T and Arai Y (1993). "Highly polysialylated neural cell adhesion molecule (NCAM-H) is expressed by newly generated granule cells in the dentate gyrus of the adult rat." *J Neurosci* 13(6): 2351-8.

Sheen VL, Arnold MW, Wang Y and Macklis JD (1999). "Neural precursor differentiation following transplantation into neocortex is dependent on intrinsic developmental state and receptor competence." *Exp Neurol* 158(1): 47-62.

Shingo T, Gregg C, Enwere E, Fujikawa H, Hassam R, Geary C, Cross JC and Weiss S (2003). "Pregnancy-stimulated neurogenesis in the adult female forebrain mediated by prolactin." *Science* 299(5603): 117-20.

Shors TJ, Miesegaes G, Beylin A, Zhao M, Rydel T and Gould E (2001). "Neurogenesis in the adult is involved in the formation of trace memories." *Nature* 410(6826): 372-6.

Song H, Stevens CF and Gage FH (2002). "Astroglia induce neurogenesis from adult neural stem cells." *Nature* 417(6884): 39-44.

Song JH, Wang CX, Song DK, Wang P, Shuaib A and Hao C (2005). "Interferon gamma induces neurite outgrowth by up-regulation of p35 neuron-specific cyclin-dependent kinase 5 activator via activation of ERK1/2 pathway." *J Biol Chem* 280(13): 12896-901.

Spulber S, Oprica M, Bartfai T, Winblad B and Schultzberg M (2008). "Blunted neurogenesis and gliosis due to transgenic overexpression of human soluble IL-1ra in the mouse." *Eur J Neurosci* 27(3): 549-58.

Stoll G and Jander S (1999). "The role of microglia and macrophages in the pathophysiology of the CNS." *Prog Neurobiol* 58(3): 233-47.

Streit WJ, Graeber MB and Kreutzberg GW (1988). "Functional plasticity of microglia: a review." *Glia* 1(5): 301-7.

Streit WJ, Walter SA and Pennell NA (1999). "Reactive microgliosis." *Prog Neurobiol* 57(6): 563-81.

Sun L, Lee J and Fine HA (2004). "Neuronally expressed stem cell factor induces neural stem cell migration to areas of brain injury." *J Clin Invest* 113(9): 1364-74.

Sun Y, Jin K, Childs JT, Xie L, Mao XO and Greenberg DA (2006). "Vascular endothelial growth factor-B (VEGFB) stimulates neurogenesis: evidence from knockout mice and growth factor administration." *Dev Biol* 289(2): 329-35.

Suslov ON, Kukekov VG, Ignatova TN and Steindler DA (2002). "Neural stem cell heterogeneity demonstrated by molecular phenotyping of clonal neurospheres." *Proc Natl Acad Sci U S A* 99(22): 14506-11.

Suzumura A, Marunouchi T and Yamamoto H (1991). "Morphological transformation of microglia in vitro." *Brain Res* 545(1-2): 301-6.

Suzumura A, Sawada M, Yamamoto H and Marunouchi T (1990). "Effects of colony stimulating factors on isolated microglia in vitro." *J Neuroimmunol* 30(2-3): 111-20.

Svendsen CN (2002). "The amazing astrocyte." *Nature* 417(6884): 29-32.

Taupin P (2008). "Adult neurogenesis, neuroinflammation and therapeutic potential of adult neural stem cells." *Int J Med Sci* 5(3): 127-32.

Thored P, Arvidsson A, Cacci E, Ahlenius H, Kallur T, Darsalia V, Ekdahl CT, Kokaia Z and Lindvall O (2006). "Persistent production of neurons from adult brain stem cells during recovery after stroke." *Stem Cells* 24(3): 739-47.

Thored P, Heldmann U, Gomes-Leal W, Gisler R, Darsalia V, Taneera J, Nygren JM, Jacobsen SE, Ekdahl CT, Kokaia Z and Lindvall O (2009). "Long-term accumulation of microglia with proneurogenic phenotype concomitant with persistent neurogenesis in adult subventricular zone after stroke." *Glia* 57(8): 835-49.

Vallieres L, Campbell IL, Gage FH and Sawchenko PE (2002). "Reduced hippocampal neurogenesis in adult transgenic mice with chronic astrocytic production of interleukin-6." *J Neurosci* 22(2): 486-92.

Vazey EM, Chen K, Hughes SM and Connor B (2006). "Transplanted adult neural progenitor cells survive, differentiate and reduce motor function impairment in a rodent model of Huntington's disease." *Exp Neurol* 199(2): 384-96.

Vernadakis A, Mangoura D, Sakellaridis N and Linderholm S (1984). "Glial cells dissociated from newborn and aged mouse brain." *J Neurosci Res* 11(3): 253-62.

Vezzani A, Moneta D, Richichi C, Aliprandi M, Burrows SJ, Ravizza T, Perego C and De Simoni MG (2002). "Functional role of inflammatory cytokines and antiinflammatory molecules in seizures and epileptogenesis." *Epilepsia* 43 Suppl 5: 30-5.

Vukicevic V, Jauch A, Dinger TC, Gebauer L, Hornich V, Bornstein SR, Ehrhart-Bornstein M and Muller AM (2010). "Genetic instability and diminished differentiation capacity in long-term cultured mouse neurosphere cells." *Mech Ageing Dev* 131(2): 124-32.

Walton NM, Sutter BM, Laywell ED, Levkoff LH, Kearns SM, Marshall GP, 2nd, Scheffler B and Steindler DA (2006). "Microglia instruct subventricular zone neurogenesis." *Glia* 54(8): 815-25.

Wang Y, Sheen VL and Macklis JD (1998). "Cortical interneurons upregulate neurotrophins in vivo in response to targeted apoptotic degeneration of neighboring pyramidal neurons." *Exp Neurol* 154(2): 389-402.

Wegiel J, Wisniewski HM, Dziewiatkowski J, Tarnawski M, Kozielski R, Trenkner E and Wiktor-Jedrzejczak W (1998). "Reduced number and altered morphology of microglial cells in colony stimulating factor-1-deficient osteopetrotic op/op mice." *Brain Res* 804(1): 135-9.

Whitney NP, Eidem TM, Peng H, Huang Y and Zheng JC (2009). "Inflammation mediates varying effects in neurogenesis: relevance to the pathogenesis of brain injury and neurodegenerative disorders." *J Neurochem* 108(6): 1343-59.

Wollmer MA, Lucius R, Wilms H, Held-Feindt J, Sievers J and Mentlein R (2001). "ATP and adenosine induce ramification of microglia in vitro." *J Neuroimmunol* 115(1-2): 19-27.

Wong G, Goldshmit Y and Turnley AM (2004). "Interferon-gamma but not TNF alpha promotes neuronal differentiation and neurite outgrowth of murine adult neural stem cells." *Exp Neurol* 187(1): 171-7.

Wu J, Ohlsson M, Warner EA, Loo KK, Hoang TX, Voskuhl RR and Havton LA (2008). "Glial reactions and degeneration of myelinated processes in spinal cord gray matter in chronic experimental autoimmune encephalomyelitis." *Neuroscience* 156(3): 586-96.

Xu Y, Tamamaki N, Noda T, Kimura K, Itokazu Y, Matsumoto N, Dezawa M and Ide C (2005). "Neurogenesis in the ependymal layer of the adult rat 3rd ventricle." *Exp Neurol* 192(2): 251-64.

Yamamoto S, Yamamoto N, Kitamura T, Nakamura K and Nakafuku M (2001). "Proliferation of parenchymal neural progenitors in response to injury in the adult rat spinal cord." *Exp Neurol* 172(1): 115-27.

Yoshikawa K (2000). "Cell cycle regulators in neural stem cells and postmitotic neurons." *Neurosci Res* 37(1): 1-14.

Zhang J, Shi XQ, Echeverry S, Mogil JS, De Koninck Y and Rivest S (2007). "Expression of CCR2 in both resident and bone marrow-derived microglia plays a critical role in neuropathic pain." *J Neurosci* 27(45): 12396-406.

Zhang RL, Zhang L, Zhang ZG, Morris D, Jiang Q, Wang L, Zhang LJ and Chopp M (2003). "Migration and differentiation of adult rat subventricular zone progenitor cells transplanted into the adult rat striatum." *Neuroscience* 116(2): 373-82.

Zhao M, Momma S, Delfani K, Carlen M, Cassidy RM, Johansson CB, Brismar H, Shupliakov O, Frisen J and Janson AM (2003). "Evidence for neurogenesis in the adult mammalian substantia nigra." *Proc Natl Acad Sci U S A* 100(13): 7925-30.

Zigova T, Pencea V, Betarbet R, Wiegand SJ, Alexander C, Bakay RA and Luskin MB (1998). "Neuronal progenitor cells of the neonatal subventricular zone differentiate and disperse following transplantation into the adult rat striatum." *Cell Transplant* 7(2): 137-56.

7

Immune System Modulation of Germinal and Parenchymal Neural Progenitor Cells in Physiological and Pathological Conditions

Chiara Rolando, Enrica Boda and Annalisa Buffo
Department of Neuroscience
Neuroscience Institute Cavalieri Ottolenghi, NICO
University of Turin
Italy

1. Introduction

Historically, the Central Nervous System (CNS) was considered as an immune privileged site (Billingham and Boswell, 1953), being viewed as a territory physiologically out of the competence of immune cells. This notion has developed on initial studies showing that: (i) CNS unrelated antigens (i.e. foreign grafts, bacteria, viruses) evade an immune recognition when delivered to the brain parenchyma (Galea et al., 2007); (ii) no infiltrating immune cells nor antigen presenting cells (APCs, i.e. dendritic cells, DCs, see Table 1) can be detected in the CNS parenchyma in physiological conditions (Engelhardt and Ransohoff, 2005); (iii) CNS cells do not constitutively express major histocompatibility complex (MHC)I and MHCII molecules (Fabry et al., 1994); (iv) neural cells express apoptosis inductors for immune cells (Bechmann et al., 1999); (v) the CNS does not possess lymphatic vessels (Engelhardt and Ransohoff, 2005). The segregation between nervous and immune cells appeared tightly preserved by the anatomical separations offered by the Blood Brain Barrier (BBB) and the blood-cerebrospinal fluid barrier (Choi and Benveniste, 2004). Over time, on the basis of the association between immune inflammation and neurodegeneration, the concept of immune privilege further acquired the connotation of a defence mechanism against the detrimental effects of immune activation within the CNS.

However, during the last ten years evidence for an extensive and continuous bi-directional communication between the CNS and the immune system has accumulated, changing the traditional view of the CNS as an immune privileged site into an immune specialised site (Engelhardt and Ransohoff, 2005). Under physiological conditions, the CNS strictly controls circulating immune cell entry across its barriers by allowing a regulated exchange of factors between the nervous tissue and immune elements. Such exchange provides an incessant scavenging for self (host) and pathological antigens occurring in the CNS (immunosurveillance) and is at the basis of the newly recognised functions of immune cells in neural stem cell (NSC) activity, hippocampal neurogenesis, learning and stress-mediated responses (see below). In case of pathology, when the BBB is damaged or altered and immune attractive signals are released within the CNS, lymphocytes and macrophages penetrate into the CNS parenchyma. This invasion has now lost the former exclusively detrimental flavour in view of newly unveiled effects supportive for neuroprotection and reparative responses (Schwartz et al., 2009).

Studies on the interplay between the immune system and NSCs/progenitors in both health and disease have particularly contributed to this conceptual revolution in neuroimmunology. These studies are the actual focus of this chapter. We shall present them after having overviewed the main players and mechanisms involved in the CNS-immune system crosstalk.

1.1 Routes and modes of immunosurveillance in the healthy CNS

Main players in immunosurveillance are microglia cells residing within the CNS parenchyma, circulating monocytes and lymphocytes that mostly remain located at the outer anatomical borders of the CNS (Table 1, Schwartz and Shechter, 2010). These borders are defined by several structures: the outermost dural membrane, the arachnoid membrane and the innermost pial membrane. The subarachnoid space settles between the arachnoid and pial membrane and it is filled with the cerebrospinal fluid (CSF), which is continuously produced by the choroid plexus epithelium in the ventricular system. It circulates from the ventricle to the subarachnoid space and it is reabsorbed by the arachnoid villi that extend in the venous sinuses. The nervous artery supply follows the CNS surface in the subarachnoid space. As vessels enter the CNS parenchyma, they are surrounded by a perivascular space, the Virchow-Robin space, connected to the subarachnoid space. Moreover, the BBB separates the blood from the CNS parenchyma and is formed by highly specialized endothelial cells surrounded by basement membranes and astroglial end feet.

In the healthy CNS, immune reactivity is strictly controlled by limiting the presentation of neuroantigens outside the CNS and by tightly regulating the trafficking of immunocompetent cells. The BBB avoids leaking of neuroantigens into the systemic circulation, while within the nervous tissue microglia cells continuously survey the parenchyma with highly dynamic processes and protrusions that may clear accumulated metabolites and cell debris, thereby regulating microenvironmental homeostasis (Nimmerjahn et al., 2005). This microglial function is proposed to be directly influenced by T cell-derived soluble factors, at least at specific CNS sites (see section 2.1; Ziv et al., 2006a). T cells normally do not enter the healthy nervous tissue, but can reach the CSF together with monocytes (about 3000 leukocytes per ml can be found in the CSF of healthy individuals) from both vessels of the choroid plexi and post-capillary venules surrounded by the Virchow-Robin space. Soluble proteins and cells constitutively move from the CNS parenchyma into the CSF through the choroid plexi and ependymal cells and are transported up to peripheral lymph nodes, where they are presented to naïve CD4+ T lymphocytes (afferent arm of immunosurveillance) to achieve their first activation (see Table 1). In the efferent route of this loop, activated CD4+ T cells get to the CNS via the blood stream, and there, moving into the CSF, flow back to the systemic circulation (Ransohoff et al., 2003). The CSF is the site of secondary activation of CD4+ T cells that there encounter monocytes presenting neuroantigens and contribute to immunosurveillance without being encephalitogenic.

Very few if any leukocytes can directly access the healthy CNS parenchyma by crossing the BBB and the endothelial basal lamina. Of note, the few T cells entering the parenchyma have undergone the first activation with neuroantigens, while resting lymphocytes fail to penetrate even after stimulation with inflammatory cues (Ransohoff et al., 2003). The involvement of lymphocyte populations other than CD4+ T (CD8+ T, B cells and NKs) in CNS immunosurveillance has so far been considered poorly relevant, as they comprise neglectable fractions in the healthy CNS/CSF (Ransohoff et al., 2003). During pathology the scenario depicted so far can undergo dramatic changes that compromise the CNS specialised status. Dangerous antigens can be sensed locally within the CNS or directly drained to the periphery to stimulate further recruitment of immune cells. The accompanying massive release of cytokines and chemokines by immune and neural cells mediates the initiation of an immune reaction aimed at promoting CNS defence and restoring tissue homeostasis.

1.2 Innate and adaptive immune responses in the diseased CNS

To effectively exert its defensive functions, the immune system has developed two different reaction modes: a relatively fast and generic action against external agents (innate response), and a specific and targeted action that requires plasticity and memory (adaptive or acquired immunity). Innate and adaptive responses operate in strict collaboration and undergo distinct levels of activation depending on the type of pathology. The innate response is the first line of CNS defence, preceding and stimulating the adaptive reaction (Nguyen, 2002), and relies on microglia cells and on astrocytes. Both cell types constitutively express phagocytic and scavenger receptors (pattern-recognition receptors, PPRs) capable of distinguishing self (host) from non-self (i.e. pathogens, toxic agents and molecules released by damaged/dying cells). Peripheral macrophages/monocytes can also participate in this initial activation when lesions such as traumatic or vascular injury induce BBB breakdown and allow direct CNS parenchyma-blood interactions. Amongst PPRs are Toll-like receptors (TLRs, Table 1) that activate phagocytosis and, via the nuclear transcription factor NFkB pathway, promote the production of pro-inflammatory signals, including cytokines (Interleukin1β, IL1β; Tumor Necrosis Factor-α, TNFα; IL6) and chemokines (Becher et al., 2000; Farina et al., 2007), modulating the nervous tissue response to damage (Buffo et al., 2010) and triggering adaptive immunity (Becher et al., 2000). Notably, several CNS intrinsic mechanisms operate to avoid uncontrolled or hyperactive innate responses: (i) neurons, endothelial and ependymal cells express neuroimmune regulatory proteins (NIRegs) to protect CNS cells from the phagocytic activity of macrophages and microglia and attenuate inflammatory cytokine secretion by lymphocytes (Griffiths et al., 2007); (ii) gliotic astrocytes limit blood leukocyte infiltration (Voskuhl et al., 2009).

Initiation of an adaptive immune response requires time after the initial appearance of pathogenic signals, and implies the participation of numerous cell types and signalling molecules. Adaptive immunity can be either cell-mediated (major effectors are T cells), or humoral (with the involvement of B cells, see Table 1). Although humoral immune responses are most important for the organism's defence, their role in the regulation of neural stem cells and parenchymal progenitor activity is so far unknown. Thus, we shall leave them aside and focus on cell-mediated immune responses.

During CNS damage (e.g. traumatic and neurovascular injuries such as stroke) the integrity of the BBB is primarily disrupted, leading to increased and often deregulated communication between the CNS and the immune system, including the entry of immune cells. In other cases, however, an increased exchange of cellular elements and signals between the two systems occurs while the gross anatomy of the BBB is preserved, thereby implying more subtle functional alterations (Kaur and Ling, 2008). In some cases, such as the initial phase of Multiple Sclerosis (MS), deregulated autoimmune cellular elements find their way into the CNS where they trigger an acute inflammatory reaction to myelin components that can progress into a chronic phase of neurodegeneration. In general, after a CNS insult, resident microglia, astrocytes and DCs that can migrate from the perivascular space into the CNS parenchyma if the BBB is disrupted, present antigens to CD4+ and CD8+ T cells in association with co-stimulatory molecules. After priming with APCs, both T cell types become activated and proliferate: CD8+ T cells exert their cytotoxic activity inducing the apoptosis of antigen-bounded MHCI expressing cells, whereas CD4+ T cells produce pro- or anti-inflammatory cytokines, depending on their subtypes (Th1, Th2, see Table 1, Becher et al., 2000). Th1 cells release pro-inflammatory molecules that sustain and potentiate microglial activation in a feed-forward loop, and stimulate MHCII expression on astrocytes and endothelial cells (see Table 1). In turn, chemokines and cytokines from microglia and activated astrocytes such as interferon-γ (INFγ) and TNFα can both attract and activate immune cells (Carpentier et al., 2005). Conversely, Th2 cells exert anti-inflammatory effects through the production of IL4 and IL10, reducing macrophage and microglia activation (see Table 1). The balance between Th1/Th2 phenotypes is finely tuned by cytokines themselves (Goverman, 2009), and requires a tight regulation to avoid detrimental hyperinflammation: for instance, IL12 produced by activated microglia promotes Th1 type, while astrocytes are known to counteract this phenomenon (Becker et al., 2000).

A further modulatory mechanism of T cell activity involves a specific subclass of T cells, the CD4+ CD25+ Foxp3 T regulatory cells (Tregs, see Table1, Walsh and Kipnis, 2010). Tregs act by suppressing autoimmunity (T cells directed against self-antigens) and terminating immune responses. They exert their inhibitory action mostly through Transforming Growth Factor-β (TGFβ) signalling and IL10 production, which suppresses auto-reactive T cells (Vignali et al., 2008).

Further mechanisms participate in terminating immune reactions: (i) activated T cells themselves express receptors (i.e. CTLA-4) that reduce their proliferation and production of cytokines after interaction with microglia; (ii) T cells after cytokine exposure upregulate receptors that induce their apoptosis (i.e. CD95); (iii) IL2 potentiates CD95-mediated apoptosis. Thus, immune responses are self-limited and decline with time after antigenic stimulation, leaving functionally quiescent memory lymphocytes as indicators of previous antigen exposure (Parijis and Albas, 1998). Acute immune response and inflammation may therefore be soon resolved, and the damage circumscribed by astroglial scarring and microglia cells with poor replacement of lost cells and transected axons (Bush et al., 1999; Donnelly and Popovich, 2007). Yet, an involvement of abnormal autoimmunity or the persistence of pro-inflammatory stimuli can protract the inflammatory/immuno response into a chronic status and exacerbate the destructive effects of immune activation (McFarland and Martin, 2007).

Despite the described mechanisms of immune response have evolved primarily as a defence from infectious agents, they take place in all types of CNS injuries. In the following sections we will not deal with infectious diseases, but instead focus on traumatic, vascular, autoimmune damage and chronic neurodegeneration, where loss or malfunctioning of cellular elements is followed by activation and recruitment of NSCs and parenchymal progenitors, engaged for the most in replacing lost myelin rather then neurons, and in the production of scarring astrocytes (see below).

	Features	Functions	Molecular Signals	References
Microglia	• Invade the CNS parenchyma during late embryogenesis and perinatal stage • Myeloid cells • APC upon activation	• Immunosurveillance • Innate immunity • Cytokine secretion (IL1, IL6, IL12, TNFα) • Phagocytic and cytotoxic activity • T cell stimulation and apoptosis (Fas ligand mediated) • Neurogenesis control	• Upregulation MHCI and II and CD40, CD86 to activate T cells • TLR expression • Upregulation of complement receptor (CR1, CR3, CR4)	Yang et al., 2010 Aloisi et al., 2000
Astrocyte	• Most abundant glial cells in the CNS • Neuroectodermal origin	• Brain homeostasis • BBB formation • Scar formation • APC function induced by Th1 cytokines • Cytokine production (TNFα, IL6, IL12, IL1) • Polarization of T cell cytokine responses • B cell survival and differentiation • Microglia activation • Neurogenesis	• Upregulation MHCII, TLRs (TLRs1-6, TLR9), ICAM1 and VCAM1, chemokines (CCL2, CCL5) • Expression of BAFF (B cell activating factor) • Neurotrophic factor release (BDNF, NGF, IGF1, LIF)	Carpentier et al., 2005 Farina et al., 2007
CD4+ T	• Helper T cells (Th) • Antigen recognition bound to MHCII through T cell Receptor (TCR) • Th1 pro-inflammatory phenotype (INFγ, TNFα production) • Th2 anti-inflammatory phenotype (IL4 and IL10 production)	• Adaptive cell-mediated immune response • Autoimmunity • Activation of B cells	• BDNF production • IL2 production for T cell survival	Goverman, 2009 Dittel, 2008
CD8+ T	• Cytotoxic T cells • Antigen recognition bound to MHCI through TCR	• Cytolysis (perforin mediated) • CNS autoimmunity	• Cytokine production (INFγ and TNFα, IL10, IL17)	Goverman, 2009
Treg	• CD4 positive • Foxp3 positive (forkhead box P3) that controls their development and function and it is induced by TGFβ • CD25 expression (IL2R)	• Avoidance of autoimmune disease and tumoral autoimmunity (peripheral tolerance) • Suppression by cytokine inhibition, cytolysis, by metabolic disruption, by targeting DCs	• Release of TGFβ, IL10, IL35, Granzime B, Adenoside nucleoside, cAMP	Vignali et al., 2008; Walsh and Kipnis, 2010

	Features	Functions	Molecular Signals	References
		• Control CD8+ T cell invasion		
Th17	• Pro-inflammatory lineage • Autoimmune disease	• Cytokine production (TGFβ, IL6, IL23) • Suppression Treg differentiation (IL21 mediated)	• Activation of the STAT3 pathway • Activation of RORα/RORγ	Fabry et al., 2008
B cells	• Rarely detected in the healthy CSF • Four different developmental states (mature B cells, memory B cells, plasmablast, plasma cells)	• Humoral immune response • T cell activation • Ig production • APCs • Ig CNS autoantigen production that induce complement activation, MBP proteolysis, macrophages stimulation	• Upregulation of CXCR12/13 and CCR1,2,4 • Cytokine production (IL6, IL10, IL12, TGFβ) • Neurotrophic factor release (NGF and BDNF)	Meinl et al., 2006
DCs	• APCs • Lymphoid and myeloid origin • Localized in the meninges and chroid plexi in the healthy brain • During inflammation, autoimmune diseases and neurodegeneration they reach the CNS parenchyma	• Immunosurveillance • T cell stimulation, tolerance induction, T cell polarization, phagocytosis, cytokine secretion (IL1b, IL6, IL10, IL12, TNFα, INFγ)	• MHC class II, costimulatory proteins (CD40, CD80, CD86), chemokine receptor (CCR7)	McMahon et al., 2006
Toll like Receptors (TLR)	• Expressed on APCs including microglia and DCs • Surface recognition of PAMPs • Expression on resting and activated microglia and astrocytes (TLR3 on astrocytes, TLR2 and TLR4 on microglia) • Extracellular portion with multiple leucine-rich repeats	• Recognition of exogenous components of the bacterial membrane and flagella, bacterial DNA and viral dsRNA • Neurogenesis	• NFkB activation • Cytokine and chemokine production	Farina et al., 2007 Rolls et al., 2007

Table 1. Immunoplayers.

Main cellular types and molecular signals that regulate the interplay between the immune system and the CNS. This process involves the participation of CNS resident cells (microglia and astrocytes), immune system cells and numerous molecular signals.

2. Immune-based regulation of adult Neural Stem Cell activities and neurogenesis

In the adult brain NSCs displaying astrocytic features reside in two anatomically defined germinal niches, namely the subventricular zone (SVZ) of the lateral wall of the lateral ventricles and the subgranular zone of the hippocampus (SGZ). Adult NSCs of the SVZ (also termed Type-B cells) retain the capability to asymmetrically divide, giving rise to actively proliferating intermediate neural progenitors defined as transit amplifying cells or Type-C cells. These latter cells symmetrically divide to produce neuroblasts (Type-A cells) that migrate through the Rostral Migratory Stream (RMS) into the olfactory bulb, where they eventually differentiate in interneurons. *In vivo* type-B cells can also generate oligodendroglial cells of the corpus callosum and fimbria fornix, although to a lesser extent compared to neurons (Kriegstein and Alvarez-Buylla, 2009). NSCs residing within the hippocampal SGZ divide asymmetrically to give rise to neuroblasts that locally differentiate into mature granular neurons (Kriegstein and Alvarez-Buylla, 2009). Numerous studies indicate that continuous neurogenesis in the olfactory bulb and hippocampus is instrumental for memory acquisition, learning and mood regulation (Zhao et al., 2008), while both physiological (i.e. life experiences, such as learning, physical activity, environmental or olfactory enrichment, stress) and pathological (i.e. brain insults or pathologies, local or systemic inflammation) stimuli affect NSCs and their derivatives.

Surprisingly, a number of recent studies have provided evidence that local and systemic immune-mediated mechanisms, including both innate and adaptive factors, exert a key role in modulating neuro/oligodendrogenic events within the germinal niches in healthy and pathological conditions. Such immune-based regulation takes place at many levels, including (i) proliferation of NSCs and intermediate progenitors; (ii) neuronal vs. glial specification of NSC-derivatives; (iii) migratory ability of the new-born elements; and (iv) their survival, maturation and integration in the adult brain parenchyma. Since the identity of immune system players and the level of their recruitment/activation/production are dramatically different in distinct brain conditions (i.e. healthy vs. acutely injured vs. chronically diseased), immune modulation displays complex and context-dependent effects on the functioning and survival of NSCs and their derivatives (see below). For the sake of simplicity and brevity, in the following text we will refer to germinal functions as "neuro/oligodendrogenesis" or "neuro/oligodendrogenic activity", while the specific effects of immune elements on the diverse germinal components and activities will be dissected in Table 2 (see also Figure 1).

2.1 Immune regulation of adult germinal niche functioning under physiological conditions

Among all immune elements, microglial cells are reportedly crucial modulators of neurogenic niche activities in both the healthy and injured adult CNS. They populate both adult SVZ and SGZ, where they localize in close proximity to NSCs. Interestingly, germinal microglia displays phenotypes and behaviours (i.e. higher levels of activation, proliferation and phagocytic activity; Goings et al., 2006; Ziv et al., 2006a; Sierra et al., 2010) distinct from both their resting counterparts in the non-neurogenic CNS parenchyma, and fully activated and phagocytic microglia detected upon injury or in inflammatory conditions. *In vitro* experiments suggest that such basal germinal activated (BGA) phenotype is maintained through interactions with components of the niche environment, including matrix molecules (e.g. Tenascin-R; Liao et al., 2008), low levels of inflammatory molecules (e.g. IL4 and IFNγ), and elements of adaptive immunity (see below; Ziv et al., 2006a). Notably, various studies report a positive correlation between the persistence of the BGA microglial state and basal levels of neurogenesis and oligodendrogenesis both *in vivo* and *in vitro* (see also Table 2), with blockade of any microglial activation by minocycline resulting in decreased numbers of newborn neurons (Carpentier and Palmer, 2009 and references therein). *In vitro* studies suggest that, although microglial cells are abundantly distributed within the germinal niches in the adult CNS, direct contacts between microglia and NSCs/precursors/ neuroblasts may not be required for facilitating neurogenesis (Aarum et al., 2003; Walton et al., 2006). Notably, microglia cells residing within the germinal niches constitutively secrete a plethora of soluble mediators, including growth factors (e.g. Brain Derived Neurotrophic Factor BDNF and Insulin-like Growth Factor IGF1; Liao et al., 2008; Ziv et al., 2006a) and low levels of inflammatory molecules (e.g. TGFβ, TNFα, IL1β; Battista et al., 2006; Liao et al., 2008; Carpentier and Palmer, 2009; Yirmiya and Goshen, 2011). Both categories of mediators are importantly implicated in neurogenesis, as attested by the negative outcomes on constitutive NSC functioning of genetically- or pharmacologically-driven ablation of growth factor- or inflammatory cytokine-mediated signalling pathways (see also Table 2; Ziv et al., 2006a; Butovsky et al., 2006; Carpentier and Palmer, 2009 and references therein). Moreover, microglia-derived inflammatory molecules can directly influence basal NSC/progenitor functions, as these cells express a set of cytokine receptors, including those for IFNγ (Li et al., 2010), TNFα (Carpentier and Palmer, 2009), IL1β (Yirmiya and Goshen, 2011) and IL6 (Monje et al., 2003). Moreover, pioneer studies reported that adult NSCs basally display a set of features typical of immune cells, including the expression of MHC-related molecules, TLRs and complement receptors, whose activation may allow NSCs themselves to (i) act as antigen-presenting cells; (ii) directly sense alterations in tissue integrity and immune system activity upon injury; and (iii) plastically modulate their own neuro/oligodendrogenic activity in response to environmental alterations (see Table 2; Popa et al., 2011; Rolls et al., 2007; Moriyama et al., 2011; Rahpeymai et al., 2006).

Further novelty in the field has been provided by the unexpected discovery that, in addition to resident microglia and derived soluble factors, T cells contribute to maintain the neurogenic homeostasis in the adult CNS. By using nude or SCID (severe combined immune deficiency) mice, lacking respectively either only mature T cells or both T and B cell populations, Michal Schwartz and colleagues in 2006 demonstrated that T cell deficiency is correlated with impaired NSC/progenitor proliferation and neuronal differentiation of new born derivatives in both SGZ and SVZ, accompanied by a defective spatial learning ability (Ziv et al., 2006a). Such effect on SGZ progenitor cells is specifically exerted by T helper lymphocytes, as repopulation with CD4+, but not CD8+ or B cells, rescues defective neurogenesis (Wolf et al., 2009). Notably, antigenic specificity to CNS autoantigens and the consequent lymphocyte homing to the CNS appear required for the expression of these T cell supportive effects on neurogenesis. Consistently, transgenic (tg) mice in which the majority of the T cell population is directed to an irrelevant antigen (i.e. ovalbumin) show impaired hippocampal neurogenesis, while, conversely, tg mice in which the majority of the T cells is directed to a CNS-specific antigen, such as certain peptides of the myelin basic protein (MBP), display increased hippocampal neurogenesis (Ziv et al., 2006a). Interestingly, data collected so far allow to propose a model in which the homeostatic role of T cells on germinal niche functions includes both a direct action on NSCs and their derivatives via release of BDNF, and an indirect effect mediated by modulation of the microglial BGA state and increased BDNF production induced in surrounding neurons (Ziv et al., 2006a; Hohlfeld et al., 2006). In line with this scenario, minocycline treatment results in a reduced hippocampal neurogenesis even in tg mice where T cells are directed to MBP antigens, while BDNF levels are reduced in immune deficient mice and elevated in tg mice enriched with T cells directed to MBP antigens (Ziv et al., 2006a; Wolf et al., 2009).

The participation of immune cells in the regulation of hippocampal NSCs/progenitors is further supported by experiments showing that while wild type mice respond to enriched housing conditions (including social, sensory and motor stimulation) by increased neurogenesis, SCID animals do not show any change in NSC activity (Ziv et al., 2006a). Notably, in the same experimental condition it has been reported the appearance of T cells in the hippocampal hilus and an increased number of SGZ microglial cells upregulating MHCII molecules and IGF1 (Ziv et al., 2006a). Since this microglia phenotype is typically promoted by Th2-derived IL4 (Butovsky et al., 2005), it can be speculated that these changes are stimulated by defined T cell activities occurring as a consequence of the organism-environment interactions. In addition, based on the capability of microglia stimulated by either IL4 or low levels of INFγ (which is known to be produced by T cells) to promote neurogenesis and oligodendrogenesis in hippocampal progenitor cell/microglia co-cultures, (Butovsky et al., 2006), one may claim that the observed microglia changes contribute to the occurring increased neurogenesis. Stress and elevated levels of circulating glucocorticoid hormones can also affect the BGA microglial state (Song and Wang, 2011). Accordingly, the surgical removal of the adrenal gland and the consequent suppression of glucocorticoid production result in a moderately higher activation of microglial cells, whose density increase again correlates with a higher number of dividing cells and of newly generated neurons in the SGZ. Such microglial activation is accompanied by the upregulation of inflammatory cytokines, such as TGFβ (Battista et al., 2006). Taken together, these data indicate that T lymphocytes and microglia cells take part in the homeostatic regulation of adult neurogenesis, comprising the mediation of part of the pro-and anti-neurogenic effects of experience/emotional stimuli.

Another study confirmed the contribution of immune cells to the plastic regulation of adult neurogenesis. Wolf and colleagues in 2009 showed that when the effect of voluntary wheel running on neurogenesis is assessed in CD4 knock-out mice or in mice treated with anti-CD4 neutralizing antibodies, both wild type and CD4-depleted/deficient mice respond by increased hippocampal proliferation (although starting from different basal levels), while such expected effect is absent only in mice devoid of functional T, B and NK cells. This latter finding suggests that while CD4+ T cells are the major player in controlling constitutive neurogenesis, the entire pool of adaptive immune cells may contribute to induce a response to neurogenic stimuli. Only one study so far excluded a role for T cells and microglia activation in activity-induced increase of adult hippocampal neurogenesis (Olah et al., 2009). Whether differences in experimental paradigms applied (voluntary physical activity vs. enriched environment) or in animal models used (mice vs. rats) account for such different results remains to be assessed.

To sum up, data collected so far provide evidence that in non-pathological conditions both resident microglia and T cells have a prominent role in maintaining and plastically modulating the basal levels of neurogenesis within the adult CNS (see Figure 1). Microglia residing within the neurogenic niches displays a germinal-specific basally activated phenotype, characterized by the expression of defined pro-neurogenic inflammatory mediators (e.g. TGFβ, TNFα, IL1β) and growth factors (e.g. BDNF and IGF1). The maintenance of such BGA microglial phenotype depends on the interaction with local elements and with CNS-directed T cells, and positively correlates with the neurogenic activity of adult germinal niches.

2.2 Immune system regulation of germinal niche functioning after injury

The discovery of the retention of NSCs within the mature CNS has inspired two decades of intense investigations aimed at assessing whether such endogenous source of new neurons and oligodendrocytes could be exploited for the repopulation of lost neuronal populations and the restoration of damaged myelin sheaths. However, it is now well established that adult germinal niche activity has a very limited ability to mediate a long-lasting cell replacement and to support a complete repair of the injured CNS cytoarchitecture and functions. Many studies have shown that early after acute insults (e.g. stroke, trauma, single epileptic attacks, acute phase of relapsing-remitting experimental autoimmune encephalomyelitis EAE) endogenous neurogenesis and oligodendrogenesis are stimulated. However, in most cases reactive neurogenesis is eventually abortive, since the majority of the newly generated neurons are not recruited to the lesion site but remain within the germinal areas, nor are integrated into the parenchyma, and ultimately undergo cell death (Carpentier and Palmer, 2009). Moreover, in chronic pathologies (e.g. neurodegenerative diseases, recurrent seizures, chronic progressive EAE) and stress conditions (e.g. mouse isolation), neurogenesis and oligodendrogenesis appear impaired (Carpentier and Palmer, 2009; Pluchino et al., 2008; Rasmussen et al., 2011). Studies using ablation of single immune cell populations or molecular pathways have revealed that upon injury immune system elements exert a dual role, contributing to both the early neuro/oligodendrogenic reaction and the subsequent establishment of a milieu non-permissive for NSC activities. Major players in such regulation are again microglia and T cells (see below).

Early after acute damage, cell debris, nucleotides released from dying cells and reactive glial cells, and extracellular matrix protein fragments serve as ligands for the TLRs expressed by microglia residing within the germinal niches, and trigger its full activation, with subsequent release of high levels of pro-inflammatory cytokines (i.e. TNFα, INFγ, IL6 and IL1β) and growth factors (e.g. IGF1; Ekdahl, 2009 and references therein; Deierborg et al., 2010). Various studies reported that such early microglial activation is *per se* needed to induce the post-injury increase of neurogenesis. In fact, minocycline inhibition of activated microglial cells exposed to injury (i.e. stroke) abolishes the increase in NSC proliferation both *in vivo* and *in vitro* (Kim et al., 2010; Deierborg et al., 2010). Consistently, genetically- or pharmacologically-driven ablation of IL1β- or TNFα-mediated signalling pathways negatively affects neurogenesis after seizures and stroke (Spulber et al., 2008; Carpentier and Palmer, 2009 and references therein), indicating that, in addition to growth factors, these microglial-derived mediators contribute to post-injury reactive neurogenesis. Notably, similar to the healthy conditions, defined subpopulations of T cells contribute to modulate germinal niche functioning at early stages after injury. Removal of the whole CD4+ T cell population results in increased precursor/neuroblast generation few days after stroke, while depletion of the only Treg lymphocytes suppresses neurogenesis and reduces functional recovery (Saino et al., 2010). In contrast, promotion of Treg homing to the ischemic brain enhances NSC and neuroblast survival (Ishibashi et al., 2009). At variance with non-pathological conditions, post-injury T cell effects appear to modulate pro-inflammatory cytokine secretion by activated endothelial cells rather than being mediated by microglial functions (Saino et al., 2010; Ishibashi et al., 2009).

When persistent and uncontrolled microglial activation occurs, the same molecular players appear to switch their acute stimulating function into detrimental effect on germinal niche activity. For instance, when minocycline is administered in the chronic phase of CNS injuries or diseases, such treatment results in increased generation of neurons and oligodendrocytes (Carpentier and Palmer, 2009; Yirmiya and Goshen, 2011 and references therein; Rasmussen et al., 2011). Whether such phenomenon is due to a beneficial-to-detrimental switch in the microglial phenotype is still highly debated. It remains also unresolved whether changes in the intrinsic responsiveness to immuno/inflammatory mediators of NSCs and their derivatives may account for these harmful effects. Although data are not completely consistent (Ekdahl, 2009), transcriptional profiling of isolated SVZ microglia cells reveals that microglia exhibits disease phase-specific gene expression signatures (Starossom et al., 2011). Moreover, *in vitro* evidence suggests that while early-activated microglia displays pro-neurogenic features, it acquires a non-supportive phenotype at delayed time point after injury (Deierborg et al., 2010). Moreover, inflammatory cytokines can act through different receptors, thereby triggering distinct effects. This is the case of TNFα that can activate both the TNFα receptor 1 (TNFR1), mediating cytotoxic functions on NSCs and neuroblasts, and the TNFR2, activating pro-neurogenic pathways (Carpentier and Palmer, 2009). These data suggest that upon chronic damage both microglia and NSC can contribute to reduced neuro/oligodendrogenesis, by acquiring phenotypes non-supportive for germinal niche functioning and newborn cell survival.

In summary, early microglia activation is required to induce post-injury increase in NSC proliferation and neurogenesis. However, when microglial activation and inflammatory molecule secretion persist for long time, as in chronically injured CNS, adult neurogenesis and oligodendrogenesis are suppressed. At variance with what reported in physiological conditions, at early stages after injury CD4+ T cell activity negatively affects precursor/neuroblast generation through microglia-indipendent mechanisms. However, under the same conditions, the Treg subpopulation appear to exert beneficial effects on neurogenesis and functional recovery (see Figure 1).

Although still controversial, these data support the idea that anti-inflammatory treatments should be finely and temporarily calibrated in order to be beneficial for neuro/oligodendrogenesis and promote CNS regeneration following injury.

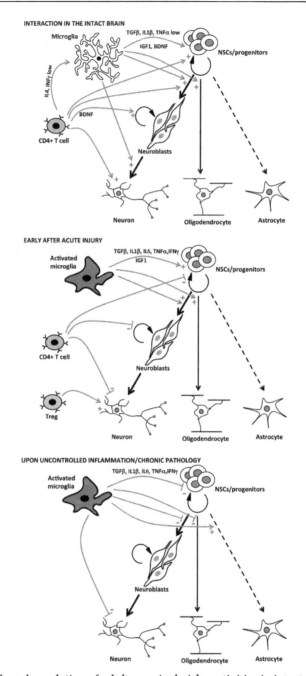

Fig. 1. Immune-based regulation of adult germinal niche activities in intact and pathological conditions. Curved arrows indicate proliferation; straight arrows indicate differentiation along cell lineages.

In the adult brain NSCs residing in the SVZ and SGZ asymmetrically divide and give rise to actively proliferating neuroblasts that eventually differentiate in mature neurons into the olfactory bulb or in the dentate gyrus. Within the adult germinal niches, oligodendrocytes and astrocytes are also produced, though to a much lesser extent. Depending on their state of activation, immune system elements can positively (+) or negatively (-) affect the generation of new neurons or glial cells within the mature CNS. Immune-mediated mechanisms include microglia- and T cell-derived soluble factors, and influence (i) NSC and neuroblast proliferation, (ii) neuronal vs. glial specification, (iii) survival and maturation of the newborn elements, thereby exerting an important role in modulating the germinal niche activities in both healthy and pathological conditions.

Immunoplayer	Proliferation	Specification	Survival	Neuroblast differentiation	Oligodendro genesis
Immune cells					
Microglia					
in physiological conditions	+ (NSCs/ precursors)	n.r.	n.r.	+	+
early after acute injury	+ (NSCs/ precursors)	+ neurogenesis + oligodendro-genesis	n.r.	n.r.	+
in chronic pathology/ uncontrolled immuno-activation	- (NSCs/ precursors)	- neurogenesis	- (neurobl.)	n.r.	-
CD4+ T cells					
in physiological conditions	+ (NSCs/ precursors/ neurobl.)	+ neurogenesis	+ (neurobl.)	+	n.r.
early after injury	- (NSCs/ precursors/ neurobl.)	n.r.	- (precursor/ neurobl.)	n.r.	n.r.
T regs	n.r.	n.r.	+ (neurobl.)	n.r.	n.r.
Inflammatory cytokines					
TGFβ	n.r.	+ neurogenesis	n.r.	+	
IL4	n.r.	n.r.	n.r.	+	+
IL1β	- (*in vitro*; NSCs/ precursors); + (*in vivo*; NSCs/ precursors)	n.r.	n.r.	n.r.	n.r.
IL6	- (NSCs/ precursors/ neurobl.)	+ astroglio-genesis - neurogenesis	-	n.r.	n.r.

Immunoplayer	Proliferation	Specification	Survival	Neuroblast differentiation	Oligodendro genesis
TNFα	- (>200ng/ml; precursors); + (1 ng/ml; NSCs/ precursors/ neurobl.)	n.r.	- (10-100 ng/ml; NSC/ precursors); + (1ng/ml; NSCs/ precursors/ neurobl.)	+ (1ng/ml); No effect (10ng/ml)	n.r.
IFNγ	- (NSCs/ precursors)	+ neurogenesis - oligodendro- genesis (*in vivo*); - astroglio- genesis (*in vitro*); - neurogenesis - oligodendro- genesis + astroglio- genesis (neurosphere assay)	- (neurobl.)	+ (20 ng/ml)	-
Receptors on NSCs and derivatives					
TLR2	n.r.	+ neurogenesis	n.r.	+	n.r.
TLR4	- (NSCs)	n.r.	+ (neurobl.)	+	n.r.
CR2 complement receptor	- (NSCs/ precursors/ neurobl.)	n.r.	n.r.	n.r.	n.r.
C3aR complement receptor	n.r.	n.r.	n.r.	+	n.r.
RAE-1 (MHCI – related)	+ (NSCs/ precursors)	n.r.	n.r.	n.r.	n.r.

Table 2. Major immune factors regulating the adult germinal niche activity.

Data were obtained from studies in which genetically- or pharmacologically-driven ablation of single cell populations or molecular pathways allows to unveil a causal relationship between the activity of a defined cell type or molecule and a specific effect on NSC or derivatives. References can be found in the text. Note that the effects of inflammatory cytokines are often context- or dose-dependent. Abbreviations: NSCs, Neural Stem Cells; neurobl., neuroblasts; +, increased; -, decreased; n.r., not reported.

3. Immune system regulation of parenchymal neural progenitors

Studies over the last decades have revealed that glia cells residing in the nervous parenchyma outside the neurogenic areas can display progenitor functions (Boda and Buffo, 2010), in addition to absolving supportive roles for neurons and contributing to information processing (Kettenmann and Verkhratsky, 2008; Bakiri et al., 2009). Typically, cells expressing the proteoglycan NG2 comprise the vast majority of cycling elements outside the germinal areas (Horner et al., 2000; Dawson et al., 2003) and respond to a variety of lesion conditions by an increased cytogenic activity and hypertrophy (Keirstead et al., 1998; Reynolds et al., 2002; Hampton et al., 2004). Conversely, mature parenchymal astrocytes remain quiescent in the healthy CNS, but can re-enter the cell cycle and assume features of progenitor cells upon injury (Buffo et al., 2008, 2010). Numerous approaches including proliferation studies, expression analysis, grafting experiments and Cre-lox based fate-mapping investigations (revised in Trotter et al., 2010; Richardson et al., 2011) have consolidated the view of NG2 positive cells as endogenous reservoir of mature and myelinating oligodendrocytes during development, adulthood and in most pathological conditions. Therefore, these cells are generally termed oligodendrocyte precursor cells (OPCs), despite the names 'polydendrocytes' or 'synanthiocytes' have been recently adopted in view of their morphology and contiguity to neurons. A controversial issue, dawned by seminal experiments showing that OPCs *in vitro* can revert to a stem cell-like state and differentiate along all the three neural lineages (Kondo and Raff, 2000), is whether *in vivo* these cells can undergo low levels of neurogenesis and generate glial cells other than oligodendrocytes at specific CNS sites or in specific conditions. Data on this issue are conflicting, although the prevailing view agrees that some astrogliogenesis (and generation of Schwann cells in the spinal cord) can occur in defined injury conditions and developmental ages (embryonic astrogliogenesis). Production of new neurons has also been reported, but remains to be further confirmed (see Boda and Buffo, 2010; Richardson et al., 2011; Fröhlich et al., 2011 for review). Recent studies on CNS lesions have also attributed precursor properties to reactive astrocytes and spinal cord ependymal cells. During anisomorphic gliosis, parenchymal astrocytes dedifferentiate and acquire progenitor features, which are not expressed *in vivo*, likely inhibited by a plethora of injury-evoked restrictive signals such as inflammatory molecules, but can be disclosed *ex vivo* (Buffo et al., 2008; 2010). Spinal cord ependymal cells appear instead able to undergo astrogliogenesis and oligodendrogenesis upon injury directly *in vivo* (Barnabè-Heider et al., 2010).

3.1 Protective and destructive effects of immune activation in the nervous tissue

As presented above (see also Table 2), poor survival of progenitor cells as well as restriction of their differentiation potentials to astrogliogenesis, blockade of maturational programs and induction of cell death have been long ascribed to immuno-mediated inflammatory signals released at sites of lesions. This purely negative view of immunity and inflammation has also extended to parenchymal progenitor functioning, based on the established detrimental inflammatory burden of immune (e.g. MS), traumatic, neurovascular and neurodegenerative (Alzheimer's Disease, Parkinson disease, Amyotrophic Lateral Sclerosis) pathologies. However, recent studies have highlighted a positive contribution of immunity to repair of neural damage. Thus, while nothing is known on whether and how both local microglia and peripheral immune cells physiologically modulate the proliferation and differentiation rates of OPCs and/or affect the progenitor potentials of other glial cells, it is increasingly clear that the concept of immune activation as purely harmful to CNS repair is too simplistic. Accordingly, well-defined features, levels and timing of immune activity appear to promote neuroprotection and post-injury plasticity in the forms of axon regrowth, replacement of degenerated cells and functional recovery.

This emerging view suggests that supportive functions for tissue repair and functional recovery can be exerted by defined populations or functional states of macrophages/microglia and T cells. For instance, infiltrating blood-derived macrophages have been shown to promote recovery at sub-acute stages in rodents with spinal cord injury (Rapalino et al., 1998; Shechter et al., 2009). This action appears related to the production of immunomodulatory (anti-inflammatory IL10) and neurotrophic molecules (BDNF), which is triggered by exposure to self-antigens or by the actions of T cells responding to neuroantigens ('protective autoimmunity', Schechter et al., 2009; see also Schwartz and Yoles, 2006; Schwartz and Shechter, 2010). A similar modulatory function would be exerted by T cells on local microglia that, upon proper stimulation, can become beneficial to the nervous tissue (Butovsky et al., 2005, 2006; Shaked et al., 2005). According to this view, autoimmune T cells sensibilised against CNS antigens (and in particular myelin components) (Moalem et al., 1999; Hauben et al., 2000; Kipnis et al., 2002; Fisher et al., 2001; Beers et al., 2008) have been proposed to play a crucial role in the recovery from acute CNS insults. These cells would enhance cellular and molecular mechanisms responsible of cleaning up the injured area and creating a milieu favourable to tissue remodelling and function restoration. Yet, in autoimmune neuropathologies such as EAE Tregs have been primarily implicated in neuroprotection and inflammation control (Liu et al., 2006; Huang et al., 2009; Reddy et al., 2004), where they would partly contribute to limiting the overactivation of cytotoxic autoimmune cells. A similar function for Tregs in non-autoimmune CNS damage has been confirmed by a further study on a stroke model (Liesz et al., 2009). The important novelty of these findings resides on the identification of physiological reparative mechanisms mediated by innate and adaptive immunity that, in the natural state may remain too weak or abortive to express their full neuroprotective and reparative potential, and could therefore be implemented for therapeutic purposes (Schwartz and Yoles, 2006; Walsh and Kipnis, 2011). In other words, with distinct timings and modalities, defined immune cell populations can be proposed as an endogenous therapeutic target to restrain or modulate self-checking mechanisms on the part of beneficial immunity activated spontaneously in response to CNS injury (Walsh and Kipnis, 2011). However, any immediate extension of this view to all types of CNS injury, including chronic neurodegenerative diseases, requires further confirmations and disclosure of the specific mechanisms of immune cell actions in distinct disease conditions (Walsh and Kipnis, 2011).

3.2 Immune-mediated control of parenchymal progenitor functioning

Whereas the above presented findings referred to nervous tissue protection and recovery from damage in general terms, in this section we will take a closer look on how and when innate and adaptive cells and inflammatory cues influence the activity and survival of OPCs and parenchymal progenitors. Oligodendrocyte produce myelin sheaths that allow fast conduction of electrical signals along axons. These cells undergo primary degeneration due to genetic causes (leukodistrophies) and are highly vulnerable to noxious signals produced during traumatic and ischemic events and inflammatory/autoimmune pathologies. In many instances their replacement with subsequent remyelination of temporary demyelinated axons occurs spontaneously. However, if oligodendrocyte death is particularly extended or in defined damage conditions such as traumatic compressive injuries, stroke and MS, this process remains incomplete or blocked. Neo-oligodendrogenesis and remyelination are not operated by spared mature oligodendrocytes but by OPCs. To attain remyelination, these progenitors have to become activated, undergo hyperthrophic changes, activate fast proliferation, migrate to the site of demyelination, start a complex differentiation process including the establishment of contacts with the denudated axons, expression of myelin genes, generation of the myelin membranes that wrap the axons and form the sheath. It is unquestionably true that OPCs respond to a variety of insults other than demyelination. Amongst these, compelling evidence supports a role for inflammatory/immune components in OPC proliferation, recruitment and differentiation.

In a mouse model of traumatic injury, Rhodes and colleagues have established that, amongst early factors capable to induce immediate reactivity in OPC in the form of NG2 upregulation, hypertrophy and increase in OPC cell number, are blood-derived macrophages in a defined activation state including the release of the inflammatory cytokines TNFα, IL1α, TGFβ, INFγ (Rhodes et al., 2006). Furthermore, specific macrophage/microglia activation phenotypes have been proposed to differentially affect OPC proliferation and regenerative capabilities through the selective activation of specific microglia/macrophage TLRs (Lehenardt et al., 2002; Glezer et al., 2006; Schonberg et al., 2007; Taylor et al., 2010). Despite data presented in distinct studies are not completely consistent (perhaps due to different experimental conditions), the consensus view is that defined microglia/macrophage activation states, correlated with specific pattern of cytokine production, act by either triggering or hampering OPC proliferation and differentiation. For instance, IL4-stimulated microglia has been shown to promote oligodendrogenesis from local progenitors in an autoimmune demyelination models, whereas INFγ-stimulated microglia had no or very limited effects (Butovsky et al., 2005). The role of innate immunity in OPC functioning in damage has further been substantiated by studies on non-immunity-mediated toxin-induced models of focal demyelination. In these models, genetic-based depletion or pharmacological inhibition of macrophages leads to an impairment of remyelination (Kotter et al., 2001, 2005), indicating a defective OPC response in an injury condition that normally leads to complete regeneration of myelinating oligodendrocytes by local reactive OPCs (Woodruff and Franklin, 1999). In the same experimental lesion, enhancing TLR4 mediated microglia activation by LPS infusion increases OPC reactivity, promotes a more efficient removal of myelin debris and triggers a faster appearance of remyelination markers (Glezer et al., 2006). It is clear that one key aspect of the innate immunity contribution to the full expression of the OPC regenerative potential is the removal of myelin debris. In vitro and in vivo data support the notion that myelin components dampen OPC differentiation (Miller, 1999). In line with these findings, anti-inflammatory drugs attenuating microglia/macrophage activity can affect OPC responses by delaying their differentiation in experimental demyelination (Li et al., 2005; Chari et al., 2005).

A similar role in the modulation of OPC reaction to demyelination has been attributed to T cells (both CD4+ and CD8+) indicating that also adaptive immunity is required for the correct OPC regenerative response (Bieber et al., 2003). Indeed, lack or depletion of either

CD4+ or CD8+ is associated with reduced remyelination in focal demyelination. Interestingly, the disease-delaying drug Glatiramer acetate (GA) adopted for therapy in MS, may promote remyelination by potentiating a specific T cell mediated effects. Indeed, it has been shown *in vitro* that GA increases the production of Th2 cells, IGF1, and that the conditioned medium from GA-reactive T cells promotes the formation of OPCs from embryonic brain-derived forebrain cell culture. These findings are confirmed *in vivo*, where GA increases the OPC number and the extent of remyelinaton in toxin-mediated focal demyelination (Skihar et al., 2009).

Moving from cells to molecular signals, a wide range of pro-inflammatory cytokines (e.g. IL1β and TNFα, along with lymphotoxin-β receptor and MHCII) have been implicated as mediators of remyelination in non-autoimmune remyelination, implying that they promote the reactivity and the reparative behaviour of OPCs (revised in Franklin and ffrench-Costant, 2008). Another cytokine, INFγ, has instead been shown to inhibit remyelination (Franklin and ffrench-Costant, 2008). In turn, upon INFγ stimulation glial precursors with features of OPCs have been shown to produce a variety of immunomodulators, trophic factors, microglia attractive factors, and activate the expression of specific TLRs (Cassiani-Ingoni et al., 2006), indicating that OPC participate in active and bidirectional interplay with immune cells. Finally, cytokines have also been proposed as capable to instruct alternative OPC fates: *in vitro* exposure to INFγ diverted glial progenitor from oligodendrogenesis to astrogliogenesis. Despite this finding is consistent with the capability of INFγ to block remyelination, astrogliogenesis from OPCs *in vivo* remains debated (see above).

Moving to injury models distinct from demyelination, spinal cord contusions offer an example of a traumatic injury where intense OPC proliferation is not accompanied by complete glial repopulation of the lesioned area. In this specific immuno-inflammatory condition, activated microglia/macrophages have been shown to secrete inhibitory factors (i.e. TNFα, and extracellular matrix modifiers) hampering survival and growth of OPC *ex vivo*, and impeding their migration into the lesioned demyelinated area (Wu et al., 2010). Opposite effects of activated microglia on tissue repair in different lesion models may indeed be explained by different timing of recruitment of T cells in this process ensuing distinct microglia activation states (following Schwartz and Yoles, 2006).

Immuno-inflammatory levels have also been suggested to affect the neurogenic potential of parenchymal precursors, independent on their identity. Low levels of inflammation or specific immuno/inflammatory states have been proposed to allow the disclosure of neurogenic potentialities. In the cerebral cortex, selective cortical neuron damage mediated by apoptotic events and very low levels of inflammatory/immune activation has been associated with the appearance of glial cells with radial progenitor traits and rare immature neurons, suggesting that injury-induced de-differentiatiation of resident astrocytes to a radial glia state may subserve local neurogenesis (Leavitt et al., 1999; Chen et al., 2004). Also mild ischemic damage has been reported to allow neurogenesis from parenchymal sources: viral-based tracing revealed that layer I cortical progenitors can give birth to a low number of GABAergic cortical interneurons (Ohira et al., 2010).

A further support to the contention that local immune response strongly influences the behaviour of local precursors was provided by the observation in a model of spinal cord lesion that combined modulation of T cell activation by myelin-derived peptide vaccination and transplantation of immunomodulatory adult NSCs correlated with the appearance of neurogenic attempts from local progenitors accompanied by modulation of parenchymal T cell response and microglia activation, and, increased BDNF and noggin expression (Ziv et al., 2006b). Pioneering studies have also started investigating the influence of T cells on astrocytes, showing that T-cell derived signals modify the astrocytic metabolic state *in vitro*. Namely, glutamate released by T cells promotes the acquisition of a neuroprotective phenotype and potentiates their capability to clear glutamate (Garg et al., 2008). Astroglial dysfunctions appear instead induced by LPS-activated microglia *in vivo*, resulting in defect of the BBB and subsequent myelin damage (Sharma et al., 2010). Astrocytes are obviously intensely involved in any kind of response to noxious stimuli, given their essential functions in the maintenance of tissue homeostatis, scavenging of toxic molecules, production of trophic support to neurons and oligodendrocytes, and cytogenic glial scarring to prevent the spreading of potential secondary damage to the healthy tissue (Buffo et al., 2010). The astrocytic reaction is directly or indirectly induced by various inflammatory cytokines and, in turn, reactive astrocytes produce pro-inflammatory molecules that modulate their own activation state and that of immune cells (Buffo et al., 2010; Kostianovsky et al., 2008). Whether and how inflammatory/immune factors specifically affect the progenitor potential of reactive astroglia is not known. What is well accepted is that extended damage is associated with high levels of inflammation and immune activation that are generally unfavourable to the disclosure of progenitor properties and regeneration (see also above). Accordingly, controlled microlesions to the CNS and associated low levels of inflammatory/immuno activation were reported to induce immature/progenitor phenotypes associated with rare neurogenic events as well as the establishment of a microenvironment more prone to support axon growth (Leavitt et al., 1999; Chen et al., 2004). It remains to be established whether specific components or modalities of innate/adaptive immune activation can boost such pro-reparative changes in resident astroglia in case of extended damage. On the whole, these data indicate that the expression of the reparative potentials of parenchymal progenitors can be supported by immune mechanisms directed at both removing debris and toxic molecules, and performing immunomodulation to avoid the overactivation of the immune response.

4. Concluding remarks

Recent discoveries have profoundly changed the perception of CNS–immune interactions. In particular, the novel roles of immune cells in the maintenance and plastic regulation of adult NSC functions have revealed an unexpected exchange of signals between the nervous and immune systems, opening the possibility that immune malfunction may have relevance in so far unsuspected CNS diseases. Furthermore, a decade of investigations has dissected components of the immune response to CNS injury that potentiate or dampen CNS reparative activities. While more research is needed to disclose the influence of immune factors on the properties of parenchymal sources of progenitor cells, on the whole immune cells can be proposed as an endogenous therapeutic target to modulate immune mechanisms on the part beneficial to foster CNS repair and function restoration.

5. Acknowledgments

Chiara Rolando' s fellowship and work in our laboratory are supported by Compagnia di San Paolo, GLIAREP project.

6. References

Aarum, J., Sandberg, K., Haeberlein, S.L.B., Persson, M.A.A. (2003). Migration and differentiation of neural precursor cells can be directed by microglia. *Proceedings of the National Academy of Sciences USA*, Vol.100, No.26 (Dec 2003), pp. 15983-15988, ISSN 1091-6490.

Aloisi, F., Ria, F., & Adorini, L. (2000). Regulation of T-cell responses by CNS antigen-presenting cells: different roles for microglia and astrocytes. *Immunology today*, Vol.21, No.3 (Mar 2000), pp. 141-147, ISSN 0167-5699.

Bakiri, Y., Attwell, D,. & Káradóttir, R. (2009). Electrical signalling properties of oligodendrocyte precursor cells. *Neuron Glia Biology*, Vol.5, No.1-2 (May 2009), pp. 3-11, ISSN 1740-925X.

Barnabé-Heider, F., Göritz, C., Sabelström, H., Takebayashi, H., Pfrieger, F.W., Meletis, K., & Frisén, J. (2010). Origin of new glial cells in intact and injured adult spinal cord. *Cell Stem Cell*. Vol.7, No.4 (Oct 2010), pp. 470-82, ISSN 19345909.

Battista, D., Ferrari, C.C., Gage, F.H., & Pitossi, F.J. (2006). Neurogenic niche modulation by activated microglia: transforming growth factor β increases neurogenesis in the adult dentate gyrus. *European Journal of Neuroscience*, Vol.23, No.1 (Jan 2006), pp. 83-93, ISSN 1460-9568.

Becher, B., Prat, A., & Antel, J.P. (2000). Brain-immune connection: immuno-regulatory properties of CNS-resident cells. *Glia*, Vol.29, No.4 (Feb 2000), pp. 293-304, ISSN 1098-1136.

Bechmann, I., Mor, G., Nilsen, J., Eliza, M., Nitsch, R., & Naftolin, F. (1999). FasL (CD95L, Apo1L) is expressed in the normal rat and human brain: evidence for the existence of an immunological brain barrier. *Glia*, Vol.27, No.1 (Jul 1999), pp.62-74, ISSN 1098-1136.

Beers, D.R., Henkel, J.S., Zhao, W., Wang, J., & Appel, S.H. (2008). CD4+ T cells support glial neuroprotection, slow disease progression, and modify glial morphology in an animal model of inherited ALS. *Proceedings of the National Academy of Sciences USA*, Vol.105, No.40 (Oct 2008), pp. 15558-15563, ISSN 0027-8424.

Bieber, A. J., Kerr, S. & Rodriguez, M. Efficient central nervous system remyelination requires T cells. (2003). *Annals of Neurology*, Vol.53, No.5 (May 2003), pp. 680-684, 531-8249.

Billingham, R.E., Boswell, T. (1953). Studies on the problem of corneal homografts. *Proceeding of the Royal Society Biological Science*, Vol.141, No.904, pp. 392-406, ISSN 1471-2954.

Boda, E., Buffo, A. (2010) Glial cells in non-germinal territories: insights into their stem/progenitor properties in the intact and injured nervous tissue. *Archives Italiennes de Biologie*, Vol. 148, No.2 (June 2010), pp 119-136, ISSN 0003-9829.

Buffo, A., Rite, I., Tripathi, P., Lepier, A., Colak, D., Horn, A.P., Mori, T., & Götz M. (2008). Origin and progeny of reactive gliosis: A source of multipotent cells in the injured

brain. *Proceedings of the National Academy of Sciences U S A*. Vol.105, No.9 (Mar 2008),
pp. 3581-3586, ISSN 0027-8424.

Buffo, A., Rolando, C., & Ceruti, S. (2010). Astrocytes in the damaged brain: molecular and
cellular insights into their reactive response and healing potential. *Biochemical
Pharmacology*, Vol.79, No.2 (Jan 2010), pp. 77-89, ISSN 0006-2952.

Bush, T.G., Puvanachandra, N., Horner, C.H., Polito, A., Ostenfeld, T., Svendsen, C.N.,
Mucke, L., Johnson, M.H., & Sofroniew, M.V. (1999). Leukocyte infiltration,
neuronal degeneration, and neurite outgrowth after ablation of scar-forming,
reactive astrocytes in adult transgenic mice. *Neuron*, Vol.23 No.2 (Jun 1999), pp.
297-308. ISSN 0896-6273.

Butovsky, O., Talpalar, A.E., Ben-Yaakov, K., & Schwartz, M. (2005). Activation of microglia
by aggregated β-amyloid or lipopolysaccharide impairs MHC-II expression and
renders them cytotoxic whereas IFN-γ and IL-4 render them protective. *Molecular
and Cellular Neuroscience*, Vol.29, No.3 (Jul 2005), pp. 381-393, ISSN 1044-7431.

Butovsky, O., Landa, G., Kunis, G., Ziv, Y., Avidan, H., Greenberg, N., Schwartz, A.,
Smirnov, I., Pollack, A., Jung, S., & Schwartz, M. (2006). Induction and blockage of
oligodendrogenesis by differently activated microglia in an animal model of
multiple sclerosis. *Journal of Clinical Investigation*, Vol.116, No.4 (Mar 2006), pp. 905-
915, ISSN 00219738.

Carpentier, P.A., Begolka, W.S., Olson, J.K., Elhofy, A., Karpus, W.J., & Miller, S.D. (2005).
Differential activation of astrocytes by innate and adaptive immune stimuli. *Glia*,
Vol.49, No.3 (Feb 2005), pp. 360-374, ISSN 1098-1136.

Carpentier, P.A., & Palmer, T.D. (2009). Immune Influence on Adult Neural Stem Cell
Regulation and Function. *Neuron*, Vol.64, No.1 (Oct 2009), pp. 79-92, ISSN 0896-
6273.

Cassiani-Ingoni, R., Coksaygan, T., Xue, H., Reichert-Scrivner, S.A., Wiendl, H., Rao, M.S., &
Magnus, T. (2006). Cytoplasmic translocation of Olig2 in adult glial progenitors
marks the generation of reactive astrocytes following autoimmune inflammation.
Experimental Neurology, Vol.201, No.2 (Oct 2006), pp. 349-58, ISSN 0014-4886.

Chari, D. M., Zhao, C., Kotter, M. R., Blakemore, W. F. & Franklin, R. J. M. (2006).
Corticosteroids delay remyelination of experimental demyelination in the rodent
central nervous system. *Journal of Neuroscience Research*, Vol.83, No.4 (Mar 2006),
pp. 594-605, ISSN 1097-4547.

Chen, J., Magavi, S.S., & Macklis, J.D. (2004). Neurogenesis of corticospinal motor neurons
extending spinal projections in adult mice. *Proceedings of the National Academy of
Sciences U S A*, Vol.101, No.46 (Nov 2004), pp. 16357-16362, ISSN 0027-8424.

Choi, C., Benveniste, E.N. (2004). Fas ligand/Fas system in the brain: regulator of immune
and apoptotic responses. *Brain Research Review*, Vol.44, No.1 (Jan 2004), pp. 65-81,
ISSN 0165-0173.

Dawson MR, Polito A, Levine JM, & Reynolds, R. (2003). NG2-expressing glial progenitor
cells: an abundant and widespread population of cycling cells in the adult rat CNS.
Molecular Cellular Neuroscience, Vol.24, No.2 (Oct 2003), pp.476-88, ISSN 1044-7431.

Deierborg, T., Roybon, L., Inacio, A.R., Pesic, J., & Brundin, P. (2010). Brain injury activates
microglia that induce neural stem cell proliferation ex vivo and promote
differentiation of neurosphere-derived cells into neurons and oligodendrocytes.
Neuroscience, Vol.171, No.4 (Dec 2010), pp. 1386-1396, ISSN 03064522.

Dittel, B.N. (2008). CD4 T cells: Balancing the coming and going of autoimmune-mediated inflammation in the CNS. *Brain, Behavior, and Immunity,* Vol.22, pp. 421-430, ISSN 0889-1591.

Donnelly, D.J., Popovich, P.G. (2007). Inflammation and its role in neuroprotection, axonal regeneration and functional recovery after spinal cord injury. *Experimental Neurology,* Vol.209, No.2 (Feb 2008), pp. 378-388, ISSN 0014-4886.

Ekdahl, C.T., Kokaia, Z., & Lindvall, O. (2009). Brain inflammation and adult neurogenesis: The dual role of microglia. *Neuroscience,* Vol.158, No.3 (Feb 2009), pp. 1021-1029, ISSN 03064522.

Engelhardt, B., Ransohoff, R.M. (2005). The ins and outs of T-lymphocyte trafficking to the CNS: anatomical sites and molecular mechanisms. *Trends in Immunology,* Vol.26, No.9 (Sep 2005), pp. 485-495, ISSN 1471-4906.

Fabry Z, Raine CS, & MN, H. (1994). Nervous tissue as an immune compartment: the dialect of the immune response in the CNS. *Immunology Today,* Vol.15, No.5 (May 1994), pp. 218-224, ISSN 0167-5699.

Fabry, Z., Schreiber, H.A., Harris, M.G., & Sandor, M. (2008). Sensing the microenvironment of the central nervous system: immune cells in the central nervous system and their pharmacological manipulation. *Current Opinion in Pharmacology,* Vol.8, pp. 496-507, ISSN 1471-4892.

Farina, C., Aloisi, F., & Meinl, E. (2007). Astrocytes are active players in cerebral innate immunity. *Trends in Immunology,* Vol.28, No.3 (Feb 2007), pp. 138-145, ISSN 1471-4906.

Fisher, J., Levkovitch-Verbin, H., Schori, H., Yoles, E., Butovsky, O., Kaye, J.F., Ben-Nun, A., & Schwartz, M. (2001). Vaccination for neuroprotection in the mouseoptic nerve: implications for optic neuropathies. *Journal of Neuroscience,* Vol.21, No.1 (Jan 2001), pp. 136–142, ISSN 0270-6474.

Franklin, R.J., & Ffrench-Constant, C. (2008). Remyelination in the CNS: from biology to therapy. *Nature Reviews Neuroscience,* Vol.9, No.11 (Nov 2008), pp. 839-55, ISSN 1471-003X.

Fröhlich, N., Nagy, B., Hovhannisyan, A., & Kukley, M. (2011). Fate of neuron-glia synapses during proliferation and differentiation of NG2 cells. *Journal of Anatomy,* Vol.219, No.1 (Jul 2011), pp. 18-32, ISSN 1469-7580.

Galea, I., Bechmann, I., & Perry, V.H. (2007). What is immune privilege (not)? *Trends in Immunology,* Vol.28, No.1 (Jan 2007) pp. 12-18, ISSN 1471-4906.

Garg, S.K., Banerjee, R., & Kipnis, J. (2008). Neuroprotective immunity: T cell-derived glutamate endows astrocytes with a neuroprotective phenotype. *Journal of Immunology,* Vol.180, No.6 (Mar 2008), pp. 3866-3873, ISSN 0022-1767.

Glezer, I., Lapointe, A., & Rivest, S. (2006). Innate immunity triggers oligodendrocyte progenitor reactivity and confines damages to brain injuries. *FASEB Journal,* Vol.20, No.6 (Apr 2006), pp.750-2, ISSN 0892-6638.

Goings, G.E., Kozlowski, D.A., & Szele, F.G. (2006). Differential activation of microglia in neurogenic versus non-neurogenic regions of the forebrain. *Glia,* Vol.54, No.4 (Sept 2006), pp. 329-342, ISSN 1098-1136.

Goverman, J. (2009). Autoimmune T cell responses in the central nervous system. *Nature Review Immunology,* Vol.9, No.6 (Jun 2009), pp. 393-407, ISSN 1474-1733.

Griffiths, M., Neal, J.W., Gasque, P., Giacinto Bagetta, M.T.C., & Stuart, A.L. (2007). Innate Immunity and Protective Neuroinflammation: New Emphasis on the Role of Neuroimmune Regulatory Proteins. *International Review of Neurobiology*, Vol.82, pp. 29-55, ISSN 0074-7742.

Hampton, D.W., Rhodes, K.E, Zhao, C., Franklin, RJ, Fawcett, J.W. (2004) The responses of oligodendrocyte precursor cells, astrocytes and microglia to a cortical stab injury, in the brain. *Neuroscience*. Vol.127, No.4 (Jul 2004), pp. 813-20, ISSN 0306-4522.

Hauben, E., Butovsky, O., Nevo, U., Yoles, E., Moalem, G., Agranov, E., Mor, F., Leibowitz-Amit, R., Pevsner, E., Akselrod, S., Neeman, M., Cohen, I.R., &Schwartz, M. (2000). Passive or active immunization with myelin basic protein promotes recovery from spinal cord contusion. *Journal Neuroscience*, Vol.20, No.17 (Sep 2000), pp. 6421-30, ISSN 0270-6474.

Hohlfeld, R., Kerschensteiner, M., Stadelmann, C., Lassmann, H., & Wekerle, H. (2000). The neuroprotective effect of inflammation: implications for the therapy of multiple sclerosis. *Journal of Neuroimmunology*, Vol.107, No.2 (Jul 2000), pp.161-166, ISSN 0165-5728.

Horner ,P.J., Power, A.E., Kempermann. G., Kuhn, H.G., Palmer, T.D., Winkler, J., Thal, L.J., & Gage, FH. (2000). Proliferation and differentiation of progenitor cells throughout the intact adult rat spinal cord. *Journal of Neuroscience*, Vol.20, No.6 (Mar 2000), pp. 2218-2228, ISSN 0270-6474.

Huang, X.Y., Reynolds, A.D., Mosley, R.L., & Gendelman, H.E. (2009). CD 4+T cells in the pathobiology of neurodegenerative disorders. *Journal of Neuroimmunology*, Vol.211, No.1-2, pp. 3–15, ISSN 0165-5728.

Ishibashi, S., Maric, D., Mou, Y., Ohtani, R., Ruetzler, C., & Hallenbeck, J.M. (2008). Mucosal tolerance to E-selectin promotes the survival of newly generated neuroblasts via regulatory T-cell induction after stroke in spontaneously hypertensive rats. *Journal Cerebral Blood Flow Metabolism*, Vol.29, No.3 (Mar 2009), pp. 606-620, ISSN 0271-678X.

Kaur, C., Ling, E.A. (2008). Blood brain barrier in hypoxic-ischemic conditions. *Current Neurovascular Research*, Vol.5, No.1 (Feb 2008), pp. 71-81, ISSN 1567-2026.

Keirstead, H.S., Levine, J.M., & Blakemore, W.F. (1998). Response of the oligodendrocyte progenitor cell population (defined by NG2 labelling) to demyelination in the adult spinal cord. *Glia*, Vol.22, No.2 (Feb 1998), pp.161-170, ISSN 1098-1136.

Kettenmann H., & Verkhratsky, A. (2008). Neuroglia: the 150 years after. *Trends Neuroscience*, Vol.31, No.12 (Dec 2008), pp.653-659, ISSN 0166-2236.

Kim, D.H., Kim, J.M., Park, S.J., Lee, S., Yoon, B.H., & Ryu, J.H. (2010). Early-activated microglia play a role in transient forebrain ischemia-induced neural precursor proliferation in the dentate gyrus of mice. *Neuroscience Letters*, Vol.475, No.2 (May 2010), pp. 74-79, ISSN 0304-3940.

Kipnis, J., Mizrahi, T., Hauben, E., Shaked, I., Shevach, E., & Schwartz, M. (2002). Neuroprotective autoimmunity: naturally occurring CD4+CD25+ regulatory T cells suppress the ability to withstand injury to the central nervous system. *Proceedings of the National Academy of Sciences U S A.* Vol. 99, No. 24 (Nov 2002), pp. 15620-5, ISSN 0027-8424.

Kondo T., & Raff, M. (2000). Oligodendrocyte precursor cells reprogrammed to become multipotential CNS stem cells. *Science*, Vol.289, No.5485 (Sep 2000), pp. 1754-1757, ISSN 0036-8075.

Kostianovsky, A.M., Maier, L.M., Anderson, R.C., Bruce, J.N., & Anderson, D.E. (2008). Astrocytic regulation of human monocytic/microglial activation. *Journal of Immunology*, Vol.181, No.8 (Oct 2008), pp. 5425-5432, ISSN 0022-1767.

Kotter, M. R., Setzu, A., Sim, F. J., van Rooijen, N. & Franklin, R. J. M. (2001). Macrophage depletion impairs oligodendrocyte remyelination following lysolecithin induced demyelination. *Glia*, Vol.35, No.3 (Sep 2001), pp. 204–212, ISSN 1098-1136.

Kotter, M. R., Zhao, C., van Rooijen, N. & Franklin, R. J. M. (2005). Macrophage-depletion induced impairment of experimental CNS remyelination is associated with a reduced oligodendrocyte progenitor cell response and altered growth factor expression. *Neurobiology of Disease*, Vol.18, No.1 (Feb 2005), pp. 166–175, ISSN 0969-9961.

Kriegstein, A., & Alvarez-Buylla, A. (2009). The glial nature of embryonic and adult neural stem cells. *Annual Review of Neuroscience*, Vol.32, pp. 149-184, ISSN 1545-4126.

Leavitt, B.R., Hernit-Grant, C.S., & Macklis, J.D. (1999). Mature astrocytes transform into transitional radial glia within adult mouse neocortex that supports directed migration of transplanted immature neurons. *Experimenal Neurology*, Vol.157, No.1 (May 1999), pp. 43-57, ISSN 0022-3069.

Lehnardt, S., Lachance, C., Patrizi, S., Lefebvre, S., Follett, P.L., Jensen, F.E., Rosenberg, P.A., Volpe, J.J., & Vartanian, T. (2002). The toll-like receptor TLR4 is necessary for lipopolysaccharide-induced oligodendrocyte injury in the CNS. *Journal of Neuroscience*, Vol.22, No.7 (Apr 2002), pp. 2478-86, ISSN 0270-6474.

Li, L., Walker, T.L., Zhang, Y., Mackay, E.W., & Bartlett, P.F. (2010). Endogenous Interferon-γ Directly Regulates Neural Precursors in the Non-Inflammatory Brain. *The Journal of Neuroscience, Vol.30*, No.27 (Jul 2010) pp. 9038-9050, ISSN 0270-6474.

Li, W.W., Setzu, A., Zhao, C. & Franklin, R. J. M. (2005). Minocycline-mediated inhibition of microglia activation impairs oligodendrocyte progenitor cell responses and remyelination in a non-immune model of demyelination. *Journal of Neuroimmunology*, Vol.158, No.1-2 (Jan 2005), pp. 58–66, ISSN 0165-5728.

Liao, H., Huang, W., Niu, R., Sun, L., & Zhang, L. (2008). Cross-talk between the epidermal growth factor-like repeats/fibronectin 6–8 repeats domains of Tenascin-R and microglia modulates neural stem/progenitor cell proliferation and differentiation. *Journal of Neuroscience Research*, Vol.86, No.1 (Jan 2008), pp. 27-34, ISSN 0360-4012.

Liesz, A., Suri-Payer, E., Veltkamp, C., Doerr, H,. Sommer, C., Rivest, S., Giese, T., & Veltkamp, R. (2009). Regulatory T cells are key cerebroprotective immunomodulators in acute experimental stroke. *Nature Medicine*, Vol.15, No.2 (Feb 2009) pp. 192-199, ISSN 1078-8956.

Liu, Y.W., Teige, I., Birnir, B., & Issazadeh-Navika, S. (2006). Neuron-mediated generation of regulatory T cells from encephalitogenic T cells suppresses EAE. *Nature Medicine*, Vol.12, No.5 (May 2006), pp. 518–525, ISSN 1078-8956.

McFarland, H.F., Martin, R. (2007). Multiple sclerosis: a complicated picture of autoimmunity. *Nature Immunology*, Vol.8, No.9 (Sep 2007), pp. 913-919, ISSN 1529-2908.

McMahon, E.J., Bailey, S.L., & Miller, S.D. (2006). CNS dendritic cells: critical participants in CNS inflammation? *Neurochemistry International*, Vol.49, No.2, pp. 195-203, ISSN 0197-0186.

Meinl, E., Krumbholz, M., & Hohlfeld, R. (2006). B lineage cells in the inflammatory central
    nervous system environment: Migration, maintenance, local antibody production,
    and therapeutic modulation. *Annals of Neurology*, Vol.59, No.6 (Jun 2006), pp. 880-
    892, ISSN 0364-5134.

Miller, R.H. (1999). Contact with central nervous system myelin inhibits oligodendrocyte
    progenitor maturation. *Developmental Biology*, Vol.216, No.1 (Dec 1999), pp. 359–
    368, ISSN 0012-1606.

Moalem, G., Leibowitz-Amit, R., Yoles, E., Mor, F., Cohen, I.R., & Schwartz, M. (1999).
    Autoimmune T cells protect neurons from secondary degeneration after central
    nervous system axotomy. *Nature Medicine*, Vol.5, No.1 (Jan 1999), pp. 49-55, ISSN
    1078-8956.

Monje, M.L., Toda, H., & Palmer, T.D. (2003). Inflammatory Blockade Restores Adult
    Hippocampal Neurogenesis. *Science*, Vol.302, No.5651 (Dec 2003), pp. 1760-1765,
    ISSN 1095-9203.

Moriyama, M., Fukuhara, T., Britschgi, M., He, Y., Narasimhan, R., Villeda, S., Molina, H.,
    Huber, B.T., Holers, M., & Wyss-Coray, T. (2011). Complement receptor 2 is
    expressed in neural progenitor cells and regulates adult hippocampal
    neurogenesis. *The Journal of Neuroscience*, Vol.31, No.11 (Mar 2011), pp. 3981-3989,
    ISSN 0270-6474.

Nguyen, M.D., Julien, J.P., & Rivest, S. (2002). Innate immunity: the missing link in
    neuroprotection and neurodegeneration? *Nature Review Neuroscience*, Vol.3, No.3
    (Mar 2002), pp. 216-227, ISSN 1471-0048.

Nimmerjahn, A., Kirchhoff, F., & Helmchen, F. (2005). Resting microglial cells are highly
    dynamic surveillants of brain parenchyma in vivo. *Science*, Vol.308, No.5726 (May
    2005), pp. 271314-271318.

Ohira, K., Furuta, T., Hioki, H., Nakamura, K.C., Kuramoto, E., Tanaka, Y., Funatsu, N.,
    Shimizu, K., Oishi, T., Hayashi, M., Miyakawa, T., Kaneko, T., & Nakamura, S.
    (2010) Ischemia-induced neurogenesis of neocortical layer 1 progenitor cells. *Nature
    Neuroscience*, Vol.13, No.2 (Feb 2010), pp. 173-179, ISSN 1097-6256.

Olah, M., Ping, G., De Haas, A.H., Brouwer, N., Meerlo, P., Van Der Zee, E.A., Biber, K., &
    Boddeke, H.W.G.M. (2009). Enhanced hippocampal neurogenesis in the absence of
    microglia T cell interaction and microglia activation in the murine running wheel
    model. *Glia*, Vol.57, No.10 (Aug 2010), pp. 1046-1061, ISSN 1098-1136.

Parijs, L.V., Abbas, A.K. (1998). Homeostasis and self-tolerance in the immune system:
    turning lymphocytes off. *Science*, Vol.280, No.5361 (Apr 1998), pp. 243-248, ISSN
    1095-9203.

Pluchino, S., Muzio, L., Imitola, J., Deleidi, M., Alfaro-Cervello, C., Salani, G., Porcheri, C.,
    Brambilla, E., Cavasinni, F., Bergamaschi, A., Garcia-Verdugo, J.M., Comi, G.,
    Khoury, S.J., & Martino, G. (2008). Persistent inflammation alters the function of the
    endogenous brain stem cell compartment. *Brain*, Vol.131, No.10 (Oct 2010), pp.
    2564-2578, ISSN 1460-2156.

Popa, N., Cedile, O., Pollet-Villard, X., Bagnis, C., Durbec, P., Boucraut, J.E. (2011). RAE-1 is
    expressed in the adult subventricular zone and controls cell proliferation of
    neurospheres. *Glia*, Vol.59, No.1 (Jan 2011), pp. 35-44, ISSN 1098-1136.

Rahpeymai, Y., Hietala, M.A., Wilhelmsson, U., Fotheringham, A., Davies, I., Nilsson, A.-K.,
    Zwirner, J., Wetsel, R.A., Gerard, C., Pekny, M., & Pekna, M. (2006). Complement: a

novel factor in basal and ischemia-induced neurogenesis. *EMBO Journal*, Vol.25, No.6 (Mar 2006), pp. 1364-1374, ISSN 1460-2075.

Ransohoff, R.M., Kivisakk, P., & Kidd, G. (2003). Three or more routes for leukocyte migration into the central nervous system. *Nature Review Immunology*, Vol.3, No.7 (Jul 2007), pp. 569-581, ISSN 1474-1733.

Rapalino, O., Lazarov-Spiegler, O., Agranov, E., Velan, G.J., Yoles, E., Fraidakis, M., Solomon, A., Gepstein, R., Katz, A., Belkin, M., Hadani, M., & Schwartz, M. (1998). Implantation of stimulated homologous macrophages results in partial recovery of paraplegic rats. *Nature Medicine*, Vol.4, No.7 (Jul 1998), pp. 814-21, ISSN 1078-8956.

Rasmussen, S., Imitola, J., Ayuso-Sacido, A., Wang, Y., Starossom, S.C., Kivisäkk, P., Zhu, B., Meyer, M., Bronson, R.T., Garcia-Verdugo, J.M., & Khoury, S.J. (2011). Reversible neural stem cell niche dysfunction in a model of multiple sclerosis. *Annals of Neurology*, Vol.69, No.5 (May 2011), pp. 878-891, ISSN 1531-8249.

Reddy, J., Illes, Z., Zhang, X., Encinas, J., Pyrdol, J., Nicholson, L., Sobel, R.A., Wucherpfennig, K.W., & Kuchroo, V.K. (2004). Myelin proteolipid protein-specific CD4+CD25+ regulatory cells mediate genetic resistance to experimental autoimmune encephalomyelitis. *Proceedings of the National Academy of Sciences U S A*, Vol.101, No.43 (Oct 2004), pp. 15434-15439, ISSN 0027-8424.

Reynolds, R., Dawson, M., Papadopoulos, D., Polito, A., Di Bello, I.C., Pham-Dinh, D., & Levine J. (2002) The response of NG2-expressing oligodendrocyte progenitors to demyelination in MOG-EAE and MS. *Journal Neurocytology*, Vol.31, No.6-7 (Jul-Aug 2002), pp.523-536, ISSN 0300-4864.

Rhodes, K.E., Raivich, G, & Fawcett, J.W. (2006). The injury response of oligodendrocyte precursor cells is induced by platelets, macrophages and inflammation-associated cytokines. *Neuroscience*, Vol.14, No.1 (Jun 2006), pp. 87-100, ISSN 03064522.

Richardson, WD, Young, K.M., Tripathi, R.B., & McKenzie, I. (2011). NG2-glia as multipotent neural stem cells: fact or fantasy? *Neuron*. Vol.70, No.4 (May 2011), pp. 661-673, ISSN 0896-6273.

Rolls, A., Shechter, R., London, A., Ziv, Y., Ronen, A., Levy, R., & Schwartz, M. (2007). Toll-like receptors modulate adult hippocampal neurogenesis. *Nature Cell Biology*, Vol.9, No.9 (Sep 2007), pp. 1081-1088, ISSN 1465-7392.

Saino, O., Taguchi, A., Nakagomi, T., Nakano-Doi, A., Kashiwamura, S.I., Doe, N., Nakagomi, N., Soma, T., Yoshikawa, H., Stern, D.M., Okamura, H., & Matsuyama, T. (2010). Immunodeficiency reduces neural stem/progenitor cell apoptosis and enhances neurogenesis in the cerebral cortex after stroke. *Journal of Neuroscience Research*, Vol.88, No.11 (Aug 2011), pp. 2385-2397, ISSN 0360-4012.

Schonberg, D.L., Popovich, P.G., & McTigue, D.M. (2007). Oligodendrocyte generation is differentially influenced by toll-like receptor (TLR) 2 and TLR4-mediated intraspinal macrophage activation. *Journal Neuropathology Experimental Neurology* Vol.66, No.12 (Dec 2007), pp. 1124-35, ISSN 0022-3069.

Schwartz, M., & Yoles, E. (2006). Immune-based therapy for spinal cord repair: autologous macrophages and beyond. *Journal Neurotrauma*, Vol.23, No.3-4 (Apr 2006), pp. 360-370, ISSN- 1557-9042.

Schwartz, M., A., & Shechter, R. (2009). Boosting T-cell immunity as a therapeutic approach for neurodegenerative conditions: the role of innate immunity. *Neuroscience*, Vol.158, No.3 (Febr 2009), pp. 1133-1142, ISSN 03064522.

Schwartz, M., & Shechter, R. (2010). Systemic inflammatory cells fight off neurodegenerative disease. *Nature Review in Neurology*, Vol.6, No.7 (Jul 2010) pp. 405-10, ISSN 1759-4758.

Shaked, I., Tchoresh, D., Gersner, R., Meiri, G., Mordechai, S., Xiao, X., Hart, R.P., & Schwartz, M. (2005). Protective autoimmunity: interferon-gamma enables microglia to remove glutamate without evoking inflammatory mediators. *Journal of Neurochemistry*, Vol.92, No.5 (Mar 2005), pp. 997-1009, ISSN 0022-3042.

Sharma, R., Fischer, M.T., Bauer, J., Felts, P.A., Smith, K.J., Misu, T, Fujihara, K., Bradl, M., & Lassmann, H. (2010). Inflammation induced by innate immunity in the central nervous system leads to primary astrocyte dysfunction followed by demyelination. *Acta Neuropathologica*, Vol.120, No.2 (Aug 2010), pp. 223-236, ISSN 0001-6322.

Shechter, R., London, A., Varol, C., Raposo, C., Cusimano, M., Yovel, G., Rolls, A., Mack, M., Pluchino, S., Martino, G., Jung, S., & Schwartz, M. (2009). Infiltrating blood-derived macrophages are vital cells playing an anti-inflammatory role in recovery from spinal cord injury in mice. *PLoS Medicine*, Vol.6, No.7 (Jul 2009), ISSN 1549-1676.

Sierra, A., Encinas, J.M., Deudero, J.J.P., Chancey, J.H., Enikolopov, G., Overstreet-Wadiche, L.S., Tsirka, S.E., & Maletic-Savatic, M. (2010). Microglia Shape Adult Hippocampal Neurogenesis through Apoptosis-Coupled Phagocytosis. (2010). *Cell Stem Cell*, Vol.7, No.4 (Oct 2010), pp. 483-495, ISSN 1934-5909.

Skihar, V., Silva, C., Chojnacki, A., Döring, A., Stallcup, W.B., Weiss, S., Yong, V.W. (2009). Promoting oligodendrogenesis and myelin repair using the multiple sclerosis medication glatiramer acetate. *Proceedings of the National Academy of Sciences U S A.* Vol.106, No.42 (Oct 2009), pp. 17992-17997, ISSN 0027-8424.

Song, C., & Wang, H. Cytokines mediated inflammation and decreased neurogenesis in animal models of depression. (2011). *Progress in Neuro-Psychopharmacology and Biological Psychiatry*, Vol.35, No.3 (Apr 2011) pp. 760-768, ISSN 0278-5846.

Spulber, S., Oprica, M., Bartfai, T., Winblad, B., & Schultzberg, M. (2008). Blunted neurogenesis and gliosis due to transgenic overexpression of human soluble IL-1ra in the mouse. *European Journal of Neuroscience*, Vol.27, No.3 (Feb 2008), pp. 549-558, ISSN 1460-9568.

Starossom, S.C., Imitola, J., Wang, Y., Cao, L., Khoury, S.J. (2011). Subventricular zone microglia transcriptional network. *Brain Behaviour Immunology*, Vol.25, No.5 (Nov 2010), pp. 991-999, ISSN 0889-1591.

Taylor, D.L., Pirianov, G., Holland, S., McGinnity, C.J., Norman, A.L., Reali, C., Diemel, L.T., Gveric, D., Yeung, D., & Mehmet, H. (2010). Attenuation of proliferation in oligodendrocyte precursor cells by activated microglia. *Journal of Neuroscience Research*, Vol.88, No.8 (Jun 2010), pp.1632-44, ISSN 1097-4547.

Trotter, J., Karram, K., & Nishiyama, A. NG2 cells: Properties, progeny and origin. (2003). *Brain Research Reviews, Vol.63*, No.1-2 (May 2003), pp. 72-82, ISSN 0165-0173.

Vignali, D.A.A., Collison, L.W., & Workman, C.J. (2008). How regulatory T cells work. *Nature Review Immunology*, Vol.8, No.7 (July 2008), pp. 523-532, ISSN 1474-1733.

Voskuhl, R.R., Peterson, R.S., Song, B., Ao, Y., Morales, L.B., Tiwari-Woodruff, S., & Sofroniew, M.V. (2009). Reactive astrocytes form scar-like perivascular barriers to leukocytes during adaptive immune inflammation of the CNS. *Journal of Neuroscience*, Vol.29, No.37 (Sep 2009), pp. 11511-11522, ISSN 0270-6474.

Walsh, J.T., Kipnis, J. (2010). Regulatory T cells in CNS injury: the simple, the complex and the confused. *Trends in Molecular Medicine, In Press, Corrected Proof,* ISSN 1471-4914.

Walton, N.M., Sutter, B.M., Laywell, E.D., Levkoff, L.H., Kearns, S.M., Marshall, G.P., Scheffler, B., & Steindler, D.A. (2006). Microglia instruct subventricular zone neurogenesis. *Glia*, Vol.54, No.8 (Dec 2006), pp. 815-825, ISSN 1098-1136.

Wolf, S.A., Steiner, B., Akpinarli, A., Kammertoens, T., Nassenstein, C., Braun, A., Blankenstein, T., & Kempermann, G. (2009). CD4-Positive T Lymphocytes Provide a Neuroimmunological Link in the Control of Adult Hippocampal Neurogenesis. *The Journal of Immunology*, Vol.182, No.7 (Apr 2009), pp. 3979-3984, ISSN 0165-5728.

Woodruff, R.H., & Franklin, R.J. (1999). Demyelination and remyelination of the caudal cerebellar peduncle of adult rats following stereotaxic injections of lysolecithin, ethidium bromide, and complement/anti-galactocerebroside: a comparative study. *Glia*, Vol.25, No.1 (Feb 1999), pp. 216-228, ISSN 1098-1136.

Wu, J., Yoo, S., Wilcock, D., Lytle, J.M., Leung, P.Y., Colton, C.A., & Wrathall, J.R. (2010). Interaction of NG2(+) glial progenitors and microglia/macrophages from the injured spinal cord. *Glia*, Vol.58, No.4 (Mar 2010), pp. 410-22, ISSN 1098-1136.

Yang, I., Han, S.J., Kaur, G., Crane, C., & Parsa, A.T. (2010). The role of microglia in central nervous system immunity and glioma immunology. *Journal of Clinical Neuroscience*, Vol.17, No.1, pp. 6-10, ISSN 0967-5868.

Yirmiya, R., & Goshen, I. Immune modulation of learning, memory, neural plasticity and neurogenesis. (2011). *Brain, Behavior, and Immunity*, Vol.25, No.2 (Feb 2011), pp. 181-213, ISSN 0889-1591.

Zhao, C., Deng, W., & Gage, F.H. (2008). Mechanisms and functional implications of adult neurogenesis. *Cell*, Vol.132, No.4 (Feb 2008), pp. 645-660.

Ziv, Y., Ron, N., Butovsky, O., Landa, G., Sudai, E., Greenberg, N., Cohen, H., Kipnis, J., & Schwartz, M. (2006a). Immune cells contribute to the maintenance of neurogenesis and spatial learning abilities in adulthood. *Nature Neuroscience*, Vol.9, No.2 (Feb 2006), pp. 268-275, ISSN 1097-6256.

Ziv, Y., Avidan, H., Pluchino, S., Martino, G., & Schwartz, M. (2006b). Synergy between immune cells and adult neural stem/progenitor cells promotes functional recovery from spinal cord injury. *Proceedings of the National Academy of Sciences U S A*. Vol.103, No.35 (Aug 2006), pp. 13174-13179, ISSN 0027-8424.

8

Mesenchymal Stromal Cells and Neural Stem Cells Potential for Neural Repair in Spinal Cord Injury and Human Neurodegenerative Disorders

Dasa Cizkova et al*

Institute of Neurobiology, Center of Excellence for Brain Research,
Slovak Academy of Sciences, Kosice,
Slovakia

1. Introduction

Spinal cord injury represents a serious neurodegenerative condition mostly characterized by inflammation, demyelination, loss of neurons and glial cells. Patients who suffer from spinal cord trauma show limited functional recovery, which frequently leads to deficit of multiple sensory, motor and autonomic systems resulting to clinical signs of partial or complete paralysis with prominent spasticity and rigidity (Cizkova et al. 2007). Because of the limited regenerative capacity of the adult CNS due to the inhibitory molecules, decrease of trophic factor support and scar tissue formation, the current functional treatments for SCI are not successful (Rowland et al. 2008). However, emerging research evidences on regenerative medicine involving adult and neural stem cells has put much attention on the development of cell based therapies which could promote regeneration of lesioned CNS (Barnabe-Heider & Frisen, 2008; Goldman, 2005). One of the most important factors for the stem cells candidates that are being used in transplantation strategies, is their compatibility with the host tissue. Therefore, preferential criteria for stem cells transplantation in clinical trials are their ability to be used as autologous transplant to avoid moral and ethical dilemma as well as immunosuppressive therapy. Mesenchymal stem cells (MSCs) fulfill all these criteria and can be easily isolated from patient's bone marrow or adipose tissue. However, in many cases their beneficial effect in regard to the treatment of neurodegenerative disorders is most likely due to paracrine (Zacharek et al. 2007) or immunomodulatory effects (Djouad et al. 2003), rather than by direct cell replacement (Jorgensen, 2009). Therefore, other sources of autologous stem cells, such as „Schwann cells" derived from peripheral nerve, „Olfactory ensheating cells" (OECs) (Papastefanaki et al. 2007; Raisman et al. 2011) from olfactory bulb, or even allogenic

*Norbert Zilka[3], Zuzana Kazmerova[3], Lucia Slovinska[1], Ivo Vanicky[1], Ivana Novotna-Grulova[1],
Viera Cigankova[2], Milan Cizek[2] and Michal Novak[3]
[1]Institute of Neurobiology, Center of Excellence for Brain Research, Slovak Academy of Sciences, Kosice, Slovakia
[2]University of Veterinary Medicine and Pharmacy , Kosice, Slovakia
[3]Institute of Neuroimunology, Center of Excellence for Brain Research, Slovak Academy of Sciences, Bratislava,
Slovakia*

embryonic or neural stem cells have been involved in different studies to replace lost/impaired neural population. Particularly, rapidly improving neural stem cells (NSCs) research has been providing encouraging evidence that stem cells derived from nerve tissue can repair CNS structure and perhaps even function which is impaired by various neurodegenerative disorders. NSCs that can self-renew, are multipotent cells committed to generate a neural phenotype, thus making them easier to differentiate into the desired sources of neuronal or pro-oligodendroglial cells that may be applied for further transplantation strategies. The accuracy of both autologous vs allogenic cell based approaches was confirmed in recent studies where application of adult and neural stem cells into injured spinal cord or to a wide variety of neurodegenerative diseases led to improvement of functional outcome in animal models through replacement of damaged or dead motor neurons and thereby remyelination of spared axons and modulation of inflammation (Louro & Pearse, 2008; Kim & de Vellis, 2009; Nandoe Tewarie et al. 2009). As with any cell therapy in CNS, it is important to realize that more complex issues need to be considered, such as: the selection of cell source, effective delivery strategies, optimal dosing of stem cells, proper timing and safety guarantees of stem cells based treatment.

Here we have tried to outline the most important basic issues of MSC, NSC research in regard to their therapeutic potential to repair or enhance plasticity in neurodegenerative disorders, with main focus on SCI. The following sections summarize the MSCs and NSCs fundamental biological properties, their potential sources and perspective advantages in cell-based therapies.

2. Mesenchymal stem cells

Mesenchymal stem cells, also called bone marrow stromal cells represent a heterogeneous population of the cells derived from the non-blood forming fraction of bone marrow . They are able to differentiate into bone, tendon, cartilage and fat (Pittenger et al. 1999) or under specific condition into neuronal, muscle, liver cells (Keilhoff et al. 2006; Yu et al. 2007; Greco & Rameshwar, 2008) as well as epithelial cells of lung, skin, kidney and gastrointestinal tract (Herzog et al. 2003). The first evidence for the existence of non-hematopoietic stem cells derived from bone marrow has been available from Friedenstein's work in 1970s (Friedenstein et al. 1976). Friedenstein isolated cells from bone marrow and plated them on plastic culture dish. After 4 hours, he removed the medium with non-adherent cells (mostly containing hematopoietic stem cells) and observed that a small number of cells with spindle-shape morphology remained adhered to the Petri dish and form foci of two or four cells. After the 2-4 days, the adherent cells started to multiply and attained spindle-shaped morphology (Friedenstein et al. 1976). From a physiological point of view, MSCs represent a major population of bone marrow stromal cells, that by the continuous release of EPO (erythropoietin-EPO) and granulocyte-colony formation stimulating factor (granulocyte colony stimulating factor G-CSF), promote survival, division and differentiation of hematopoietic precursor/stem cells (Cui et al. 2009). Since then non-hematopoietic stem cells have been identified in many other organs and tissues including skin, skeletal muscle, teeth, adipose tissue, testis, gut, liver and ovarian epithelium (Kerkis et al. 2006; Guan et al. 2006; Zuk et al. 2002).

2.1 Isolation of MSCs from bone marrow and adipose tissue

MSCs can be isolated by aspiration of bone marrow from the diaphysis of the tibia or femur
in rats, mice, which represent only 0,001-0,01% of the total population of nucleated cells
(Pittenger et al. 1999). In humans, bone marrow derived MSCs (BM-MSCs) are mainly
obtained from superior iliac crest of pelvis (Digirolamo et al. 1999). *In-vitro* cultivation of
MSCs is very simple because of their plastic adherence, their extensive proliferative capacity
and ability to create single-cell-derived colonies (Colter et al. 2000). There is a possibility for
MSCs exploitation in autologous transplantations to prevent immunological response or
rejection of implanted cells. Compared to embryonic stem cells, MSCs have reportedly low
tumorigenic potential and they are capable to migrate toward tumors (Loebinger et al. 2009)
and into the sites of neural lesions (Chen et al. 2008). Another source of mesenchymal stem
cells represents the adipose tissue. Adipose tissue-derived mesenchymal stem cells (AT-
MSCs) are also multipotent, plastic adherent, have similar CD markers as BM-MSCs and
under specific condition they are able to differentiate into cells of the mesodermal,
osteogenic, chondrogenic, adipogenic and myogenic lineages and even into cells with
neuron-like morphology (Zuk et al. 2002). Moreover, isolation of AT-MSCs is easier (by
liposuction); less painful and number of obtained cells is much higher in comparison to BM-
MSCs (Lin et al. 2008). In spite of this, MSCs obtained from bone marrow represent the main
source of stem cells in preclinical and clinical studies until now.

2.1.1 Morphology and phenotype of MSCs

According to the morphology, MSCs are classified into two groups: spindle-shaped type,
also called very small rapidly self-renewal round cells (RSCs) (Colter et al. 2001) and
flattened type (Mets & Verdonk, 1981) known as a mature MSCs (mMSCs). RSCs are
characterised by rapid rate of replication after low density plating, potential for multilineage
differentiation and by the presence of specific cell surface epitopes which are not found at
mMSCs stage, such as: vascular endothelial growth factor receptor-2 (FLK-1), TRK (a nerve
growth factor receptor), transferrin receptor and annexin II (lipocortine 2) (Colter et al.
2001). Unlike, mMSCs are characterised by large-scale and flatted morphology, lower
property of replication and higher ratio of cytoplasm-to-nucleus when compared to RSCs.
Moreover, MSCs express several positive cell surface molecules that allow us to distinguish
them from the hematopoietic stem cells such as: β-integrins (CD29), CD44, α-integrins
(CD49a, CD49b), CD61, P-selectin (CD62), CD90 (thy-1), CD105, CD106 (VCAM-1) and
CD166 (Majumdar et al. 2003; Docheva et al. 2007), collagen type I and IV, laminin,
fibronectin; chemokine receptors: CXCR5,6-R, CCR1,7,9-R; CX3CL1-R; growth factor
receptors: TGFβ-R, PDGF-R, NGF-R, FGF-R; and cytokine receptors: IL1,3,4,6,7,15-R, TNFα-
R (Dominici et al. 2006; Stagg, 2007). The immune phenotype of cultured MSCs is described
as MHC class I+, MHC class II-, CD40-, CD80- and CD86-. This phenotype is regarded as
non-immunogenic and suggests that MSCs might be effective in inducing tolerance (Javazon
et al. 2001). It has been documented that during aging, MSCs undergo several changes and
thereby lose their differentiation capacity and decrease production of specific proteins and
factors responsible for cell differentiation such as bone morphogenic protein (BMP-7),
alkaline phosphatase, G-CSF (granulocyte colony-stimulating factor), LIF (leukemia
inhibitory factor) and stem cell factor (SCF). Moreover, differentiation potential of MSCs is

down regulated from the 6th passage on and the mean length of telomeres is shortened after 9th passage revealing morphological abnormalities typical of the Hayflick model of cellular aging (Bonab et al. 2006). According to these evidences it is very important to realize the fact that mesenchymal stem cells which are applied in regenerative medicine should be used in early passages where currently their rapid proliferation and increased differentiation capacity are utilized.

2.1.2 Trophic properties of MSCs

Several reports suggest that application of MSCs in neurodegenerative disorders led to neuroprotective effect and to the replacement of diseased and damaged cells and tissues in the most affected area. Profuse scientific investigations revealed that the main effect of the neuroprotection and neuroregeneration is mediated by specific neurotrophic molecules and cytokines that are directly produced by MSCs. It has been also shown that these factors can support neuronal cell survival and regenerate nerve fibers at the lesion sites (Mahmood et al. 2004). In vitro studies have confirmed the presence of various neurotrophic factors produced by MSCs, including nerve growth factor (NGF), brain-derived neurotrophic factor (BDNF), glial cell line-derived neurotrophic factor (GDNF), ciliary neurotrophic factor (CNTF) and neurotrophin-3 (NT-3) (Chen et al. 2005; Kurozumi et al. 2005). Measurement of 56 separate subclones derived from human MSCs showed that differences in neurotrophin's production between single cell clones can vary in a huge range (from 167 to 2000-fold) and expression of these neuro-regulatory molecules was able to promote survival and neurite outgrowth in the SH-SY5Y neuroblastoma cell line. Consecutive selection of the most producing single cell derived clones can lead to better exploitation of MSCs in regenerative and cell replacement medicine (Crigler et al. 2006). Moreover, MSCs also constitutively express several interleukins including IL-6, IL-7, IL-8, IL-11, IL-12, IL-14, IL-15, macrophage or granulocyte-macrophage colony stimulating factor (M-CSF, GM-CSF), stromal cell-derived factor 1α (SDF-1α) (Crigler et al. 2006), Flt-3 ligand and stem cell factor (Majumdar et al. 1998) that can play an important role in immunomodulatory processes.

2.1.3 Immunomodulatory effect of MSCs

Recent studies demonstrate that MSCs command with the ability to modulate an immune response depending on the stimulus to which they are exposed. Their dual ability, to suppress and/or activate immune responses, can lead to modulation of the reaction of broad range of immune cells, including T cells, B cells, NK cells and antigen-presenting cells (Stagg, 2007). It is assumed that the main effect of immunosuppresion is evoked by soluble factors that are produced by MSCs or immune cells, such as: hepatocyte growth factor, indoleamine 2, 3-dioxygenase (IDO), prostaglandin E2, TGF-β1, nitric oxide and IL10. It has been also observed that MSCs use different mechanisms that are responsible for inhibition of function and proliferation of immune cells (Nauta & Fibbe, 2007). INFγ play a crucial role in regulation of MSC-mediated immunosuppresion. INFγ induce MSCs to release prostaglandins and IDO, which causes depletion of tryptophan, an essential factor for lymphocyte proliferation (Aggarwal & Pittenger, 2005). The similar suppressive effect on T-cell proliferation was also suggested in the presence of TGF-β and hepatocyte growth factor, which are constitutively produced by MSCs (Di Nicola et al. 2002). Cocultivation of MSCs with lymphocytes revealed that MSCs don't constitutively secrete suppressive factors but provide a dynamic cross-talk between MSCs and lymphocytes (Augello et al. 2005). MSCs can interfere with dendritic cells (DCs) differentiation, maturation and function. It has been observed that MSCs had an inhibitory effect on differentiation of monocytes and CD34+ progenitors into CD1a+-DCs by skewing of their differentiation property toward macrophages (Nauta & Fibbe, 2007). At the same time, immature DCs were unable to induce T cells activation in the presence of MSCs. Cocultivation of MSCs with NK cells showed that allogeneic MSCs could inhibit IL-2 and IL-15-induced proliferation of resting NK cells and either MSCs are able to suppress the proliferation and cytokine production of IL-15 stimulated NK cells via soluble factors. Suggesting that there is also the existence of different mechanisms for MSC-mediated NK cell suppression demonstrated experiments where after inhibition of both soluble factors - PGE2 and TGF-β produced by MSCs complete restoration of proliferation capacity of NK cells was observed (Sotiropoulou et al. 2006).

3. Application of MSCs in neurodegenerative diseases

Transplantation of autologous or allogenic mesenchymal stem cells has been considered as a potential therapeutic approach to a wide variety of neurodegenerative diseases such as Alzheimer's disease (AD), Parkinson disease (PD), sclerosis multiplex (SM), amyotrophic lateral sclerosis (ALS), spinal cord injury (SCI) or stroke.

3.1 Utilization of MSCs in therapy for SCI

Traumatic injury to the spinal cord initiates a cascade of reactive changes, which results in permanent damage and loss of neurological function below the lesion site (Rowland et al., 2008). The inflammatory events, together with ischemia, Ca2+ influx into cells, edema, and progressive hemorrhagic necrosis significantly contribute to secondary injury, which causes progressive cavitation and loss of spinal tissue (Kwon et al. 2010). The expression of adverse neurite growth-inhibitory molecules in the extracellular matrix (Fawcett, 2006; Schwab, 2004) together with lack of trophic factor support and the discontinuity of axonal projections caused by progressive tissue cyst formation pose multifactor obstacles contributing to the loss of spinal cord regeneration and inability to find an effective therapy (Nagahara & Tuszynski, 2011). However, by addressing aspects, such as neutralization of growth inhibitors Nogo-A, CSPGs, delivery of various trophic factors or utilizing stem cells/progenitors, a considerable progress has been made in enhancing the growth of injured adult axons (Bradbury et al. 2002). The widespread use of stem cell therapy has shown that transplantation of MSCs can improve recovery after stroke (Chopp & Li, 2002), promote remyelination (Akiyama et al. 2002), as well as contribute to partial recovery of locomotor function in animal models of spinal cord injury (SCI) (Cizkova et al. 2006) (Sykova & Jendelova, 2005; Arboleda et al. 2011; Forostyak et al. 2011). Thus, achieved progress in animal SCI models utilizing MSCs made it possible for translating preclinical findings to human clinical trials. For example, transplantation of unmanipulated autologous bone marrow in patients with subacute and chronic SCI resulted into improvement of motor/or sensory functions within 3 months. Although, implantation of autologous bone marrow cells appears to be safe, it is necessary to follow up patients outcome data, for more than 2 years (Sykova et al. 2006; Pal et al. 2009; Moviglia et al. 2009). While there is evidence that MSCs can give rise to cells with neural characteristics in vitro (Kim et al. 2002) and in vivo (Jendelova et al. 2004), it is more likely that production of neurotrophic or vascular factors (Zhong et al. 2003; Hamano et al. 2000) together with immunomodulatory effects (Aggarwal & Pittenger, 2005) have a dominant influence on recovery of function following spinal cord trauma. Particularly, suggested hypoimmunologic nature of MSCs, imply for unique MSCs immunomodulatory approaches, that could be used for immunosuppression to induce allotransplantation tolerance or even to attenuate autoimmune, inflammatory responses (Le Blanc & Ringden, 2005). Although some experimental studies in animals or pre-clinical human studies demonstrate the effectiveness and safety of MSCs therapy, there are still many questions to be answered regarding the mechanisms of engraftment, homing, inter-cellular interactions, immunological profiles, in vivo differentiation as well as long-term safety.

3.1.1 MSCs therapy for Parkinson disease

Parkinson disease (PD) is the second most common neurodegenerative disorder in the world characterized by progressive loss of nigrostriatal dopaminergic neurons leading to deficiency of dopamine in striatum which is responsible for control of movement. The characteristic symptoms in patients suffering from PD are rigidity, akinesia, tremor and balance problems (Pechadre et al. 1976). Number of studies investigated whether transplantation of human mesenchymal stem cells (hMSCs) can lead to protective effect on progressive dopaminergic neuronal loss in vitro or in vivo conditions. Intravenous injection of hMSCs into the PD transgenic rat models showed strong protective effect on progressive loss of dopaminergic neurons in substantia nigra. Human MSCs reduced the caspase-3 activity and increased survival of TH-immunoreactive cells in substantia nigra in comparison with the control group. Moreover, a significant improvement in behavioral motor tests in hMSCs treated group has also been observed (Park et al. 2008). *In vitro* study demonstrated that SDF-α-1, chemokine constitutively produced by MSCs increased dopamine release and led to suppression of cell death induced by 6-OHDA administration compared to untreated group (Wang et al. 2010). Neuroprotective effect of hMSCs on dopaminergic neurons mediated by anti-inflammatory properties of MSCs and their modulation of microglial activation were uncovered (Kim et al. 2009). Transplantation of GDNF-transduced MSCs into the PD animal model supported the evidence, that they are capable to induce a local trophic effect in the denervated striatum and sprouting from remaining dopaminergic terminals toward neurotrophic milieu. Exploitation of new optogenetic technique demonstrated for the first time that intrastriatally grafted stem cell-derived dopamine neurons become functionally integrated in the dopamine-denervated striatum (Tonnesen et al. 2011). Noninvasive intranasal delivery of MSCs to the unilaterally 6-hydroxydopamine - lesioned rat brains showed decreasing concentrations of inflammatory cytokines, increasing of tyrosine hydroxylase level in the lesioned ipsilateral striatum and substancia nigra, and prevented any decrease of dopamine in the lesioned hemisphere. Simultaneously, significant improvement of motor function of forepaw in PD rat model was observed (Danielyan et al. 2011).

3.1.2 MSCs therapy for Alzheimer disease

Alzheimer disease (AD), the most common form of dementia, is characterized as a progressive neurodegenerative disorder (Berchtold & Cotman, 1998). Degeneration and dysfunction of the neurons and decline of synaptic function and plasticity mostly in brain regions responsible for memory and learning, as hippocampus, entorhinal cortex, basal forebrain and neocortical association cortices, are the most incident symptoms that generally characterize AD (DeKosky et al. 1996). There is no cure or early preclinical diagnostic assay available for Alzheimer's disease. Currently, most prevalent is symptomatic therapy, which is not able to stop the progression of the disease. Therefore, Alzheimer's disease is still being recognized as an unmet medical need. In 1906, Dr. Alois Alzheimer, identified two specific features that are mostly figured in AD human brain, neurofibrillary tangles and amyloid plaques. Deep investigation in the study of the main structural components responsible for the creation of two pathological hallmarks in AD brain, uncovered inherence of tau protein in NFT and amyloid beta peptide in amyloid plaques. Several years later, it was demonstrated that strong neuroinflammation occurs in AD brain (Novak et al. 1993) (Dickson et al. 1988; Zilka et al. 2006; Zilkova et al. 2006).

Application of stem cells in AD preclinical studies brought in last years several positive results. Taking advantage of stem cells immunomodulatory and trophic properties and their transplantation into AD transgenic animal models showed that they are the most appropriate tool for the achievement of functional restoration of damaged cells and in the same manner for the replacement by healthy one (Blurton-Jones et al. 2009; Hampton et al. 19 2010; Lee et al. 2010). Recent developments in stem cell technology raise the prospect of cell therapy for human neurodegenerative tauopathies. Transplantation of the neural stem cells or administration of mesenchymal stem cells isolated either from human umbilical cord or from the bone marrow has produced beneficial effects in several independent animal models of AD (Blurton-Jones et al. 2009). Above mentioned reports have shown that the neuroprotective effect of stem cells may be mediated 1) by their ability to produce various trophic factors that contribute to functional recovery or 2) by activation of neuroinflammatory pathways. *In vitro* studies show that MSCs can prevent tau mediated cell death in the Alzheimer's cell model. It has been confirmed that MSCs have significant impact on tau cell death cascade and can ameliorate toxic effect of misfolded truncated tau that is considered to be driving force behind neurofibrillary degeneration. Therefore it may be suggested that the cell neuroprotective therapy rather than cell replacement therapy represents prospective strategy for treatment of Alzheimer's disease and related tauopathies (Zilka et al. 2011).

4. Neural stem cells

The human brain contains roughly 100 billion neurons, of which several thousands die every day, representing the loss of millions of nerve cells across the life span. For this reason, it has been believed for a long time, that adult mammalian central nervous system (CNS) is rather rigid structure, unable to repair itself following diseases or injury. However, in some brain regions dead neurons could be replaced and potentially could contribute to the regeneration of damaged nerve tissue (Graziadei & Graziadei, 1979). Therefore, a number of controversial issues concerning possible CNS plasticity was raised and broadly discussed. Finally, in the 1960s and 1970s, most of the uncertainties were addressed and neuroscience's central tenets the 'no new neurons' doctrine, was reconsidered following the key-revolutionary discovery of Joseph Altman (Altman, 1962; Altman & Das, 1965), documenting thymidine-H_3-labelled neurons and neuroblasts in the adult rat brain. From now on a huge effort has gone into unraveling and understanding the fundamental mechanisms of adult CNS regeneration in mammals.

4.1 Neural stem cells definition and origin

It took almost twenty years of dedicated research involving a large number of scientific experiments which clearly confirmed ongoing neurogenesis not only in songbirds (Nottebohm, 1981), but also in rodents, non-human primates and humans, in whom new imaging techniques, such as bromodeoxyuridin (BrdU) labeling, etc, enabling identification of proliferating cells were applied (Eriksson et al. 1998). All these studies jointly confirmed that new functional neurons are generated in the adult mammalian, including human CNS in two discrete areas: i) in the hippocampus, the subgranular zone (SGZ) of the dentate gyrus, which is an important center of our memory (Gage, 2000; Alvarez-Buylla et al. 2002) and, ii) in subventricular zone (SVZ), representing a thin layer of cells lining along the lateral cerebral ventricles, where a nerve cells essential for olfaction are generated (Gage, 2000; Lledo et al. 2006). In both areas, neurogenesis progresses as a complex multi-stage process, which starts with the proliferation, followed by migration and terminal differentiation (Abrous et al. 2005). The current knowledge of self-renewing and multipotent neural stem cells is largely defined by in vitro, as well as *in vivo* evidences documenting their ability to generate the main progeny of the nervous system: neurons, astrocytes and oligodendrocytes (Gage, 2000). NSCs reside in specific anatomical microenvironments that are called neurogenic niches; small islands where neurons and glial cells are continuously generated (Doetsch et al. 1999). However, neurogenic regions (SVZ, SGZ) must meet following criteria: 1) contain neural precursors (NPCs) that are generated in, 2) neurogenic niches, providing cell-cell contacts and diffusible factors for terminal neural differentiation, and 3) provide neurogenic potential (thus, ability of NPCs that are implanted in a neurogenic areas to generate neurons, while when implanted into other brain location they give rise to glia). Another interesting pool of neural precursor cells is represented by astrocytes found within the germinal layers of the adult brain. It has been broadly documented that these astrocytes retain the stem cell properties throughout the life span, and are involved in both neuro- and glio-genesis (Alvarez-Buylla et al. 2001; Gotz & Huttner, 2005; Mori et al. 2005).

4.1.1 Neurogenesis mediated by pathological conditions; Properties of non-neurogenic areas

Normal adult neurogenesis produces a limited number of newly generated functional cells that primarily serves to maintain physiological tissue homeostasis in specific CNS systems. Initially, the neurogenic processes have been expected to be rather stable, moreover insensitive to external stimuli. However, this view has been changed, due to the growing evidence documenting that SVZ and SGZ are responding to a various local or global signals generated from nerve tissue damage. For example, neurogenesis in both neurogenic zones is increased in animal experimental models of ischemia/stroke (Zhang et al. 2008) as well as in humans suffering from stroke (Curtis et al. 2007), epileptic seizures (Grote & Hannan, 2007) and multiple sclerosis (Nait-Oumesmar et al. 2007). Furthermore, neurogenesis is increased in human cases and animal models of Huntington's disease while it is reduced in Alzheimer's and Parkinson's disease as well as in depression and stress (Elder et al. 2006; Grote & Hannan, 2007). Stem cells with the potential to generate new neurons that could replace dying neurons in neurodegenerative diseases or CNS injuries reside also in other areas of the adult CNS, indicating to the possibility that endogenous sources of NSCs can be mobilized also from non-neurogenic regions (Minger, 2007). These NSCs have been demonstrated in brain areas such as septum, striatum or even in the spinal cord, but so far it was not clearly established whether these stem cells are capable of differentiation to the final functional neurons (Liu & Martin, 2003; Wiltrout et al. 2007). Furthermore, it has been suggested that ependymal cells (ECs) adjacent to the SVZ of the lateral ventricles, may mimic the characteristics of NSCs (Johansson et al. 1999; Doetsch et al. 1999). A study by Coskun et al. (Coskun et al. 2008) documented that this may be the case, because the subpopulation of ependymal cells, CD133+/CD24-, exhibited features of quiescent NSCs *in vitro*, i.e., self-renewal and multipotency as well as participation in neurogenesis *in vivo* after injury. In this relation, the occurrence of ependymal cell layer covering CNS ventricular system including the areas around the third, fourth ventricles, and the central canal (CC) of the spinal cord supports suggestion, that also these regions may retain similar quiescent NSCs as those which were identified in the lateral ventricles (Weiss et al. 1996).

4.1.2 Neurogenic potential in the spinal cord and stimulatory factors

There is increasing evidence that the CC ependymal cell region, which is regarded as presumptive neurogenic area of adult spinal cord, contains a limited number of neural stem cells. Once implanted in the animals, they differentiate into oligodendrocytes and astrocytes (Mothe & Tator, 2005) while, under *in vitro* conditions, they give rise to both neurons and glia (Yamamoto et al. 2001). On the other hand, neuronal or glial fate of grafted ECs is highly depended on the host neurogenic/non–neurogenic microenvironment (Shihabuddin et al. 2000). These contradictory findings are often explained in regard to beneficial (*in vitro*) or inhibitory (*in vivo*) conditions directly influencing neuronal or glial fate (Weiss et al. 1996). Furthermore, after pathological condition such as spinal cord injury, most of the newly dividing intrinsic ependymal stem cells migrate toward damaged tissue, where they develop into macroglial cells, while only few cells retain primitive nestin-like phenotype (Johansson et al. 1999; Cizkova et al. 2009a). Likewise, a significant number of neural progenitors could be activated also in other regions of the parenchyma (Horner et al. 2000) (Kehl et al. 1997). However, it remains unclear whether these progenitors develop into functional neurons.

A stimulatory effect on spinal progenitors may be obtained also after physiological stimulation, when experimental animals are exposed to an enrichment environment or physical activity. Previous experiments have shown that mice providing systematic exercise in a running wheel had twice more new hippocampal neurons than controls (Gomez-Pinilla et al. 2001). Beside this, it has been confirmed that voluntary exercise can increase levels of brain-derived neurotrophic factor (BDNF) and other growth factors, which stimulate neurogenesis, improve learning, mental performance (Gomez-Pinilla et al. 2001) and may mobilize gene expression profiles that could be beneficial for CNS plasticity processes (Neeper et al. 1995). These data were further confirmed in latter studies showing that enhanced physical activity in adult rats induces an endogenous ependymal cell response leading to increased proliferation, although in more attenuated manner if compared with

SCI (Cizkova et al. 2009b) (Fig.1). Indeed, there is one group of studies that favor the fact that ECs might contribute to *de novo* neuronal differentiation following CNS injury (Ke et al. 2006; Danilov et al. 2006), while others refuse this suggestion (Zai & Wrathall, 2005). Based on these findings, it is un-doubtful that the adult spinal cord retain a certain reservoir of neural precursors, which can under various specific conditions stimulate and promote the recovery of injured spinal cord.

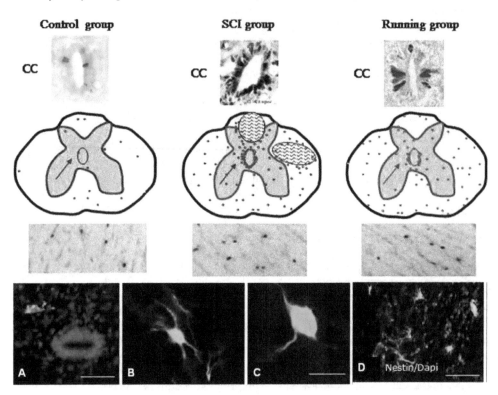

Fig. 1. Schematic illustration of BrdU IR in the thoracic spinal cord section (Th8) of the control, SCI or Running group. Note, the highest BrdU expression in the CC canal, and around the lesion site of SCI group, different distribution patterns of BrdU positive nuclei in the ependyma between SCI and Running group, and increased BrdU response in the parenchyma of the SC in both groups. Below each schematic drawing, a panel revealing BrdU–IR in the corresponding ventral white matter is performed. (A-D) Fluorescence microscopy images of occasionally occurring nestin-positive cell bodies (green) with processes, found in the close vicinity to the CC gray matter, dorsal horn or adjacent to lesion site.

4.1.3 Molecular mechanisms of neurogenesis

Neurogenesis is understood as a complex process that is regulated by a wide variety of important signaling molecules such as: growth factors, cytokines, and neurotransmitters.

Their primary function is to mediate a balance between proliferation, migration and survival of NSCs within the neurogenic niche. The most important growth factors affecting cell division are: FGF (fibroblast growth factor), VEGF (vascular endothelial growth factor), EGF (epidermal growth factor / epidermal growth factor), PDGF (platelet-derived growth factor) and BDNF (brain derived neurotrophic factor). Therefore, endogenous neurogenesis can be stimulated by intraventricular infusion of mitogenic factors such as EGF, bFGF, TGFβ (transforming growth factor β) that stimulate the proliferation activity in the SVZ and thus restore the nervous tissue (Kuhn et al. 1997). Nitric oxide (NO), erythropoietin, bone morphogenetic protein (BMP Bone Morphogenetic Protein) and Wnt proteins (Wiltrout et al. 2007) also play an important role in regulating neurogenesis. BMP and its receptor that are expressed by the SVZ cells promoting differentiation of the NSCs toward glial phenotype are blocked by Noggin, which is produced by ECs and in contrast drives differentiation into neurons (Lim et al. 2000). The most important regulatory neurotransmitters include GABA (γ-aminobutyric acid) and glutamate, which maintain homeostasis of newly formed neurons (Platel et al. 2007). GABA decreases the proliferation of neuroblasts and NSCs, whereas glutamate stimulates their division. It is noteworthy that in all types of damaged nerve tissue which is associated with glutamate excitotoxicity an increased neurogenesis, is documented. GABA is synthesized and released by neuroblasts and activates $GABA_A$ receptor, causing loss of proliferation of neuroblasts and astrocytes. We can conclude that GABA acts as a negative modulator inhibiting cell division, which means that with increased number of neuroblasts there is a higher amount of released of GABA and more $GABA_A$ receptors are activated (Bordet et al. 2007).

5. Transplantation strategies utilizing NSCs

Neural progenitors isolated from vertebrate central nervous system (CNS) represent valuable source of cells that hold particular promise for treating a variety of human neurological diseases such as spinal cord injury (Goldman, 2005). Due to the pathological events and limited ability of the spinal cord to repair itself, therapeutic approaches are focused either on: i) stimulation of endogenous neuronal plasticity and mobilization of oligodendroglial progenitors (Azari et al. 2005; Fawcett, 2006; Yang et al. 2006) or ii) development of an effective cell selection techniques to gain desired NSCs progeny used for cell-replacement therapy (Faulkner & Keirstead, 2005; Hofstetter et al. 2005; Keirstead et al. 2005). However, an important issue due to the pathological nature of spinal cord damage it is important to select the most convenient strategy involving desired cellular pools for transplantation. For example, spinal ischemia-induced spastic paraplegia which is associated with a selective loss of small inhibitory interneurons, would necessarily involve implantation of neuronal progenitors. On the other hand, diseases or spinal cord trauma, with different pathological outcome, resulting in demyelination of axons followed by destruction of long descending tracts would rather require transplantation of myelin-producing cells such as oligodendroglial cells, Schwann cells or Olfactory ensheating cells (Keirstead et al. 2005; Keilhoff et al. 2006; Pearse et al. 2007; Raisman, 2007). Since a well-documented repertoire of specific surface markers for cells of NSCs at different developmental stages have been identified, it may be possible to identify factors which affect their commitment to oligodendroglial cells or neurons and combine this with optimal sorting methods (Deng & Poretz, 2003; Pruszak et al. 2007; Uchida et al. 2000). In particular, magnetic cell separation using specific monoclonal antibodies (e.g. A2B5, PSA-NCAM) conjugated to nanoparticles allowing positive retention or negative dilution of selected cells provide a feasible approach for experimental cell enrichment of desired oligodendroglial progeny, which may be used in future trials for cell-based therapies to treat spinal cord injury (Cizkova et al. 2009a). These studies have shown that MACs technology enable us to gain about a 5 to 9 fold increase of immature, mature oligodendrocytes content (NG2+, RIP+, MBP+) when compared to amount of oligodendroglial cells acquired from unseparated population (Fig.2). A great deal of attention has been given to NSCs isolated from various regions of CNS, including embryonic and adult spinal cord, that could differentiate into desired oligodendrocytes and myelinate host axons in various pre-clinical animal models of SCI (Tarasenko et al. 2007; Kakinohana et al. 2004). For example, NSCs derived from human fetal brain improved recovery after contusion SCI either in severe combined immunodeficiency (SCID) or myelin–deficient shivered mice (Cummings et al. 2005). Highly purified oligodendrocyte progenitors could be generated also from human embryonic stem cells (hESCs) (Nistor et al. 2005; Cloutier et al. 2006). Based on their remyelination properties described in preclinical animal SCI models, the Geron Corporation has initiated a first clinical trial (Phase I) by transplanting hESC-derived oligodendrocyte

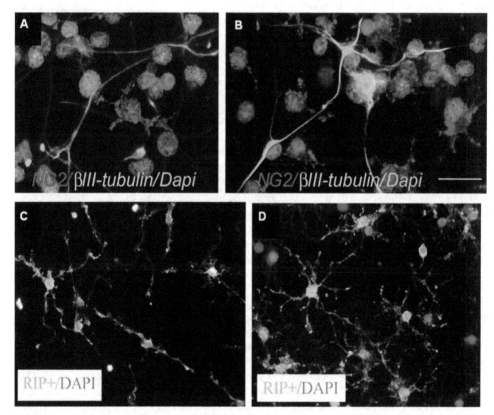

Fig. 2. Immature neurons expressing βIII-tubulin (green) occurred in both, unseparated (A) and separated NSC population (B), but higher number of immature NG2+ oligodendrocytes (red, A, B) and mature RIP+ oligodendrocytes (green C, D) was found after MACs (B, D) (compare A with B and C with D).

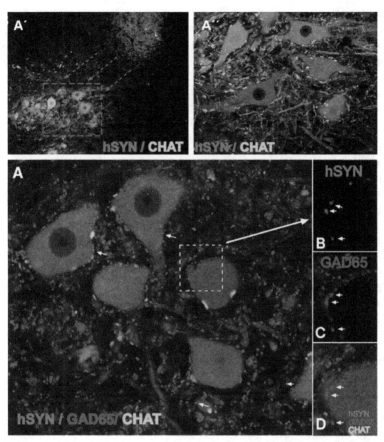

Fig. 3. Fluorescent microscopy images (A´, A´´) and single confocal optical images (A–D) of transverse spinal cord sections taken at 3 months after grafting and stained with human specific hSYN antibody (B, red), CHAT antibody (A, green) and GAD65 antibody (C, blue) antibodies. The majority of hSYN terminals showed co-localization with GAD65 (B–D, yellow arrows).

Progenitor cells in patients with spinal cord injuries. Their preliminary data showed a very good safety profile, with no serious adverse events, no evidence of cavitation at the injury site and no immune responses to the transplanted cells even after complete withdrawal of immunesuppression. One of the most important properties of NSCs is their ability to generate functional neurons, which could potentially rebuild altered local neuronal network following spinal injury. Thus, implanting NSCs-derived neuronal pools in animals subjected to spinal ischemia-induced paraplegia, where selective loss of small local inhibitory interneurons, with persisting α-motoneurons occurs, could meet the needs and expectations to reconstruct impaired local inhibitory neuronal circuits. Although, the precise mechanism leading to spastic paraplegia and rigidity is not certain, the neuropathological features of a selective degeneration of GABA, GAD immunopositive inhibitory neurons are well defined. In addition, the loss of these specific inhibitory pools localized in the intermediate zone of the spinal grey matter, ultimately leads to an increase in the monosynaptic reflex and near-complete loss in spinal polysynaptic activity. A challenging study done in collaboration with anesthesiology research laboratory at University of California San Diego, has shown that NSCs derived from human fetal spinal cord grafted into a rat model of ischemic spastic paraplegia resulted into a progressive recovery of motor function with correlative improvement in motor evoked potentials (Cizkova et al. 2007). Of note, transplanted NSCs became integrated into host neuronal circuits and displayed an extensive axo-dendritic outgrowth and active rostrocaudal/dorsoventral migration for about 8-12 weeks. Furthermore, intense hSYN immunoreactivity was identified within the grafts and in the vicinity of persisting α-motoneurons. These hSYN immunoreactive synaptic terminals expressed GAD65 immunoreactivity in 40-45% of human grafted cells, referring to their inhibitory fate (Fig. 3). All together, these data conclude that functional recovery was associated with long term survival of grafted neurons with GABAergic phenotype that most probably contributed to suppression of spasticity (Cizkova et al. 2007). Similarly, human hNT neurons (teratocarcinoma cell line) or rat spinal neuronal precursors (SNPs), grafted into ischemic spinal segments depleted of inhibitory neurons, restore local inhibitory tone and ameliorate spasticity (Marsala et al. 2004). In addition, when human derived NSCs were treated with a cocktail of growth factors and later transplanted into the injured spinal cord, they differentiated preferentially into cholinergic neurons (Wu et al. 2009). Although, it seems that NSCs are a powerful source of neural progenitors that are constitutively secreting a variety of growth stimulating factors (NGF, BDNF, GDNF), they are often genetically modified to further enhance their potential and secrete additional factors such as neurotrophin 3 (NT-3), or are combined with antibodies that neutralize ciliary neurothrophic factor (CNTF), in an attempt to attenuate astrocytic differentiation (Ishii et al. 2006).

6. Acknowledgments

We acknowledge the financial support given by MVTS-COST BM-1002- NANONET, the Grant Agency of the Slovak Academy of Sciences VEGA 2/0114/11 and the Center of Excellence for Brain Research Slovak Academy of Sciences and the project No 26110230036 University of Veterinary Medicine and Pharmacy (Nove studijne programy a vzdelavanie na Univerzite veterinarneho lekarstva v Kosiciach, Operacny program Vzdelavanie).

7. References

Abrous, D. N.; Koehl, M.& Le Moal, M. (2005). Adult neurogenesis: from precursors to network and physiology. *Physiol Rev*, Vol. 85, No. 2, (April 2005), pp 523-569, ISSN 0031-9333

Aggarwal, S .& Pittenger, M. F. (2005). Human mesenchymal stem cells modulate allogeneic immune cell responses. *Blood*, Vol. 105, No. 4, (February 2005), pp 1815-1822, ISSN 0006-4971

Akiyama, Y.; Radtke, C.; Honmou, O.& Kocsis, J. D. (2002). Remyelination of the spinal cord following intravenous delivery of bone marrow cells. *Glia*, Vol. 39, No. 3, (September 2002), pp 229-236, ISSN 0894-1491

Altman, J. (1962). Are new neurons formed in the brains of adult mammals? *Science*, Vol. 135, (March 1962), pp 1127-1128, ISSN 0036-8075

Altman, J.&Das, G. D. (1965). Autoradiographic and histological evidence of postnatal hippocampal neurogenesis in rats. *J Comp Neurol,* Vol. 124, No. 3, pp 319-335, ISSN 0021-9967

Alvarez-Buylla, A.; Garcia-Verdugo, J. M.& Tramontin, A. D. (2001). A unified hypothesis on the lineage of neural stem cells. *Nat Rev Neurosci,* Vol. 2, No. 4, (April 2001), pp 287-293, ISSN 1471-0048

Alvarez-Buylla, A.; Seri, B.& Doetsch, F. (2002). Identification of neural stem cells in the adult vertebrate brain. *Brain Res Bull,* Vol. 57, No. 6, (April 2002), pp 751-758, ISSN 0361-9230

Arboleda, D.; Forostyak, S.; Jendelova, P.; Marekova, D.; Amemori, T.; Pivonkova, H.; Masinova, K.& Sykova, E. (2011). Transplantation of Predifferentiated Adipose-Derived Stromal Cells for the Treatment of Spinal Cord Injury. *Cell Mol Neurobiol,* (June 2011), ISSN 0272-4340

Augello, A.; Tasso, R.; Negrini, S. M.; Amateis, A.; Indiveri, F.; Cancedda, R.& Pennesi, G. (2005). Bone marrow mesenchymal progenitor cells inhibit lymphocyte proliferation by activation of the programmed death 1 pathway. *Eur J Immunol,* Vol. 35, No. 5, (May 2005), (May 2005), pp 1482-1490, ISSN 0014-2980

Azari, M. F.; Profyris, C.; Zang, D. W.; Petratos, S.& Cheema, S. S. (2005). Induction of endogenous neural precursors in mouse models of spinal cord injury and disease. *Eur J Neurol,* Vol. 12, No. 8, (August 2005), pp 638-648, ISSN 1351-5101

Barnabe-Heider, F. & Frisen, J. (2008). Stem cells for spinal cord repair. *Cell Stem Cell,* Vol. 3, No. 1, (Jul 2008), pp 16-24, ISSN 1875-9777

Berchtold, N. C. & Cotman, C. W. (1998). Evolution in the conceptualization of dementia and Alzheimer's disease: Greco-Roman period to the 1960s. *Neurobiol Aging,* Vol. 19, No. 3, (May-June 1998), pp 173-189, ISSN 0197-4580

Bjorklund, A. & Svendsen, C. (1999). Stem cells. Breaking the brain-blood barrier. *Nature,* Vol. 397, No. 6720, pp 569-570, ISSN 0028-0836

Blurton-Jones, M.; Kitazawa, M.; Martinez-Coria, H.; Castello, N. A.; Muller, F. J.; Loring, J. F.; Yamasaki, T. R.; Poon, W. W.; Green, K. N.& LaFerla, F. M. (2009). Neural stem cells improve cognition via BDNF in a transgenic model of Alzheimer disease. *Proc Natl Acad Sci U S A,* Vol. 106, No. 32, (August 2009), pp 13594-13599, ISSN 1091-6490

Bonab, M. M.; Alimoghaddam, K.; Talebian, F.; Ghaffari, S. H.; Ghavamzadeh, A.& Nikbin, B. (2006). Aging of mesenchymal stem cell in vitro. *BMC Cell Biol,* Vol. 7, (March 2006), pp 14, ISSN 1471-2121

Bordet, R.; Lestage, P.& Onteniente, B. (2007). [The concept of neuroprotective agents as a treatment modulator in the development of brain diseases]. *Therapie,* Vol. 62, No. 6, (November/December 2007), pp 463-472, ISSN 0040-5957

Bradbury, E. J.; Moon, L. D.; Popat, R. J.; King, V. R.; Bennett, G. S.; Patel, P. N.; Fawcett, J. W.& McMahon, S. B. (2002). Chondroitinase ABC promotes functional recovery after spinal cord injury. *Nature,* Vol. 416, No. 6881, (April 2002), pp 636-640, ISSN 0028-0836

Cizkova, D.; Cizek, M.; Nagyova, M.; Slovinska, L.; Novotna, I.; Jergova, S.; Radonak, J.; Hlucilova, J.& Vanicky, I. (2009a). Enrichment of rat oligodendrocyte progenitor cells by magnetic cell sorting. *J Neurosci Methods,* Vol. 184, No. 1, (October 2009), pp 88-94, ISSN 1872-678X

Cizkova, D.; Kakinohana, O.; Kucharova, K.; Marsala, S.; Johe, K.; Hazel, T.; Hefferan, M. P.& Marsala, M. (2007). Functional recovery in rats with ischemic paraplegia after spinal grafting of human spinal stem cells. *Neuroscience*, Vol. 147, No. 2, (June 2007), pp 546-560, ISSN 0306-4522

Cizkova, D.; Nagyova, M.; Slovinska, L.; Novotna, I.; Radonak, J.; Cizek, M.; Mechirova, E.; Tomori, Z.; Hlucilova, J.; Motlik, J.; Sulla, I., Jr. & Vanicky, I. (2009b). Response of ependymal progenitors to spinal cord injury or enhanced physical activity in adult rat. *Cell Mol Neurobiol*, Vol. 29, No. 6-7, (September 2009), pp 999-1013, ISSN 1573-6830

Cizkova, D.; Rosocha, J.; Vanicky, I.; Jergova, S.& Cizek, M. (2006). Transplants of human mesenchymal stem cells improve functional recovery after spinal cord injury in the rat. *Cell Mol Neurobiol*, Vol. 26, No. 7-8, (November 2006), pp 1165-1178, ISSN 0272-4340

Cloutier, F.; Siegenthaler, M. M.; Nistor, G.& Keirstead, H. S. (2006). Transplantation of human embryonic stem cell-derived oligodendrocyte progenitors into rat spinal cord injuries does not cause harm. *Regen Med*, Vol. 1, No. 4, (July 2006), pp 469-479, ISSN 1746-0751

Colter, D. C.; Class, R.; DiGirolamo, C. M.& Prockop, D. J. (2000). Rapid expansion of recycling stem cells in cultures of plastic-adherent cells from human bone marrow. *Proc Natl Acad Sci U S A*, Vol. 97, No. 7, (March 2000), pp 3213-3218, ISSN 0027-8424

Colter, D. C.; Sekiya, I.& Prockop, D. J. (2001). Identification of a subpopulation of rapidly self-renewing and multipotential adult stem cells in colonies of human marrow stromal cells. *Proc Natl Acad Sci U S A*, Vol. 98, No. 14, (July 2001), pp 7841-7845, ISSN 0027-8424

Coskun, V.; Wu, H.; Blanchi, B.; Tsao, S.; Kim, K.; Zhao, J.; Biancotti, J. C.; Hutnick, L.; Krueger, R. C., Jr.; Fan, G.; de Vellis, J.& Sun, Y. E. (2008). CD133+ neural stem cells in the ependyma of mammalian postnatal forebrain. *Proc Natl Acad Sci U S A*, Vol. 105, No. 3, (January 2008), pp 1026-1031, ISSN 1091-6490

Crigler, L.; Robey, R. C.; Asawachaicharn, A.; Gaupp, D.& Phinney, D. G. (2006). Human mesenchymal stem cell subpopulations express a variety of neuro-regulatory molecules and promote neuronal cell survival and neuritogenesis. *Exp Neurol*, Vol. 198, No. 1, (March 2006), (March 2006), pp 54-64, ISSN 0014-4886

Cui, X.; Chopp, M.; Zacharek, A.; Roberts, C.; Lu, M.; Savant-Bhonsale, S. & Chen, J. (2009). Chemokine, vascular and therapeutic effects of combination Simvastatin and BMSC treatment of stroke. *Neurobiol Dis*, Vol. 36, No. 1, (October 2009), pp 35-41, ISSN 09699961

Cummings, B. J.; Uchida, N.; Tamaki, S. J.; Salazar, D. L.; Hooshmand, M.; Summers, R.; Gage, F. H.& Anderson, A. J. (2005). Human neural stem cells differentiate and promote locomotor recovery in spinal cord-injured mice. *Proc Natl Acad Sci U S A*, Vol. 102, No. 39, (September 2005), pp 14069-14074, ISSN 0027-8424

Curtis, M. A.; Kam, M.; Nannmark, U.; Anderson, M. F.; Axell, M. Z.; Wikkelso, C.; Holtas, S.; van Roon-Mom, W. M.; Bjork-Eriksson, T.; Nordborg, C.; Frisen, J.; Dragunow, M.; Faull, R. L.& Eriksson, P. S. (2007). Human neuroblasts migrate to the olfactory bulb via a lateral ventricular extension. *Science*, Vol. 315, No. 5816, (March 2007), pp 1243-1249, ISSN 0036-8075

Danielyan, L.; Schafer, R.; von Ameln-Mayerhofer, A.; Bernhard, F.; Verleysdonk, S.; Buadze, M.; Lourhmati, A.; Klopfer, T.; Schaumann, F.; Schmid, B.; Koehle, C.; Proksch, B.; Weissert, R.; Reichardt, H. M.; van den Brandt, J.; Buniatian, G. H.; Schwab, M.; Gleiter, C. H.& Frey, W. H., 2nd. (2011). Therapeutic efficacy of intranasally delivered mesenchymal stem cells in a rat model of Parkinson disease. *Rejuvenation Res*, Vol. 14, No. 1, (February 2011), pp 3-16, ISSN 1557-8577

Danilov, A. I.; Covacu, R.; Moe, M. C.; Langmoen, I. A.; Johansson, C. B.; Olsson, T.& Brundin, L. (2006). Neurogenesis in the adult spinal cord in an experimental model of multiple sclerosis. Eur J Neurosci, Vol. 23, No. 2, (January 2006), pp 394-400, ISSN 0953-816X

DeKosky, S. T.; Scheff, S. W.& Styren, S. D. (1996). Structural correlates of cognition in dementia: quantification and assessment of synapse change. *Neurodegeneration*, Vol. 5, No. 4, (December 1996), pp 417-421, ISSN 1055-8330

Deng, W.&Poretz, R. D. (2003). Oligodendroglia in developmental neurotoxicity. *Neurotoxicology*, Vol. 24, No. 2, (March 2003), pp 161-178, ISSN 0161-813X

Di Nicola, M.; Carlo-Stella, C.; Magni, M.; Milanesi, M.; Longoni, P. D.; Matteucci, P.; Grisanti, S.& Gianni, A. M. (2002). Human bone marrow stromal cells suppress T-lymphocyte proliferation induced by cellular or nonspecific mitogenic stimuli. *Blood*, Vol. 99, No. 10, (May 2002), pp 3838-3843, ISSN 0006-4971

Dickson, D. W.; Farlo, J.; Davies, P.; Crystal, H.; Fuld, P.& Yen, S. H. (1988). Alzheimer's disease. A double-labeling immunohistochemical study of senile plaques. *Am J Pathol*, Vol. 132, No. 1, (July 1988), pp 86-101, ISSN 0002-9440

Digirolamo, C. M.; Stokes, D.; Colter, D.; Phinney, D. G.; Class, R.& Prockop, D. J. (1999). Propagation and senescence of human marrow stromal cells in culture: a simple colony-forming assay identifies samples with the greatest potential to propagate and differentiate. *Br J Haematol*, Vol. 107, No. 2, (November 1999), pp 275-281, ISSN 0007-1048

Djouad, F.; Plence, P.; Bony, C.; Tropel, P.; Apparailly, F.; Sany, J.; Noel, D.& Jorgensen, C., 2003. Immunosuppressive effect of mesenchymal stem cells favors tumor growth in allogeneic animals. *In: Blood*, vol. 102. no. 10, pp. 3837-3844, ISSN 0006-4971

Doetsch, F.; Caille, I.; Lim, D. A.; Garcia-Verdugo, J. M.& Alvarez-Buylla, A. (1999). Subventricular zone astrocytes are neural stem cells in the adult mammalian brain. *Cell*, Vol. 97, No. 6, pp 703-716, ISSN 0092-8674

Docheva, D.; Popov, C.; Mutschler, W.& Schieker, M. (2007). Human mesenchymal stem cells in contact with their environment: surface characteristics and the integrin system. *J Cell Mol Med*, Vol. 11, No. 1, (January/February 2007), pp 21-38, ISSN 1582-1838

Dominici, M.; Le Blanc, K.; Mueller, I.; Slaper-Cortenbach, I.; Marini, F.; Krause, D.; Deans, R.; Keating, A.; Prockop, D.& Horwitz, E. (2006). Minimal criteria for defining multipotent mesenchymal stromal cells. The International Society for Cellular Therapy position statement. *Cytotherapy*, Vol. 8, No. 4, pp 315-317, ISSN 1465-3249

Elder, G. A.; De Gasperi, R.& Gama Sosa, M. A. (2006). Research update: neurogenesis in adult brain and neuropsychiatric disorders. *Mt Sinai J Med*, Vol. 73, No. 7, (November 2006), pp 931-940, ISSN 0027-2507

Eriksson, P. S.; Perfilieva, E.; Bjork-Eriksson, T.; Alborn, A. M.; Nordborg, C.; Peterson, D. A.& Gage, F. H. (1998). Neurogenesis in the adult human hippocampus. *Nat Med*, Vol. 4, No. 11, (November 1998), pp 1313-1317, ISSN 1078-8956

Faulkner, J.&Keirstead, H. S. (2005). Human embryonic stem cell-derived oligodendrocyte progenitors for the treatment of spinal cord injury. *Transpl Immunol*, Vol. 15, No. 2, (December 2005), pp 131-142, ISSN 0966-3274

Fawcett, J. W. (2006). Overcoming inhibition in the damaged spinal cord. *J Neurotrauma*, Vol. 23, No. 3-4, (March/April 2006), pp 371-383, 0897-7151 ISSN 0897-7151

Forostyak, S.; Jendelova, P.; Kapcalova, M.; Arboleda, D.& Sykova, E. (2011). Mesenchymal stromal cells prolong the lifespan in a rat model of amyotrophic lateral sclerosis. *Cytotherapy*, (July 2011), ISSN 1477-2566

Friedenstein, A. J.; Gorskaja, J. F.& Kulagina, N. N. (1976). Fibroblast precursors in normal and irradiated mouse hematopoietic organs. *Exp Hematol*, Vol. 4, No. 5, (September 1976), pp 267-274, ISSN 0301-472X

Gage, F. H. (2000). Mammalian neural stem cells. *Science*, Vol. 287, No. 5457, (February 2000), pp 1433-1438, ISSN 0036-8075

Goldman, S. (2005). Stem and progenitor cell-based therapy of the human central nervous system. *Nat Biotechnol*, Vol. 23, No. 7, (July,2005), pp 862-871, ISSN 1087-0156

Gomez-Pinilla, F.; Ying, Z.; Opazo, P.; Roy, R. R.& Edgerton, V. R. (2001). Differential regulation by exercise of BDNF and NT-3 in rat spinal cord and skeletal muscle. *Eur J Neurosci*, Vol. 13, No. 6, (March 2001), pp 1078-1084, ISSN 0953-816X

Gotz, M.&Huttner, W. B. (2005). The cell biology of neurogenesis. *Nat Rev Mol Cell Biol*, Vol. 6, No. 10, (Pctober 2005), pp 777-788, ISSN 1471-0072

Graziadei, P. P.&Graziadei, G. A. (1979). Neurogenesis and neuron regeneration in the olfactory system of mammals. I. Morphological aspects of differentiation and structural organization of the olfactory sensory neurons. *J Neurocytol*, Vol. 8, No. 1, (February 1979), pp 1-18, ISSN 0300-4864

Greco, S. J.&Rameshwar, P. (2008). Microenvironmental considerations in the application of human mesenchymal stem cells in regenerative therapies. *Biologics*, Vol. 2, No. 4, pp 699-705, ISSN 1177-5475

Grote, H. E.&Hannan, A. J. (2007). Regulators of adult neurogenesis in the healthy and diseased brain. *Clin Exp Pharmacol Physiol*, Vol. 34, No. 5-6, (May/June 2007), pp 533-545, ISSN 0305-1870

Guan, K.; Nayernia, K.; Maier, L. S.; Wagner, S.; Dressel, R.; Lee, J. H.; Nolte, J.; Wolf, F.; Li, M.; Engel, W.& Hasenfuss, G. (2006). Pluripotency of spermatogonial stem cells from adult mouse testis. *Nature*, Vol. 440, No. 7088, (April 2006), pp 1199-1203, ISSN 1476-4687

Hamano, K.; Li, T. S.; Kobayashi, T.; Kobayashi, S.; Matsuzaki, M.& Esato, K. (2000). Angiogenesis induced by the implantation of self-bone marrow cells: a new material for therapeutic angiogenesis. *Cell Transplant*, Vol. 9, No. 3, (May/June 2000), pp 439-443, ISSN 0963-6897

Hampton, D. W.; Webber, D. J.; Bilican, B.; Goedert, M.; Spillantini, M. G.& Chandran, S. (2010). Cell-mediated neuroprotection in a mouse model of human tauopathy. *J Neurosci*, Vol. 30, No. 30, (July 2010), pp 9973-9983, ISSN 1529-2401

Herzog, E. L.; Chai, L.& Krause, D. S. (2003). Plasticity of marrow-derived stem cells. *Blood*, Vol. 102, No. 10, (November 2003), pp 3483-3493, ISSN 0006-4971

Hofstetter, C. P.; Holmstrom, N. A.; Lilja, J. A.; Schweinhardt, P.; Hao, J.; Spenger, C.; Wiesenfeld-Hallin, Z.; Kurpad, S. N.; Frisen, J.& Olson, L. (2005). Allodynia limits the usefulness of intraspinal neural stem cell grafts; directed differentiation improves outcome. *Nat Neurosci*, Vol. 8, No. 3, (March 2005), pp 346-353, ISSN 1097-6256

Horner, P. J.; Power, A. E.; Kempermann, G.; Kuhn, H. G.; Palmer, T. D.; Winkler, J.; Thal, L. J.& Gage, F. H. (2000). Proliferation and differentiation of progenitor cells throughout the intact adult rat spinal cord. *J Neurosci*, Vol. 20, No. 6, (March 2000), pp 2218-2228, ISSN 1529-2401

Chen, J. R.; Cheng, G. Y.; Sheu, C. C.; Tseng, G. F.; Wang, T. J.& Huang, Y. S. (2008).
Transplanted bone marrow stromal cells migrate, differentiate and improve motor
function in rats with experimentally induced cerebral stroke. *J Anat*, Vol. 213, No. 3,
(September 2008), pp 249-258, ISSN 1469-7580

Chen, Q.; Long, Y.; Yuan, X.; Zou, L.; Sun, J.; Chen, S.; Perez-Polo, J. R.& Yang, K. (2005).
Protective effects of bone marrow stromal cell transplantation in injured rodent
brain: synthesis of neurotrophic factors. *J Neurosci Res*, Vol. 80, No. 5, (June 2005),
pp 611-619, ISSN 0360-4012

Chopp, M.&Li, Y. (2002). Treatment of neural injury with marrow stromal cells. *Lancet
Neurol*, Vol. 1, No. 2, (June 2002), pp 92-100, ISSN 1474-4422

Ishii, K.; Nakamura, M.; Dai, H.; Finn, T. P.; Okano, H.; Toyama, Y.& Bregman, B. S. (2006).
Neutralization of ciliary neurotrophic factor reduces astrocyte production from
transplanted neural stem cells and promotes regeneration of corticospinal tract
fibers in spinal cord injury. *J Neurosci Res*, Vol. 84, No. 8, (December 2006), pp 1669-
1681, ISSN 0360-4012

Javazon, E. H.; Colter, D. C.; Schwarz, E. J.& Prockop, D. J. (2001). Rat marrow stromal cells
are more sensitive to plating density and expand more rapidly from single-cell-
derived colonies than human marrow stromal cells. *Stem Cells*, Vol. 19, No. 3, (May
2001), pp 219-225, ISSN 1066-5099

Jendelova, P.; Herynek, V.; Urdzikova, L.; Glogarova, K.; Kroupova, J.; Andersson, B.; Bryja,
V.; Burian, M.; Hajek, M.& Sykova, E. (2004). Magnetic resonance tracking of
transplanted bone marrow and embryonic stem cells labeled by iron oxide
nanoparticles in rat brain and spinal cord. *J Neurosci Res*, Vol. 76, No. 2, (April
2004), pp 232-243, ISSN 0360-4012

Johansson, C. B.; Momma, S.; Clarke, D. L.; Risling, M.; Lendahl, U.& Frisen, J. (1999).
Identification of a neural stem cell in the adult mammalian central nervous system.
Cell, Vol. 96, No. 1, (January 1999), pp 25-34, ISSN 0092-8674

Jorgensen, C. (2009). Link between cancer stem cells and adult mesenchymal stromal cells:
implications for cancer therapy. *Regen Med*, Vol. 4, No. 2, (March 2009), pp 149-152,
ISSN 1746-076X

Kakinohana, O.; Cizkova, D.; Tomori, Z.; Hedlund, E.; Marsala, S.; Isacson, O.& Marsala, M.
(2004). Region-specific cell grafting into cervical and lumbar spinal cord in rat: a
qualitative and quantitative stereological study. *Exp Neurol*, Vol. 190, No. 1,
(November 2004), pp 122-132, ISSN 0014-4886

Ke, Y.; Chi, L.; Xu, R.; Luo, C.; Gozal, D.& Liu, R. (2006). Early response of endogenous adult
neural progenitor cells to acute spinal cord injury in mice. *Stem Cells*, Vol. 24, No. 4,
(April 2006), pp 1011-1019, ISSN 1066-5099

Kehl, L. J.; Fairbanks, C. A.; Laughlin, T. M.& Wilcox, G. L. (1997). Neurogenesis in postnatal
rat spinal cord: a study in primary culture. *Science*, Vol. 276, No. 5312, (April 1997),
pp 586-589, ISSN 0036-8075

Keilhoff, G.; Goihl, A.; Langnase, K.; Fansa, H.& Wolf, G. (2006). Transdifferentiation of
mesenchymal stem cells into Schwann cell-like myelinating cells. *Eur J Cell Biol*,
Vol. 85, No. 1, (January 2006), pp 11-24, ISSN 0171-9335

Keirstead, H. S.; Nistor, G.; Bernal, G.; Totoiu, M.; Cloutier, F.; Sharp, K.& Steward, O.
(2005). Human embryonic stem cell-derived oligodendrocyte progenitor cell
transplants remyelinate and restore locomotion after spinal cord injury. *J Neurosci*,
Vol. 25, No. 19, (May 2005), pp 4694-4705, ISSN 1529-2401

Kerkis, I.; Kerkis, A.; Dozortsev, D.; Stukart-Parsons, G. C.; Gomes Massironi, S. M.; Pereira, L. V.; Caplan, A. I.& Cerruti, H. F. (2006). Isolation and characterization of a population of immature dental pulp stem cells expressing OCT-4 and other embryonic stem cell markers. *Cells Tissues Organs,* Vol. 184, No. 3-4, pp 105-116, ISSN 1422-6421

Kim, B. J.; Seo, J. H.; Bubien, J. K.& Oh, Y. S. (2002). Differentiation of adult bone marrow stem cells into neuroprogenitor cells in vitro. *Neuroreport,* Vol. 13, No. 9, pp 1185-1188, ISSN 0959-4965

Kim, S. U.&de Vellis, J. (2009). Stem cell-based cell therapy in neurological diseases: a review. *J Neurosci Res,* Vol. 87, No. 10, (August 2009), pp 2183-2200, ISSN 1097-4547

Kim, Y. J.; Park, H. J.; Lee, G.; Bang, O. Y.; Ahn, Y. H.; Joe, E.; Kim, H. O.& Lee, P. H. (2009). Neuroprotective effects of human mesenchymal stem cells on dopaminergic neurons through anti-inflammatory action. *Glia,* Vol. 57, No. 1, (January 2009), pp 13-23, ISSN 1098-1136

Krampera, M.; Cosmi, L.; Angeli, R.; Pasini, A.; Liotta, F.; Andreini, A.; Santarlasci, V.; Mazzinghi, B.; Pizzolo, G.; Vinante, F.; Romagnani, P.; Maggi, E.; Romagnani, S.& Annunziato, F. (2006). Role for interferon-gamma in the immunomodulatory activity of human bone marrow mesenchymal stem cells. *Stem Cells,* Vol. 24, No. 2, (February 2006), pp 386-398, ISSN 1066-5099

Kuhn, H. G.; Winkler, J.; Kempermann, G.; Thal, L. J.& Gage, F. H. (1997). Epidermal growth factor and fibroblast growth factor-2 have different effects on neural progenitors in the adult rat brain. J Neurosci, Vol. 17, No. 15, (August 1997), pp 5820-5829, ISSN 0270-6474

Kurozumi, K.; Nakamura, K.; Tamiya, T.; Kawano, Y.; Ishii, K.; Kobune, M.; Hirai, S.; Uchida, H.; Sasaki, K.; Ito, Y.; Kato, K.; Honmou, O.; Houkin, K.; Date, I.& Hamada, H. (2005). Mesenchymal stem cells that produce neurotrophic factors reduce ischemic damage in the rat middle cerebral artery occlusion model. *Mol Ther,* Vol. 11, No. 1, (January 2005), pp 96-104, ISSN 1525-0016

Kwon, B. K.; Okon, E. B.; Plunet, W.; Baptiste, D.; Fouad, K.; Hillyer, J.; Weaver, L. C.; Fehlings, M. G.& Tetzlaff, W. (2010). A systematic review of directly applied biologic therapies for acute spinal cord injury. *J Neurotrauma,* Vol. 28, No. 8, (August 2010), pp 1589-1610, ISSN 1557-9042

Le Blanc, K.&Ringden, O. (2005). Immunobiology of human mesenchymal stem cells and future use in hematopoietic stem cell transplantation. *Biol Blood Marrow Transplant,* Vol. 11, No. 5, (May 2005), pp 321-334, ISSN 1083-8791

Lee, J. K.; Jin, H. K.; Endo, S.; Schuchman, E. H.; Carter, J. E.& Bae, J. S. (2010). Intracerebral transplantation of bone marrow-derived mesenchymal stem cells reduces amyloid-beta deposition and rescues memory deficits in Alzheimer's disease mice by modulation of immune responses. *Stem Cells,* Vol. 28, No. 2, (February 2010), pp 329-343, ISSN 1549-4918

Lim, D. A.; Tramontin, A. D.; Trevejo, J. M.; Herrera, D. G.; Garcia-Verdugo, J. M.& Alvarez-Buylla, A. (2000). Noggin antagonizes BMP signaling to create a niche for adult neurogenesis. *Neuron,* Vol. 28, No. 3, (December 2000), pp 713-726, ISSN 0896-6273

Lin, G.; Garcia, M.; Ning, H.; Banie, L.; Guo, Y. L.; Lue, T. F.& Lin, C. S. (2008). Defining stem and progenitor cells within adipose tissue. *Stem Cells Dev,* Vol. 17, No. 6, (December 2008), pp 1053-1063, ISSN 1557-8534

Liu, Z.&Martin, L. J. (2003). Olfactory bulb core is a rich source of neural progenitor and
stem cells in adult rodent and human. *J Comp Neurol*, Vol. 459, No. 4, (May 2003),
pp 368-391, ISSN 0021-9967

Lledo, P. M.; Alonso, M.& Grubb, M. S. (2006). Adult neurogenesis and functional plasticity
in neuronal circuits. Nat Rev Neurosci, Vol. 7, No. 3, (March 2006), pp 179-193,
ISSN 1471-003X

Loebinger, M. R.; Eddaoudi, A.; Davies, D.& Janes, S. M. (2009). Mesenchymal stem cell
delivery of TRAIL can eliminate metastatic cancer. *Cancer Res*, Vol. 69, No. 10, (May
2009), pp 4134-4142, ISSN 1538-7445

Louro, J.&Pearse, D. D. (2008). Stem and progenitor cell therapies: recent progress for spinal
cord injury repair. *Neurol Res*, Vol. 30, No. 1, (February 2008), pp 5-16, ISSN 0161-6412

Mahmood, A.; Lu, D.& Chopp, M. (2004). Marrow stromal cell transplantation after
traumatic brain injury promotes cellular proliferation within the brain.
Neurosurgery, Vol. 55, No. 5, (November 2004), pp 1185-1193, ISSN 1524-4040

Majumdar, M. K.; Keane-Moore, M.; Buyaner, D.; Hardy, W. B.; Moorman, M. A.; McIntosh,
K. R.& Mosca, J. D. (2003). Characterization and functionality of cell surface
molecules on human mesenchymal stem cells. *J Biomed Sci*, Vol. 10, No. 2,
(March/April 2003), pp 228-241, ISSN 1021-7770

Majumdar, M. K.; Thiede, M. A.; Mosca, J. D.; Moorman, M.& Gerson, S. L. (1998).
Phenotypic and functional comparison of cultures of marrow-derived
mesenchymal stem cells (MSCs) and stromal cells. *J Cell Physiol*, Vol. 176, No. 1,
(July 1998), pp 57-66, ISSN 0021-9541

Marsala, M.; Kakinohana, O.; Yaksh, T. L.; Tomori, Z.; Marsala, S.& Cizkova, D. (2004).
Spinal implantation of hNT neurons and neuronal precursors: graft survival and
functional effects in rats with ischemic spastic paraplegia. *Eur J Neurosci*, Vol. 20,
No. 9, (November 2004), pp 2401-2414, ISSN 0953-816x

Mets, T.&Verdonk, G. (1981). In vitro aging of human bone marrow derived stromal cells.
Mech Ageing Dev, Vol. 16, No. 1, (May 1981), pp 81-89, ISSN 0047-6374

Minger, S. (2007). Interspecies SCNT-derived human embryos--a new way forward for
regenerative medicine. *Regen Med*, Vol. 2, No. 2, (March 2007), pp 103-106, ISSN
1746-076X

Mori, H.; Kanemura, Y.; Onaya, J.; Hara, M.; Miyake, J.; Yamasaki, M.& Kariya, Y. (2005).
Effects of heparin and its 6-O-and 2-O-desulfated derivatives with low
anticoagulant activity on proliferation of human neural stem/progenitor cells. *J
Biosci Bioeng*, Vol. 100, No. 1, (July 2005), pp 54-61, ISSN 1389-1723

Mothe, A. J.&Tator, C. H. (2005). Proliferation, migration, and differentiation of endogenous
ependymal region stem/progenitor cells following minimal spinal cord injury in
the adult rat. *Neuroscience*, Vol. 131, No. 1, pp 177-187, ISSN 0306-4522

Moviglia, G. A.; Varela, G.; Brizuela, J. A.; Moviglia Brandolino, M. T.; Farina, P.;
Etchegaray, G.; Piccone, S.; Hirsch, J.; Martinez, G.; Marino, S.; Deffain, S.; Coria,
N.; Gonzales, A.; Sztanko, M.; Salas-Zamora, P.; Previgliano, I.; Aingel, V.; Farias, J.;
Gaeta, C. A.; Saslavsky, J.& Blasseti, N. (2009). Case report on the clinical results of
a combined cellular therapy for chronic spinal cord injured patients. *Spinal Cord*,
Vol. 47, No. 6, (June 2009), pp 499-503, ISSN 1476-5624

Nagahara, A. H.&Tuszynski, M. H. (2011). Potential therapeutic uses of BDNF in
neurological and psychiatric disorders. *Nat Rev Drug Discov*, Vol. 10, No. 3, (March
2011), pp 209-219, ISSN 1474-1784

Nait-Oumesmar, B.; Picard-Riera, N.; Kerninon, C.; Decker, L.; Seilhean, D.; Hoglinger, G. U.; Hirsch, E. C.; Reynolds, R.& Baron-Van Evercooren, A. (2007). Activation of the subventricular zone in multiple sclerosis: evidence for early glial progenitors. Proc Natl Acad Sci U S A, Vol. 104, No. 11, (March 2007), pp 4694-4699, ISSN 0027-8424

Nandoe Tewarie, R. S.; Hurtado, A.; Bartels, R. H.; Grotenhuis, A.& Oudega, M. (2009). Stem cell-based therapies for spinal cord injury. J Spinal Cord Med, Vol. 32, No. 2, pp 105-114, ISSN 1079-0268

Nauta, A. J.&Fibbe, W. E. (2007). Immunomodulatory properties of mesenchymal stromal cells. Blood, Vol. 110, No. 10, (November 2007), pp 3499-3506, ISSN 0006-4971

Neeper, S. A.; Gomez-Pinilla, F.; Choi, J.& Cotman, C. (1995). Exercise and brain neurotrophins. Nature, Vol. 373, No. 6510, (January 1995), pp 109, ISSN 0028-0836

Nistor, G. I.; Totoiu, M. O.; Haque, N.; Carpenter, M. K.& Keirstead, H. S. (2005). Human embryonic stem cells differentiate into oligodendrocytes in high purity and myelinate after spinal cord transplantation. Glia, Vol. 49, No. 3, (February 2005), pp 385-396, ISSN 0894-1491

Nottebohm, F. (1981). A brain for all seasons: cyclical anatomical changes in song control nuclei of the canary brain. Science, Vol. 214, No. 4527, (December 1981), pp 1368-1370, ISSN 0036-8075

Novak, M.; Kabat, J.& Wischik, C. M. (1993). Molecular characterization of the minimal protease resistant tau unit of the Alzheimer's disease paired helical filament. Embo J, Vol. 12, No. 1, (January 1993), pp 365-370, ISSN 0261-4189

Pal, R.; Venkataramana, N. K.; Bansal, A.; Balaraju, S.; Jan, M.; Chandra, R.; Dixit, A.; Rauthan, A.; Murgod, U.& Totey, S. (2009). Ex vivo-expanded autologous bone marrow-derived mesenchymal stromal cells in human spinal cord injury/paraplegia: a pilot clinical study. Cytotherapy, Vol. 11, No. 7, pp 897-911, ISSN 1477-2566

Papastefanaki, F.; Chen, J.; Lavdas, A. A.; Thomaidou, D.; Schachner, M.& Matsas, R. (2007). Grafts of Schwann cells engineered to express PSA-NCAM promote functional recovery after spinal cord injury. Brain, Vol. 130, No. Pt 8, (August 2007), pp 2159-2174, ISSN 1460-2156

Park, H. J.; Lee, P. H.; Bang, O. Y.; Lee, G.& Ahn, Y. H. (2008). Mesenchymal stem cells therapy exerts neuroprotection in a progressive animal model of Parkinson's disease. J Neurochem, Vol. 107, No. 1, (October 2008), pp 141-151, ISSN 1471-4159

Pearse, D. D.; Sanchez, A. R.; Pereira, F. C.; Andrade, C. M.; Puzis, R.; Pressman, Y.; Golden, K.; Kitay, B. M.; Blits, B.; Wood, P. M.& Bunge, M. B. (2007). Transplantation of Schwann cells and/or olfactory ensheathing glia into the contused spinal cord: Survival, migration, axon association, and functional recovery. Glia, Vol. 55, No. 9, (July 2007), pp 976-1000, ISSN 0894-1491

Pechadre, J. C.; Larochelle, L.& Poirier, L. J. (1976). Parkinsonian akinesia, rigidity and tremor in the monkey. Histopathological and neuropharmacological study. J Neurol Sci, Vol. 28, No. 2, (June 1976), pp 147-157, ISSN 0022-510X

Pittenger, M. F.; Mackay, A. M.; Beck, S. C.; Jaiswal, R. K.; Douglas, R.; Mosca, J. D.; Moorman, M. A.; Simonetti, D. W.; Craig, S.& Marshak, D. R. (1999). Multilineage potential of adult human mesenchymal stem cells. Science, Vol. 284, No. 5411, (April 1999), pp 143-147, ISSN 0036-8075

Platel, J. C.; Lacar, B.& Bordey, A. (2007). GABA and glutamate signaling: homeostatic control of adult forebrain neurogenesis. *J Mol Histol,* Vol. 38, No. 4, (August 2007), pp 303-311, ISSN 1567-2379

Prockop, D. J. (1997). Marrow stromal cells as stem cells for nonhematopoietic tissues. *Science,* Vol. 276, No. 5309, (April 1997), pp 71-74, ISSN 0036-8075

Pruszak, J.; Sonntag, K. C.; Aung, M. H.; Sanchez-Pernaute, R.& Isacson, O. (2007). Markers and methods for cell sorting of human embryonic stem cell-derived neural cell populations. *Stem Cells,* Vol. 25, No. 9, (September 2007), pp 2257-2268, ISSN 1549-4918

Raisman, G. (2007). Repair of spinal cord injury by transplantation of olfactory ensheathing cells. *C R Biol,* Vol. 330, No. 6-7, (June/July 2007), pp 557-560, ISSN 1631-0691

Raisman, G.; Carlstedt, T.; Choi, D.& Li, Y. (2011). Clinical prospects for transplantation of OECs in the repair of brachial and lumbosacral plexus injuries: Opening a door. *Exp Neurol,* (May2011), ISSN 1090-2430

Rowland, J. W.; Hawryluk, G. W.; Kwon, B.& Fehlings, M. G. (2008). Current status of acute spinal cord injury pathophysiology and emerging therapies: promise on the horizon. *Neurosurg Focus,* Vol. 25, No. 5, pp E2, ISSN 1092-0684

Shihabuddin, L. S.; Horner, P. J.; Ray, J.& Gage, F. H. (2000). Adult spinal cord stem cells generate neurons after transplantation in the adult dentate gyrus. *J Neurosci,* Vol. 20, No. 23, (December 200), pp 8727-8735, ISSN 1529-2401

Schwab, M. E. (2004). Nogo and axon regeneration. *Curr Opin Neurobiol,* Vol. 14, No. 1, (February 2004), pp 118-124, ISSN 0959-4388

Sotiropoulou, P. A.; Perez, S. A.; Gritzapis, A. D.; Baxevanis, C. N.& Papamichail, M. (2006). Interactions between human mesenchymal stem cells and natural killer cells. *Stem Cells,* Vol. 24, No. 1, (January 2006), pp 74-85, ISSN 1066-5099

Stagg, J. (2007). Immune regulation by mesenchymal stem cells: two sides to the coin. *Tissue Antigens,* Vol. 69, No. 1, (January 2007), pp 1-9, ISSN 0001-2815

Sykova, E.; Homola, A.; Mazanec, R.; Lachmann, H.; Konradova, S. L.; Kobylka, P.; Padr, R.; Neuwirth, J.; Komrska, V.; Vavra, V.; Stulik, J.& Bojar, M. (2006). Autologous bone marrow transplantation in patients with subacute and chronic spinal cord injury. *Cell Transplant,* Vol. 15, No. 8-9, (January 2006), pp 675-687, ISSN 0963-6897

Sykova, E. &J endelova, P. (2005). Magnetic resonance tracking of implanted adult and embryonic stem cells in injured brain and spinal cord. *Ann N Y Acad Sci,* Vol. 1049, (May 2005), pp 146-160, ISSN 0077-8923

Tarasenko, Y. I.; Gao, J.; Nie, L.; Johnson, K. M.; Grady, J. J.; Hulsebosch, C. E.; McAdoo, D. J.& Wu, P. (2007). Human fetal neural stem cells grafted into contusion-injured rat spinal cords improve behavior. *J Neurosci Res,* Vol. 85, No. 1, pp 47-57, ISSN 0360-4012

Tonnesen, J.; Parish, C. L.; Sorensen, A. T.; Andersson, A.; Lundberg, C.; Deisseroth, K.; Arenas, E.; Lindvall, O.& Kokaia, M. (2011). Functional integration of grafted neural stem cell-derived dopaminergic neurons monitored by optogenetics in an in vitro Parkinson model. *PLoS One,* Vol. 6, No. 3, (March 2011), pp e17560, ISSN 1932-6203

Uchida, N.; Buck, D. W.; He, D.; Reitsma, M. J.; Masek, M.; Phan, T. V.; Tsukamoto, A. S.; Gage, F. H.& Weissman, I. L. (2000). Direct isolation of human central nervous system stem cells. *Proc Natl Acad Sci U S A,* Vol. 97, No. 26, (December 2000), pp 14720-14725, ISSN 0027-8424

Wang, F.; Yasuhara, T.; Shingo, T.; Kameda, M.; Tajiri, N.; Yuan, W. J.; Kondo, A.; Kadota, T.; Baba, T.; Tayra, J. T.; Kikuchi, Y.; Miyoshi, Y.& Date, I. (2010). Intravenous administration of mesenchymal stem cells exerts therapeutic effects on parkinsonian model of rats: focusing on neuroprotective effects of stromal cell-derived factor-1alpha. *BMC Neurosci*, Vol. 11, pp 52, ISSN 1471-2202

Weiss, S.; Dunne, C.; Hewson, J.; Wohl, C.; Wheatley, M.; Peterson, A. C.& Reynolds, B. A. (1996). Multipotent CNS stem cells are present in the adult mammalian spinal cord and ventricular neuroaxis. *J Neurosci*, Vol. 16, No. 23, (December 1996), pp 7599-7609, ISSN

Wiltrout, C.; Lang, B.; Yan, Y.; Dempsey, R. J.& Vemuganti, R. (2007). Repairing brain after stroke: a review on post-ischemic neurogenesis. *Neurochem Int*, Vol. 50, No. 7-8, (June 2007), pp 1028-1041, ISSN 0270-6474

Wu, Y.; Shatapathy, C. C.& Minger, S. L. (2009). Isolation, in vitro cultivation and characterisation of foetal liver cells. *Methods Mol Biol*, Vol. 481, pp 181-192, ISSN 1064-3745

Yamamoto, S.; Yamamoto, N.; Kitamura, T.; Nakamura, K.& Nakafuku, M. (2001). Proliferation of parenchymal neural progenitors in response to injury in the adult rat spinal cord. *Exp Neurol*, Vol. 172, No. 1, (November 2001), pp 115-127, ISSN 0014-4886

Yang, H.; Lu, P.; McKay, H. M.; Bernot, T.; Keirstead, H.; Steward, O.; Gage, F. H.; Edgerton, V. R.& Tuszynski, M. H. (2006). Endogenous neurogenesis replaces oligodendrocytes and astrocytes after primate spinal cord injury. *J Neurosci*, Vol. 26, No. 8, (February 2006), pp 2157-2166, ISSN 1529-2401

Yu, Y.; Yao, A. H.; Chen, N.; Pu, L. Y.; Fan, Y.; Lv, L.; Sun, B. C.; Li, G. Q.& Wang, X. H. (2007). Mesenchymal stem cells over-expressing hepatocyte growth factor improve small-for-size liver grafts regeneration. *Mol Ther*, Vol. 15, No. 7, (July 2007), pp 1382-1389, ISSN 1525-0024

Zacharek, A.; Chen, J.; Cui, X.; Li, A.; Li, Y.; Roberts, C.; Feng, Y.; Gao, Q.& Chopp, M. (2007). Angiopoietin1/Tie2 and VEGF/Flk1 induced by MSC treatment amplifies angiogenesis and vascular stabilization after stroke. *J Cereb Blood Flow Metab*, Vol. 27, No. 10, (October 2007), pp 1684-1691, ISSN 0271-678X

Zai, L. J.&Wrathall, J. R. (2005). Cell proliferation and replacement following contusive spinal cord injury. *Glia*, Vol. 50, No. 3, (May 2005), pp 247-257, ISSN 0894-1491

Zhang, R. L.; Zhang, Z. G.& Chopp, M. (2008). Ischemic stroke and neurogenesis in the subventricular zone. *Neuropharmacology*, Vol. 55, No. 3, (September 2008), pp 345-352, ISSN 0028-3908

Zhong, C.; Qin, Z.; Zhong, C. J.; Wang, Y.& Shen, X. Y. (2003). Neuroprotective effects of bone marrow stromal cells on rat organotypic hippocampal slice culture model of cerebral ischemia. *Neurosci Lett*, Vol. 342, No. 1-2, (May 2003), pp 93-96, ISSN 0304-3940

Zilka, N.; Ferencik, M.& Hulin, I. (2006). Neuroinflammation in Alzheimer's disease: protector or promoter? *Bratisl Lek Listy*, Vol. 107, No. 9-10, pp 374-383, ISSN 0006-9248

Zilka, N.; Zilkova, M.; Kazmerova, Z.; Sarissky, M.; Cigankova, V.& Novak, M. (2011). Mesenchymal stem cells rescue the Alzheimer's disease cell model from cell death induced by misfolded truncated tau. Neuroscience, Vol. 193, No (July 14), pp, 330-337, ISSN 1873-7544

Zilkova, M.; Koson, P.& Zilka, N. (2006). The hunt for dying neurons: insight into the neuronal loss in Alzheimer's disease. *Bratisl Lek Listy*, Vol. 107, No. 9-10, (2006), pp 366-373, ISSN 0006-9248

Zuk, P. A.; Zhu, M.; Ashjian, P.; De Ugarte, D. A.; Huang, J. I.; Mizuno, H.; Alfonso, Z. C.; Fraser, J. K.; Benhaim, P.& Hedrick, M. H. (2002). Human adipose tissue is a source of multipotent stem cells. *Mol Biol Cell*, Vol. 13, No. 12, (November 2002), pp 4279-4295, ISSN 1059-1524

Permissions

The contributors of this book come from diverse backgrounds, making this book a truly international effort. This book will bring forth new frontiers with its revolutionizing research information and detailed analysis of the nascent developments around the world.

We would like to thank Tao Sun, for lending his expertise to make the book truly unique. He has played a crucial role in the development of this book. Without his invaluable contribution this book wouldn't have been possible. He has made vital efforts to compile up to date information on the varied aspects of this subject to make this book a valuable addition to the collection of many professionals and students.

This book was conceptualized with the vision of imparting up-to-date information and advanced data in this field. To ensure the same, a matchless editorial board was set up. Every individual on the board went through rigorous rounds of assessment to prove their worth. After which they invested a large part of their time researching and compiling the most relevant data for our readers. Conferences and sessions were held from time to time between the editorial board and the contributing authors to present the data in the most comprehensible form. The editorial team has worked tirelessly to provide valuable and valid information to help people across the globe.

Every chapter published in this book has been scrutinized by our experts. Their significance has been extensively debated. The topics covered herein carry significant findings which will fuel the growth of the discipline. They may even be implemented as practical applications or may be referred to as a beginning point for another development. Chapters in this book were first published by InTech; hereby published with permission under the Creative Commons Attribution License or equivalent.

The editorial board has been involved in producing this book since its inception. They have spent rigorous hours researching and exploring the diverse topics which have resulted in the successful publishing of this book. They have passed on their knowledge of decades through this book. To expedite this challenging task, the publisher supported the team at every step. A small team of assistant editors was also appointed to further simplify the editing procedure and attain best results for the readers.

Our editorial team has been hand-picked from every corner of the world. Their multi-ethnicity adds dynamic inputs to the discussions which result in innovative outcomes. These outcomes are then further discussed with the researchers and contributors who give their valuable feedback and opinion regarding the same. The feedback is then collaborated with the researches and they are edited in a comprehensive manner to aid the understanding of the subject.

Apart from the editorial board, the designing team has also invested a significant amount of their time in understanding the subject and creating the most relevant covers. They scrutinized every image to scout for the most suitable representation of the subject and create an appropriate cover for the book.

The publishing team has been involved in this book since its early stages. They were actively engaged in every process, be it collecting the data, connecting with the contributors or procuring relevant information. The team has been an ardent support to the editorial, designing and production team. Their endless efforts to recruit the best for this project, has resulted in the accomplishment of this book. They are a veteran in the field of academics and their pool of knowledge is as vast as their experience in printing. Their expertise and guidance has proved useful at every step. Their uncompromising quality standards have made this book an exceptional effort. Their encouragement from time to time has been an inspiration for everyone.

The publisher and the editorial board hope that this book will prove to be a valuable piece of knowledge for researchers, students, practitioners and scholars across the globe.

List of Contributors

Shan Bian and Tao Sun
Department of Cell and Developmental Biology, Cornell University Weill Medical College, USA

Hedong Li, He Zhao, Xiaoqiong Shu and Mei Jiang
West China Developmental & Stem Cell Institute, Department of Obstetrics & Gynecologic/ Pediatric,
Key Laboratory of Obstetric & Gynecologic, Pediatric Diseases and Birth Defects of Ministry of Education,
West China Second University Hospital, Sichuan University, Chengdu, Sichuan Province, P.R. China

A.K. De la Herrán-Arita, A. Boronat-García, G. Maya-Espinosa, J.R. García-Montes
Departamento de Neuropatología Molecular, Instituto de Fisiología Celular, México

M. Guerra-Crespo and R. Drucker-Colín
Departamento de Neuropatología Molecular, Instituto de Fisiología Celular, México
Grupo Células Troncales Adultas, Regeneración Neuronal y Enfermedad de Parkinson
Universidad Nacional Autónoma de México, México

J.H. Fallon
Department of Psychiatry and Human Behavior, University of California, Irvine, USA

Maria Dizon
Northwestern University/Children's Memorial Hospital, USA

Takayuki Nakagomi and Tomohiro Matsuyama
Institute for Advanced Medical Sciences, Hyogo College of Medicine Hyogo, Japan

Bruno P. Carreira, Maria Inês Morte and Caetana M. Carvalho
Center for Neuroscience and Cell Biology, Neuroendocrinology and Neurogenesis Group, University of Coimbra, Coimbra, Portugal

Inês M. Araújo
Center for Neuroscience and Cell Biology, Neuroendocrinology and Neurogenesis Group, University of Coimbra, Coimbra, Portugal
Regenerative Medicine Program, Department of Biomedical Sciences and Medicine University of Algarve, Faro, Portugal

Chiara Rolando, Enrica Boda and Annalisa Buffo
Department of Neuroscience, Neuroscience Institute Cavalieri Ottolenghi, NICO, University of Turin, Italy

Dasa Cizkova
Institute of Neurobiology, Center of Excellence for Brain Research, Slovak Academy of Sciences, Kosice, Slovakia